Manual of D
and Therapeu...
for Disorders of Deglutition

Manual of Diagnostic and Therapeutic Techniques for Disorders of Deglutition

Reza Shaker
Medical College of Wisconsin, Milwaukee, Wisconsin, USA

Caryn Easterling
University of Wisconsin-Milwaukee, Wisconsin, USA

Peter C. Belafsky
University of California, Sacramento, California, USA

Gregory N. Postma
Georgia Health Sciences University, Georgia, USA

Editors

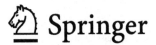 Springer

Editors
Reza Shaker
Division of Gastroenterology
and Hepatology
Medical College of Wisconsin
Milwaukee, Wisconsin, USA

Caryn Easterling
Department of Communication
Sciences and Disorders
University of Wisconsin-Milwaukee
Milwaukee, Wisconsin, USA

Peter C. Belafsky
Department of Otolaryngology/
Head and Neck Surgery
University of California
Davis Medical Center
Sacramento, California, USA

Gregory N. Postma
Center for Voice, Airway
and Swallowing Disorders
Department of Otolaryngology
Georgia Health Sciences University
Augusta, Georgia, USA

ISBN 978-1-4614-3778-9   ISBN 978-1-4614-3779-6 (eBook)
DOI 10.1007/978-1-4614-3779-6
Springer New York Heidelberg Dordrecht London

Library of Congress Control Number: 2012944370

Printed on acid-free paper

Springer is part of Springer Science+Business Media (www.springer.com)

Contents

Contributors

Jonathan E. Aviv, MD, FACS
Department of Otolaryngology, Mount Sinai Medical Center,
New York, NY, USA

Eytan Bardan, MD
Department of Gastroenterology, Sheba Medical Center, Ramat-Gan,
Tel-Hashmer, Israel

Susan G. Butler, PhD
Department of Otolaryngology, Wake Forest School of Medicine,
Winston-Salem, NC, USA

Jeffrey L. Conklin, MD
Department of Gastroenterology and Hepatology, Cedars-Sinai Medical
Center, Los Angeles, CA, USA

Caryn Easterling, PhD, CCC, BRS-S, ASHAF Fellow
Department of Communication Sciences and Disorders,
University of Wisconsin-Milwaukee, Milwaukee, WI, USA

Jacqueline A. Hind, MS/CCC-SLP, BRS-S
Department of Medicine, University of Wisconsin, Madison, WI, USA

Maggie-Lee Huckabee, PhD
Swallowing Rehabilitation Research Lab at the New Zealand
Brain Research Institute, The University of Canterbury,
Christchurch, New Zealand

Bronwyn Jones, MB, BS, FRACP, FRCR
Department of Radiology and Radiological Science,
The Johns Hopkins Hospital, Baltimore, MD, USA

Robert T. Kavitt, MD
Division of Gastroenterology, Hepatology, and Nutrition,
Vanderbilt University Medical Center, Nashville, TN, USA

Cathy Lazarus, PhD, CCC-SLP, BRS-S, ASHA Fellow
Department of Otolaryngology Head and Neck Surgery,
Albert Einstein College of Medicine of Yeshiva University,
New York, NY, USA

Susan E. Langmore, MA, PhD
Department of Otolaryngology, Boston University Medical Center,
Boston, MA, USA

Kristin Larsen, MD
Lecturer Northwestern University, Department of Communication
Sciences and Disorders, Evanston, IL, USA

Marc S. Levine, MD
Chief of Gastrointestinal Radiology, Hospital of the University
of Pennsylvania, Professor of Radiology and Advisory Dean,
Perelman School of Medicine at the University of Pennsylvania,
Philadelphia, PA, USA

Jeri A. Logemann, PhD
Department of Communication Sciences and Disorders,
Northwestern University, Evanston, IL, USA

Benson T. Massey, MD, FACP
Division of Gastroenterology and Hepatology,
Medical College of Wisconsin, Milwaukee, WI, USA

Gary H. McCullough, PhD, MA, BA
Department of Communication Sciences and Disorders,
University of Central Arkansas, Conway, AR, USA

Phoebe Macrae, BSLT (hons)
Swallowing Rehabilitation Research Lab at the Van der Veer Institute,
The University of Canterbury, Christchurch, New Zealand

Rosemary Martino, MA, MSc, PhD
Department of Speech and Language Pathology, University of Toronto,
Toronto, ON, Canada

Claire Kane Miller, PhD
Cincinnati Children's Hospital Medical Center, Cincinnati, OH, USA

Joseph Murray, PhD
VA Ann Arbor Healthcare System, Ann Arbor, MI, USA

Cathy A. Pelletier, PhD, MS, CCC-SLP
Walter Reed National Military Medical Center, Audiology and Speech
Center, Bethesda, MD, USA

Gregory N. Postma, MD
Center for Voice, Airway and Swallowing Disorders, Department
of Otolaryngology, Georgia Health Sciences University,
Augusta, GA, USA

William J. Ravich, MD
Russell H. Morgan Department of Radiology and Radiological Science,
The Johns Hopkins University School of Medicine, Lutherville,
MD, USA

JoAnne Robbins, PhD, CCC-SLP, BRS-S
Geriatric Research Education and Clinical Center (GRECC)
and Wm. S. Middleton Memorial Veterans Hospital,
University of Wisconsin, Madison, WI, USA

Kia Saeian, MD, MSc (Epi)
Division of Gastroenterology and Hepatology,
Medical College of Wisconsin, Milwaukee, WI, USA

Justine Joan Sheppard, PhD, BRS-S
Department of Biobehavioral Sciences, Columbia University,
New York, NY, USA

*Catriona M. Steele, MHSc, PhD, CCC-SLP, SLP(C), BRS-S,
Reg. CASLPO*
Department of Research, University Health Network, Toronto,
ON, Canada

Neelesh Ajit Tipnis, MD
Department of Pediatrics, University of California, San Diego, La Jolla,
CA, USA

Michael F. Vaezi, MD, PhD, MSc (Epi)
Department of Medicine, Division of Gastroenterology, Hepatology,
and Nutrition, Vanderbilt University Medical Center, Nashville,
TN, USA

J. Paul Willging, MD, FACS
Cincinnati Children's Hospital Medical Center, Cincinnati, OH, USA

Part I
General Consideration
in Evaluation of Dysphagic Patients

1. Establishing a Comprehensive Center for Diagnosis and Therapy of Swallowing Disorders

Bronwyn Jones and William J. Ravich

Abstract This chapter discuses some historical facts relating to the development of the multidisciplinary Swallowing Center concept. It also offers a perspective of the Swallowing Center concept 25 years after its original inception. The developments and changes in the world of swallowing disorders e.g. the establishment of a Journal devoted to swallowing and its disorders and the formation of a Dysphagia Research Society, to name just two of the many developments, are presented and discussed. The advantages and limitations of a multidisciplinary Swallowing Center are also discussed.

It is now 25 years since the original paper "The Swallowing Center: Concepts and Procedures" by Ravich et al. was published in *Gastrointestinal Radiology* [1]. That paper described the purpose and organization of a dedicated center at the Johns Hopkins Medical Institutions for the evaluation and management of swallowing problems. The present chapter discusses some historical facts relating to the development of the swallowing center concept and also offers a perspective of the concept 25 years later.

It also provided some information obtained by a questionnaire about the structure and function of multidisciplinary centers set up at other institutions in North America and Europe that are focused on disorders of deglutition.

The Johns Hopkins Swallowing Center was created in the hope that "the multidisciplinary approach outlined will permit a better understanding and more accurate diagnosis of the functional or organic lesions affecting the swallowing mechanisms" [1]. The concept of a "swallowing center" evolved for a number of reasons:

R. Shaker et al. (eds.), *Manual of Diagnostic and Therapeutic Techniques for Disorders of Deglutition*, DOI 10.1007/978-1-4614-3779-6_1,
© Springer Science+Business Media New York 2013

- A variety of clinical specialties have been involved in the evaluation and management of patients with swallowing disorders.
- These clinical specialties have different perspectives on, and techniques for the evaluation and management of swallowing function and patients with swallow-related complaints. The techniques of one specialty are often unfamiliar or completely unknown to other specialties involved with the care of swallowing patients.
- The symptom of dysphagia, most often described as a sensation of an obstruction to the passage of food, as well as the other common related symptoms of coughing or choking during swallowing can derive from abnormalities of function or structure of the mouth, throat, or chest, and therefore do not necessarily indicate the appropriate clinical specialty to whom the patient might best be referred. It is now well recognized that the sensation of food sticking may be referred proximal to the level of actual obstruction; the symptom, dysphagia, is not necessarily referred to the level of the disease process. For example, it is quite common for a mid or distal esophageal process to be referred proximally [2].

The impetus for the development of the Swallowing Center came from Martin W. Donner, then Chairman of Radiology, who had a background in internal medicine and a long-standing interest in the gastrointestinal tract and especially in dynamic imaging of swallowing function. Dr. Donner, with the help of Dr. James Bosma, a pediatrician who was a well-known swallowing physiologist, brought together a group of interested clinicians at the Johns Hopkins Medical Institutions including specialists in gastroenterology, otolaryngology, radiology, and rehabilitation medicine. This group met weekly on an informal basis for a number of years to discuss patients with swallowing disorders that presented issues thought to be of potential interest to other members of the group. The Johns Hopkins Swallowing Center developed from the initial experience of this group.

The formal formation of the Johns Hopkins Swallowing Center resulted from extensive discussions among this core group with a clinical and/or research interest in dysphagia. Central to the discussion were the disciplines (in alphabetical order) of gastroenterology, neurology, otolaryngology, radiology, rehabilitation medicine, and speech-language pathology, with less consistent involvement of representatives from dentistry, psychology, and thoracic surgery. The theory was to focus the attention of multiple specialties on the patient from the beginning and to expedite any necessary referrals between the disciplines, while at the same time avoiding unnecessary referrals.

Key to achieving this aim was timely communication among disciplines. This was achieved by hiring an individual, the Swallowing Center Coordinator, whose job was to receive referrals to the Swallowing Center, obtain necessary outside records, and coordinate the patient visits, under the supervision of the Swallowing Center's Clinical Director, to center-associated specialists who then saw patients in their usual clinical facilities. Because of the central role of radiology in the evaluation of swallowing disorders, most patients who came to the center had cine-fluorography (or later video-fluorography) early in the course of their evaluations, unless a previously performed radiographic study was available for review and deemed to be satisfactory.

Central to operation of the center was a weekly conference, organized by the Swallowing Center Coordinator and attended by representatives of each discipline, thus focusing the expertise of each discipline upon the individual patient. All patients referred directly to the Swallowing Center would be presented at this weekly meeting. In addition, any member of the center could request that one of their patients be listed for review.

At the weekly meeting, the patient's clinical information was presented by members who had already evaluated the patient, the radiographic study was projected, and the results of any additional testing were reviewed. This was followed by a discussion of the interpretation of the findings and possible directions for further investigations or for treatment. If not already established, a primary Swallowing Center clinician was identified who would then be responsible for incorporating the information discussed into a plan for subsequent evaluation and management. The Swallowing Center Coordinator was available to assist in the coordination of any additional consultations or tests that might be indicated.

Over time, the Center has been successful in its role as a central resource for the evaluation of common and uncommon causes of swallowing dysfunction and for straightforward and difficult management problems. In addition to clinical care, the Center, through its participating members, has contributed to the medical literature on swallowing disorders. Center members played a central role in the founding of the Dysphagia Research Society (DRS), the first multidisciplinary organization for the promotion of research in the field of swallowing disorders.

Now 30 years after its formation as an integrated clinical center, it is possible to recognize the circumstances that framed and dictated its structure. The Center was the creation of a single individual, Martin

Donner, who as Chairman of Radiology was able to support its early operation from Departmental funds without the need to seek contributions from other specialties. Although other specialties were critical to the Center's success, the directors of the other involved specialties and the hospital, when approached, were reluctant to provide additional support for the Center. An attempt to obtain funding from clinical operations by charging patients for the administrative services of the Center failed because insurance would not reimburse for these services. Billing patients directly promoted the direct referral to involved subspecialists who then, consistent with the guidelines of the Center, could list the patients for review at the weekly Swallowing Center meeting. As a result the administrative functions of the Center have remained constricted and dependent on the support of Radiology.

The Center was and remains a valuable resource for the cooperative evaluation of patients with swallowing disorders. The Center is dependent on the interests of its participating clinicians. However, as the faculty and staff in an academic institution like Johns Hopkins come and go and their areas of greatest academic and clinical interest vary over time, there is an ongoing need to bring in new members, particularly in underrepresented specialties in which the number of faculty and staff is small or the interest in swallowing disorders is not a traditional part of the specialty. In addition, there has been a steady increase on the clinical demands being placed on involved clinicians and concerns about maximizing clinical income from participating departments making it increasingly difficult for clinicians to attend scheduled meetings on a regular basis and to do multidisciplinary research in swallowing.

To provide some insights into the structure and function of multidisciplinary centers for deglutitive disorders, we distributed a questionnaire to the 328 members of the DRS during 2010. Only 11 centers returned the questionnaire and the results must therefore be considered highly selective and subject to bias. However, the results do provide some insights of possible significance. Multi-specialty centers for the evaluation and treatment of swallowing disorders are quite varied in organization. The earliest multidisciplinary center was founded in 1981 and the most recent in 2003. The number of core specialties involved ranged from 2 to 7 with the total number of involved specialties listed as either core or secondary specialties ranging from 3 to 10. The most commonly involved core specialty the one at Johns Hopkins, was speech-language pathology (8/11) with the number of core specialties involved in swallowing retraining expanding to 10 if the presence of a physiatrist and occupational therapist is included. The next most common core specialties involved are radiology and otolaryngology (6/11, each), gastroenterology (5/11), and neurology (3/11). Other core specialties mentioned include dentistry, general surgery, geriatrics, and thoracic surgery.

If both core subspecialties and secondarily involved subspecialties are included, radiology was involved in all responding centers, speech-language pathology in 10/11, gastroenterology in 10/11, otolaryngology in 9/11, neurology 8/11, thoracic surgery 5/11, psychiatry/psychology 5/11, general surgery 4/11, dentistry or oral surgery 3/11. Of note is that no center listed the involvement of a dietitian or nutritionist.

Only 2 of the 11 centers described receiving funding at any time from their institution for their administrative expenses and only a few had any extramural funding for either their clinical or research programs. Most of the extramural funding was from philanthropic sources and most of that support was not ongoing. Only 1 center described receiving an NIH grant. None of the centers were billing patients or insurance directly for their administrative services. Four of eleven directly employed at least one clinician or researcher, but only two centers billed patients directly for their clinical services. Overall, the survey gives the impression of limited financial resources under the direct control of the centers that responded.

Given the key role of the weekly multidisciplinary conference in the operation of the Johns Hopkins Swallowing Center, it was interesting to note that only 5 of the 11 centers reported a multidisciplinary conference as part of their activities, with only one other center reporting that this conference took place on a weekly basis. Others were held on a monthly or less than monthly basis.

Developments and Changes

In the last 25 years there have been many developments in the world of swallowing disorders. To list several of these:

- The establishment of a journal, *Dysphagia*, a multidisciplinary journal devoted to swallowing and its disorders.
- The formation of the DRS, a multidisciplinary society whose missions include [3]:
  - To enhance and encourage research pertinent to normal and disordered swallowing and related functions.
  - To attract new investigators to the field and to encourage interdisciplinary research.

- To promote the dissemination of knowledge related to normal and disordered swallowing.
- To provide a multidisciplinary forum for presentation of research into normal and disordered swallowing.
- To foster new methodologies and instrumentation in dysphagia research and its clinical application.

- An increasing interest in dysphagia as a symptom both within the lay community and the medical community.
- An increasing sophistication in the diagnosis and management of the dysphagic patient among many specialties including otolaryngology, gastroenterology, speech language pathology, and radiology.
- An amazing growth in the number of patients investigated with dysphagia. To give an example from radiologic studies performed at Johns Hopkins Hospital in 1985 vs. 2010. In 1985 approximately 150 videoswallowing studies were performed yearly. Today that number has multiplied to about 2,000 per year.
- The development of new technologies such as solid-state manometry and the introduction of examinations such as FEES (Fiberoptic Endoscopic Evaluation of Swallowing) and FEESST (Fiberoptic Endoscopic Evaluation of Swallowing with Sensory Testing).

Questions Relating to Swallowing Centers

Many Questions Abound

- How many specialties should be involved in a "Swallowing Center?" Can you, for example, have a swallowing center of only gastroenterologists, only otolaryngologists, only speech pathologists; or should such centers indeed be multidisciplinary by definition? Should other disciplines such as psychology and psychiatry be involved centrally or act primarily as consultants an as-needed basis?
- What about postoperative or posttreatment dysphagia (i.e., post radiation or post chemoradiation)? Should surgeons and radiation oncologists be involved or consulted as needed?
- Another question: What is the referring physician's, and equally if not more important, what is the patient's expectation of referral to a swallowing center?

Advantages and Limitations of a Multidisciplinary Swallowing Center

Advantages

- Comprehensive evaluation of the patient
- Combined expertise of several specialties focused on the patient's problems
- Expedited referral time
- Shared knowledge among involved specialists, thereby expanding each individual's expertise

Limitations and Barriers

- Different disciplines need to be recruited and retained.
- In a moving/mobile professional society individuals change institutions frequently. For example, the JHSC had a psychologist and a neurologist for many years. The psychologist retired and the neurologist developed other interests.
- So much of the activity cannot or is not reimbursable or is "bundled" by insurance carriers.
- Lack of funding from institutions for administrative personnel such as the center coordinator.
- Lack of funding for research in both clinical and basic science areas.

Conclusion

There is a definite need to raise the public and professional consciousness of the importance of having dedicated patient care and research in this emerging field of dysphagia. It should be recognized that there is a high incidence of dysphagia in many disease processes and also in the aging society. It is hoped that the formation of more multidisciplinary swallowing centers will improve knowledge and communication among specialists in this field.

References

1. Ravich WJ, Donner MW, Kashima H, Buchholz DW, Marsh B, Hendrix TR, et al. The swallowing center: concepts and procedures. Gastrointest Radiol. 1985;10:255–61.
2. Edwards DAW. History and symptoms of esophageal disease. In: Vantrappen G, Hellemans J, editors. Diseases of the esophagus. New York: Springer; 1974.
3. Dysphagia Research Society—http://www.dysphagiaresearch.org.

2. Clinical Evaluation of Patients with Dysphagia: Importance of History Taking and Physical Exam

Gary H. McCullough and Rosemary Martino

Abstract Assessment of dysphagia may include instrumental or non-instrumental measures—frequently both. The clinical evaluation is a collection of, largely, non-instrumental measures, which may include a comprehensive history, a detailed oral motor and sensory physical exam, and trial swallows of liquids and foods. Each aspect of the clinical evaluation serves a unique purpose yet contributes to a more comprehensive understanding of the swallowing problem. The findings from the clinical evaluation provide information about a patient's functional feeding and swallowing behaviors and determine the need for therapeutic intervention and/or additional instrumental testing. Patients at risk for dysphagia, and thus in need of a clinical evaluation, can be determined from screening. This chapter will describe each aspect of the clinical evaluation and screening and provide the value of each.

Introduction

Clinical assessment of swallowing should be considered an essential part of intervention for all patients with confirmed or likely dysphagia. There are several elements that comprise a clinical swallow evaluation (CSE), including a comprehensive medical history, a physical exam of oral and motor function, and assessment of food intake. In patients with confirmed dysphagia, the CSE serves to refine and update the course of intervention as the dysphagia ameliorates or potentially worsens over time. Alternatively, in patients who are suspected to have dysphagia, a CSE serves to confirm the presence of dysphagia and plan the most appropriate next steps: such as, further testing with instrumental swallow tests, consultation with other medical specialists, or tailored treatment.

R. Shaker et al. (eds.), *Manual of Diagnostic and Therapeutic Techniques for Disorders of Deglutition*, DOI 10.1007/978-1-4614-3779-6_2,
© Springer Science+Business Media New York 2013

Suspicion of dysphagia can be garnered from screening using the patient's presenting etiology and, more objectively, the clinician's findings from a standardized screening test.

Identifying Dysphagia Risk

The presence of dysphagia is highly suspect in patients with etiologies that impact the structural, neurological, or muscular aspects of the head and neck. These etiologies might include stroke [1], head and neck cancer [2], cervical spine abnormality [3], or a progressive neurological disease [4–6]. Furthermore, medical interventions aiming to maintain airway patency [7] or treat head and neck cancer [8] can also increase the risk for dysphagia. Patients with these known diseases or medical treatments should be considered high risk for dysphagia. Ideally, a Speech-Language Pathologist using a standardized CSE would assess all of these patients. Unfortunately, hospital resources are often limited and this specialized care is not available. Hence, validated screening tools serve as the next most feasible method by which to triage those patients with highest risk to a comprehensive CSE. Screening can be completed by any trained person using a brief bedside clinical test.

A brief bedside clinical test, also called a screen, differs from a CSE in purpose and scope. As previously mentioned, the CSE aims to identify possible site, severity, and prognosis of the swallowing impairment. An expert in dysphagia, typically a speech-language pathologist, administers the CSE. Information from a CSE directs the speech-language pathologist to prescribe the most appropriate dysphagia management, including further testing with instrumentation. In contrast, a nurse or other clinician not specialized in evaluation, management, and treatment of dysphagia but trained to screen administers the dysphagia screening [9]. Screening serves to identify those patients with the greatest risk of having dysphagia so that they may be referred to a dysphagia expert for a comprehensive CSE. Most importantly and unlike a CSE, screening provides no information about dysphagia severity or best management. Screening results are useful only in directing patients at greatest risk for further assessment.

The brief bedside clinical test, or screen, further differs from the CSE in accuracy. The initial swallow assessment is a two-step process whereby the screen is administered first and the CSE second. Psychometrically, a screening test aims only to identify those at greatest risk for dysphagia thus requiring a high sensitivity [10]. The sensitivity of a screen is defined as the proportion of patients with the dysphagia who are correctly identified by the screen, also known as the true positive value. The CSE is administered next and thus serves to validate the presence of dysphagia and to determine its severity as well as identify the need for further management with instrumental testing. This comprehensive assessment requires high specificity [10]. The specificity of the CSE is defined as the proportion of patients without dysphagia who are correctly ruled to not have dysphagia, also known as the true negative value. The combination of this two-step process generates an efficient and accurate way to identify dysphagia in the clinical setting.

With emerging evidence that early detection of dysphagia from screening reduces subsequent pulmonary complications, length of hospital stay, and overall health care costs for at least stroke patients [11], stroke guidelines have been developed in Canada [12], the United States [13], the United Kingdom [14], Australia [15] and elsewhere, stressing the importance of early detection of dysphagia with validated screening tools. These guidelines require that a trained clinician screen individuals admitted with stroke or suspicion of stroke for dysphagia as soon as they are alert and able. A standardized tool must be used. Those patients with a positive dysphagia screen should be kept "nil by mouth" (NPO) and seen for a CSE by a speech language pathologist within 24 h.

Several authors have systematically reviewed the literature for a properly standardized screening tool without success [16–18]. In response to the identified gap in the literature relating to availability of accurate screening tools and an effort to standardize care for stroke patients across all settings, the Toronto Bedside Swallowing Screening Test (TOR-BSST$_©$) was developed [9]. The TOR-BSST$_©$ is a brief screening tool, administered by a health care professional trained by a speech-language pathologist, that predicts the presence of dysphagia in stroke survivors. Its items include assessment of voice quality, lingual movement, and ability to manage water by teaspoon and cup. These items were derived using the best available evidence from a systematic review [16]. The TOR-BSST$_©$ is unique in that it has proven high reliability and validity with stroke patients in both acute and rehabilitation settings. This tool has yet to be validated with etiologies other than stroke in studies currently underway. Other screening tools that are available in the literature for review include those for patients with Parkinson's disease [19] and mixed etiologies [20–22].

In summary, although screening is limited to the identification of increased risk for dysphagia, there is evidence that it reduces complications such as pneumonia, tube dependency, and possibly even death [11, 16].

Needless to say, screening alone does not ensure these health benefits. Instead, the benefit is achieved from a series of events that a positive screen result initiates; namely, earlier comprehensive assessment such as that with CSE, instrumental evaluation, and, if required, earlier treatment [16].

Standardized Clinical Evaluations

Despite the high prevalence of dysphagia in patients with acute stroke [1], progressive neurological diseases such as Parkinson [23], as well with prolonged intubation [24] or head and neck carcinoma [25], there are few properly standardized dysphagia assessment tools specific for clinical evaluation [26]. Currently, there are two such swallowing clinical measures standardized with dysphagia patients, namely the Mann assessment of swallowing ability (MASA) [27] and the Functional Oral Intake Scale (FOIS) [28]. The psychometric features of these clinical swallowing measures are detailed in Table 2.1 below. The benefit of using standardized measures for aspects of the CSE is twofold; first, it ensures a systematic and more accurate capture of the targeted clinical features (detailed later in this chapter) and second, it provides an objective comparison of change over time or after therapeutic intervention.

Although these standardized measures are common in research, the literature suggests practicing clinicians do not utilize them regularly [29]. Several authors have explored the clinical assessment practice behaviors of speech language pathologists. McCullough et al. identified little consensus on what clinicians believed was most or least important; however, they reportedly had high utilization of most test maneuvers— perhaps adhering by the everything and the kitchen sink approach [30]. Likewise, Mathers-Schmidt and Kurlinski identified variability with how clinicians defined food consistencies used for the CSE [31]. Martino et al. also found variability in clinicians' reported practice and opinion of importance for a large variety of test maneuvers [29]. In this study, test maneuver utilization was greatest with the less experienced clinicians and with those working in teaching institutions. These clinicians were more likely to execute a series of bedside test maneuvers that focused on oral (e.g., lip movement and strength, drool, mastication) and pharyngeal swallowing (e.g., repeat swallows, airway protection), both with and without food. Therefore, unlike nurse screeners, speech language pathologists reportedly thoroughly assess the safety and efficiency of the swallow. In so doing, they gather useful information for proper diagnosis and individualized treatment planning.

2. Clinical Evaluation of Patients with Dysphagia…   15

Table 2.1 Standardized clinical assessment tests that measure swallowing impairment in patients with stroke.

Tools	Outcome	Domains (themes)	Validation population	Score	Test-retest reliability	Validity
Mann assessment of swallowing ability (MASA) [27]	Swallow physiology (impairment)	Dysphagia probability Aspiration probability	128 first-ever acute stroke patients	4-point ordinal scale for each domain	Dysphagia $(k) = 0.82$, Aspiration $(k) = 0.75$	Dysphagia SN = 73% SP = 89% Aspiration SN = 93% SP = 67%
Functional oral intake scale (FOIS) [28]	Oral intake (function)	Oral intake of food and liquid	302 acute stroke patients	7-point ordinal scale	Kappa from 0.86 to 0.91	Concordance $(k) = 0.90$

Clinical Swallow Evaluation: Patient History

Evaluation of a patients' medical history is a necessary precursor of the CSE. The information garnered from the patient history helps direct and tailor the rest of the clinical assessment. A comprehensive history for patients with dysphagia needs to include the following; namely, patient symptoms, past and current medical history, any previous swallowing assessments and socio-cultural status. Ideally, this information is obtained directly from the patient and validated by the family or caregivers and/or the patient's medical team. In some cases when the patient is not able due to limited cognitive status or language restrictions, these additional sources become critical to obtaining history of the swallowing problem.

Recently, properly standardized tests have been developed to systematically capture patient reported symptoms with proven accuracy. For example, the Sydney Swallow Questionnaire (SSQ) is a symptom inventory that has been developed with a neurological patient population and validated with patients pre- and post-surgery for Zenker's diverticulum [32]. It targets symptoms related to pain or discomfort during swallowing along with texture-specific restrictions. Similarly, the EAT-10 is a self-administered survey targeting patient burden from dysphagia [33]. This tool consists of ten items that, collectively, inquire about effort and pain during swallowing as well as feelings of stress and isolation. This EAT-10 has been validated broadly with a varied patient population. As with the standardized CSE tools discussed above, both the SSQ and the EAT-10 ensure a systematic and valid method by which to obtain symptom information from the perspective of the patient, and thus provide a baseline for comparison at a later point in time. The comparison over time, or after therapy intervention, will enable the clinician to ascertain functional gains in the patient's swallowing status.

There is additional patient symptom information not captured by either SSQ or EAT-10 that needs to be targeted as part of the history taking [34]. For example, it is important to inquire about the site and timing of the dysphagia symptoms. Discomfort that is reportedly experienced in the neck immediately after food intake suggests impairment at the level of the oropharynx. In contrast, symptoms that are reported to occur seconds later in the retrosternum area may suggest impairment in the esophagus. Also important is information pertaining to onset, frequency, and progression of the symptoms because it might shed light on etiology especially if it is yet unknown. Sudden onset of symptoms typically relate to etiologies such as stroke or trauma. A patient who cannot recall the start of the swallowing problem typically would suggest a slow progressive etiology such as ALS [35] or MS [36]. Details about the course of the symptoms help determine the course of the etiology, that is, typically worsening for progressive disease. However, intermittent symptoms or problems with select textures may suggest an esophageal cause [34]. The patient who indicates that the symptoms worsen only at the end of meal or end of the day, and has heightened dysphagic symptoms with "cold" temperature may suggest a neurologic dysphagia such as Myasthenia Gravis [37]. In summary, it is clear that obtaining patient symptoms is complicated, multidimensional, and somewhat exploratory. There is no one script that could be followed; hence, it requires the skill, training, and background of a dysphagia expert.

In addition to patient symptomology, a comprehensive history also includes information related to past and current medical history, previous swallowing assessments, and sociocultural status. In planning treatment it is critical to know if the etiology potentially causing the dysphagia is of neurological, structural, systemic, iatrogenic, or psychogenic origin [37]. An ameliorating etiology, such as stroke, will suggest an improvement in the swallow [38]. Likewise, a worsening disease such as ALS will suggest a poor prognosis of swallow over time [35]. Part of the medical history includes a detailed review of the patient's medications noting those that are known to cause xerostomia, GI upset, or even drowsiness [39]. Also, details from any previous swallowing assessments are useful to note if the patient has experienced change over time and determine if this change aligns with what is expected due to the presenting etiology or intervention provided. Lastly, capturing information about the patient's cultural background and environmental support will ensure that any future therapies prescribed are culturally feasible, acceptable, and appropriate given the patient's support and living situation.

Clinical Swallow Evaluation: The Physical Exam

General Observations

The physical examination begins when the clinician enters the patient's room and begins making observations [40]. Cues to three major concerns in a CSE—mental status, nutritional status, and respiratory status—can often be visually derived and may or may not concur with historical information gathered in the medical record. It is also important to draw connections between historical/medical information and the physical examination. For example, a clinician can immediately begin making observations about alertness (i.e., wakefulness and initial communication attempts) and posture of the patient. The presence of a feeding tube would indicate at least partial alternative nutritional support. The presence of suctioning equipment and/or drooling trigger concerns regarding secretion management. If the patient has a tracheostomy tube or labored breathing patterns, respiratory status is a concern. Pulse oximetry and respiratory rate may or may not be monitored for confirmation. If any concerns regarding respiratory status, nutritional status, or mental status are noted in the history and visually confirmed, the physical examination must proceed with caution; and trial swallows may not be advised.

Assessing Oral Motor and Vocal Function

When performing the physical examination, it is important to assess both structure and function. Structures at rest may provide visual clues to underlying physiologic and/or neurologic pathologies, such as lower motor neuron flaccidity. Likewise, movement of structures yields information regarding strength and speed of critical aspects to swallowing and involvement of specific cranial nerves. Most critical to deglutition are cranial nerves V, VII, IX, X, and XII. Table 2.2 provides a list of these cranial nerves and sensorimotor sites for assessment along with appropriate physical aspects to examine.

1. The face and jaw.
   Observations of the facial muscles at rest and during movement can provide information on muscle strength, tone, and mobility. For the oral stage of deglutition, we are primarily concerned with viability of the lips and cheeks for anterior bolus containment and buccal tension during bolus manipulation. These can be grossly examined by having the patient purse and retract the lips. Comparison of these muscles to upper facial muscles (i.e., raising eyebrows) can help determine and differentiate upper and lower motor neuron damage, if present, to cranial nerve VII.
   Mastication is difficult to directly assess during a physical exam as the mouth is, necessarily, closed. Jaw muscle strength and mobility as well as cranial nerve V function can be assessed by opening and closing the jaw against resistance and moving the lower jaw from side to side. Exaggerated open-mouth chewing without a bolus may also provide this information. One study [41] reported reduced bilateral

Table 2.2 Major clinical measures to assess in physical examination.

Initial observations	
Posture: upright/able to sit upright	Respiratory
	Tracheostomy tube/ventilator
	Pattern of respiration
	Monitor: rate and SpO_2
Nutritional	Mental status
Presence of feeding tube	Alertness
Type of feeding tube	Cooperation
	Communication
	Orientation
Structural/cranial nerve assessment	
CNV	Jaw mobility
	Strength open/close against resistance
	Exaggerated chewing
CNVII	Lips purse/retract
	Raise eyebrows
CNIX/CNX	Gag reflex — palatal/pharyngeal
	Cough strength
	Cough quality — wet/dry
	Voice — sustained phonation/speech
CNXII	Tongue mobility
	Strength — protrude/lateralize against resistance
	Pressure — Iowa oral performance instrument, Madison oral strength training device, other devices

Structural: note for all above structural appearance, muscle tone and laterality of deviations

Sensation: all structures can be grossly assessed with cotton-tip applicator (left/right discrimination)

Trial swallows	
Consistency/bolus size	Thin: 5 mL — 3 oz
	Puree or pudding 5 mL
	Solid: bite
Observations	Laryngeal palpation
	Timing/completeness/number of swallows
	Pre–post voice quality
	Coughing/clearing
	Oral residue
Additional observations (often best with meal)	Need for assistance
	Effects of compensations
	Amount of nutritional intake

jaw strength as one of the most robust signs of aspiration with a specificity of 99% and a positive likelihood ratio of over 17. While robust, this finding is tempered by the mere five patients who exhibited bilaterally weak jaws. In terms of being able to chew and prepare a bolus for swallowing, it would seem absurd to ignore when a patient has a weak jaw. It would seem, likewise, absurd to look at it as an exclusive clinical measure of impairment.

2. Lingual function.

Lingual function (CN XII) has been included in most clinical swallowing assessments in some form for obvious reasons. The tongue is required to not only move the bolus about and form a cohesive mass but also sequentially press the bolus through the oropharynx and into the upper esophageal segment. Lingual swallowing pressures are critical to swallowing success, and both the anterior and posterior tongue must be evaluated.

Visual observation of the tongue at rest should be conducted first. Patients with a history of oral cancer may have a partial or total glossectomy. Unilateral or bilateral atrophy and fasciculations can indicate lower motor neuron disease to cranial nerve XII, and spasticity can indicate upper motor neuron disease [42].

Clinical examination of lingual function has been accomplished with tools as crude and simple as visualization of tongue protrusion against a tongue depressor, retraction, and lateralization upon protrusion or into the cheeks. More recently, instrumental devices have been developed to assist with clinical evaluation, as well as promote rehabilitation through biofeedback. These include the Iowa Oral Performance Instrument (IOPI) [43, 44] and, more recently, the Madison Oral Strength Training device (MOST) [45], as well as a device developed in Japan—which reportedly correlated well with dysphagic tongue movements and incidence of cough [46]. The MOST measures isometric and swallowing pressures while the others are more geared toward isometric alone.

While traditional measures using a tongue blade have provided limited value in assessing for aspiration [47], measuring tongue pressures with instrumentation can differentiate individuals by age [45, 48] and separate normals from patients with disorders related to head and neck cancer [49] and stroke [50]. It has also been associated with poor lingual transfer with resulting food sticking in the pharynx [46, 51] and increased incidence of coughing. Mann and Hankey [52] reported that in conjunction with palatal weakness, tongue weakness was strongly correlated with dysphagia.

3. Oral health and dentition.

A recent review of literature [53] provides substantial reason to assess oral health and dentition in institutionalized elderly. Their review suggests strong evidence for an association between poor oral hygiene and respiratory pathogens as well as a decrease in the incidence of respiratory pathogens when oral care intervention is provided. While clinical assessment of swallowing is not exclusive to such institutions, the principles remain important. During the physical exam, clinicians should note, minimally, the number of decayed teeth and evidence of consistent or inconsistent teeth brushing [54].

Additionally, the tongue should be inspected for milky white patches which could indicate fungal infection, thrush, which could lead to oral pain [55]; and amount of saliva production should be noted, as xerostomia (dry mouth) can impair taste and swallowing function [56, 57].

4. The palate and pharynx.

The palate should be observed at rest for symmetry of structure and signs of atrophy. Palatal movement for speech and swallowing are different tasks, and palatal closure during the swallow cannot be observed without instrumentation. Regardless, having the patient repeat short "ah"s will, at least, demonstrate neuromotor ability of the palate to close. Palatal weakness and asymmetry was reported as a major predictor of dysphagia by Mann and Hankey [52].

Palatal and pharyngeal gag reflexes can be assessed. The role of assessing a gag reflex (CN IX and X) has been and remains controversial. Research by Horner and colleagues in the 1980s pointed to the absence of a pharyngeal gag reflex in stroke patients as a significant predictor of aspiration [58, 59]. Later research provided mixed results. While Daniels et al. [60] found good sensitivity and specificity for the gag reflex as a sign of aspiration, Leder [61], Linden et al. [62], and McCullough et al. [41, 47] did not. Daniels et al. [63] provided further support for the measure and suggested that the gag—as one of six signs, of which two or more had to be positive—held predictive utility for not only aspiration post-stroke but also dysphagia. Logemann et al. [64] reported observation of the absence of pharyngeal wall contraction on gag as a good sign of pharyngeal dysphagia. Even the most ardent critics of the value of testing the gag reflex rarely resist the temptation to poke their patients' soft palate and tongue base/posterior pharyngeal walls with a cotton-tip applicator. Perhaps more important than the presence or absence of the gag reflex is the patient's sensory ability to perceive "touch" on the posterior pharyngeal wall. Davies and Kidd

[65] reported that while a gag reflex was absent in 37% of healthy participants, only one demonstrated reduced pharyngeal sensation as rated by left/right distinction to touch.

Pharyngeal muscle function (CN X/Pharyngeal Plexus) is also difficult to assess during a physical exam. Endoscopy and videofluoroscopy provide better images for contraction of constrictor muscles. During the trial swallow portion of an exam, multiple swallows for small volume puree or solid boluses may indicate weak pharyngeal muscle contraction and consequential difficulty clearing the bolus [64].

5. Laryngeal Function.

Clinical measures for laryngeal function (CN X), volitional cough and a basic rating of voice quality, have received compelling yet mixed results in the literature. The clinical sign of "dysphonia" was observed to correlate with dysphagia after stroke in 1988 by Horner et al. [58]. Since then it has been associated with bilateral stroke [59] and brainstem stroke [66]. It has been reported as one of six signs, two or more of which indicate a problem, in the detection of aspiration [60] and more severe outcomes with dysphagia [63]. Most research investigating clinical signs of dysphagia cite a rating of vocal quality as useful, and rating the voice as the patient phonates "ah" appears best to make the rating [47]. Forty-seven out of 60 stroke patients had an abnormal voice quality in one study [52].

Abnormal volitional cough has, likewise, received more positive correlations with dysphagia than negative [52, 59, 60, 63, 67] and can be rated by asking the patient to cough and rating the strength as well as the quality (wet/dry) of the cough.

6. Other Measures.

In addition to the above measures, ratings of dysarthria and oral apraxia may be made. Dysarthria has received support as a correlate of swallowing function [47, 52, 60, 63, 64, 66, 67]. Logemann et al. [64] reported particular correlation with oral stage dysphagia. With the gathering of historical information and general communication with the patient, a rating of dysarthria is easily derived from a trained speech-language pathologist. Oral apraxia can be determined by asking the patient to pretend to blow out a match, cluck their tongue, or whistle, though correlations to dysphagia are not as significant. Palpating the larynx and assessing laryngeal elevation during a dry swallow (CN V, VII, XII) may also help determine the safety of continuing on to the next step, though no evidence exists to support this.

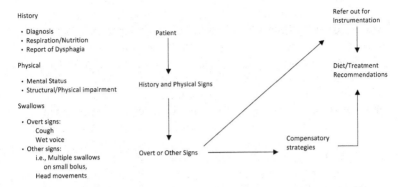

Fig. 2.1. CSE no onsite instrumentation.

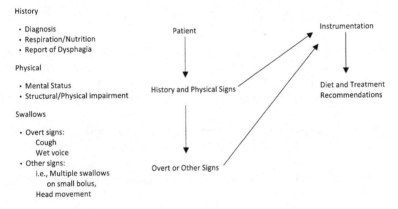

Fig. 2.2. CSE onsite instrumentation.

Trial Swallows

Not all clinical swallowing examinations should include actual swallows. Information from the historical/medical section and the physical examination of the patient should determine the need and safety for conducting trial swallows. A patient who is attentive and cooperative, has no current respiratory problems or signs of physical distress, and has at least some laryngeal elevation and function in the physical exam would be a good candidate for trial swallows. A patient with current respiratory problems and decreased mental status and cooperation may not be a good candidate—though this can be influenced by setting.

Figures 2.1 and 2.2 provide examples of how decision-making during a CSE might be influenced by setting.

In Fig. 2.1, the clinician works in a setting, such as a nursing home, with no onsite instrumentation. Red flags in the patient's history and physical exam may raise concerns regarding dysphagia. If concerns are significant enough, the clinician may deem it necessary to have the patient transported to a facility for instrumental swallowing assessment prior to oral feeding. On the other hand, the clinician may feel the benefits of trial swallows outweigh the risks and commence, cautiously, with trial swallows and even compensatory strategies to determine if overt signs can be reduced with modest manipulations of posture or the bolus.

In Fig. 2.2, the clinician works in a setting, such as a medical center, with onsite instrumental options. With red flags in the history and physical, this clinician may be much less likely to perform trial swallows without instrumentation because he can quickly and easily move to an instrumental exam before making diet or treatment recommendations.

When trial swallows are performed, they can be discontinued at any time — and should be if signs of problems occur and risks appear greater than the benefits. If the expectation is to define swallowing ability and determine course of treatment, a variety of bolus sizes and consistencies need to be evaluated. Daniels et al. [68] observed that single measures or volumes were not sufficient to define dysphagia on videofluoroscopy. It makes sense they would be insufficient in a clinical exam, as well. Different studies and protocols for CSEs exist and recommend differing volumes and consistencies, but small and larger boluses across thin liquid, puree or pudding, and solid consistencies is considered standard and necessary unless in the course of the examination signs of impairment appear. Often, if no signs of impairment are noted with boluses ranging from 1 to 20 mL, clinicians will even test the patient with multiple swallows, such as a 3 oz swallow test [69, 70]. The 3 oz swallow has also been reported to help determine the presence of aspiration when used as part of a comprehensive CSE [41, 71].

While administering trial swallows, the clinician should attend to a number of important measures. Listening to the patient's voice before and after a swallow for wetness or gurgly quality has been reported to correlate with the presence or absence of penetration/aspiration of liquids [41, 47, 60, 63, 64]. Some recommend the patient say "ah," while others prefer the patient to gently breathe in through the nares and hum to prevent the likelihood of material in the larynx from passing into the trachea. There is little doubt the presence of coughing and/or throat clearing is often a sign of laryngeal penetration/aspiration. It has been reported in two studies to be one of the most sensitive and specific signs of aspiration [41, 47] and is listed as important in many others [60, 64,

67, 72]. Due to the potential for silent aspiration, the *lack* of a cough reflex appears to provide limited information unless accompanied by other signs of swallowing impairment.

The larynx should be palpated for timing and completeness of the swallow, as well as the number of swallows. This can be accomplished by placing the index finger on the thyroid notch and remaining fingers on the thyroid cartilage [73] or by using the four finger method, where the index finger is placed submentally, the middle finger is placed on the hyoid, and the last two fingers are placed on the superior and inferior borders of the thyroid cartilage [40]. Poor laryngeal elevation on palpation may indicate reduced laryngeal elevation and closure, especially when it occurs in conjunction with other signs of dysphagia—such as coughing or a wet voice. Multiple swallows on small boluses may indicate pharyngeal weakness and inability to clear the pharynx of the bolus [64]. And examining the oral cavity before and after the swallow may help determine the patient's ability to transport the bolus effectively from the oral cavity into the pharynx.

If the clinician observes signs of dysphagia during the trial swallows but does not have access to instrumentation, he may decide it is necessary to attempt to manipulate the bolus consistency, temperature, or volume during oral intake or alter the patient's posture and/or eating behaviors to improve safety and ease of nutritional intake. Many compensatory strategies (i.e., thickening liquids, tucking the chin, turning the head) can be attempted, but safety must be paramount. If such strategies are not obviously improving the passage of the bolus, terminating the study and referring the patient out for an instrumental examination is likely necessary.

Finally, adjuncts to the CSE can include cervical auscultation [74, 75] to listen to breathing sounds during and after the swallows and/or SpO_2 levels, which has received mixed results in terms of its correlation with aspiration [76, 77]. Additional observations such as the patient's ability to feed self, level of assistance—if applicable, and ability to maintain posture and strength throughout examination should be noted. These observations can also be made very effectively with a meal observation.

Summary

The Clinical Swallowing Examination (CSE) is not a screening instrument, though determining the presence or absence of dysphagia is important. The CSE allows the speech-language pathologist to integrate information from the patient's history/medical record, physical/ neurologic/cognitive function, and, when deemed necessary, actual swallows, to develop a better overall understanding of a patient's functional feeding and swallowing ability. Many times patients will be referred on for additional instrumental testing after the CSE, and sometimes the CSE can be an endpoint in and of itself. Observation of the patient eating a meal, if applicable, is often another useful step in the evaluation process. It is critical to understand that while aspiration is of paramount importance, a dysphagia evaluation is about much more. The clinician must determine a patient's ability to safely take food and liquid in amounts appropriate for nutritional needs without compromising overall health status. A physical evaluation of these abilities is an essential part of any comprehensive evaluation for dysphagia [47, 52].

References

1. Martino R, Foley N, Bhogal S, Diamant N, Speechley M, Teasell R. Dysphagia after stroke: incidence, diagnosis, and pulmonary complications. Stroke. 2005;36:2756–63.
2. Cavalot AL, Ricci E, Schindler A, Roggero N, Albera R, Utari C, et al. The importance of preoperative swallowing therapy in subtotal laryngectomies. Otolaryngol Head Neck Surg. 2009;140:822–5.
3. Rihn JA, Kane J, Albert TJ, Vaccaro AR, Hilibrand AS. What is the incidence and severity of dysphagia after anterior cervical surgery? Clin Orthop Relat Res. 2011;469:658–65.
4. Miller N, Allcock L, Hildreth AJ, Jones D, Noble E, Burn DJ. Swallowing problems in Parkinson disease: frequency and clinical correlates. J Neurol Neurosurg Psychiatry. 2009;80:1047–9.
5. Langmore SE, Kasarskis EJ, Manca ML, Olney RK. Enteral tube feeding for amyotrophic lateral sclerosis/motor neuron disease. Cochrane Database Syst Rev. 2006;(4):CD004030.
6. Thomas FJ, Wiles CM. Dysphagia and nutritional status in multiple sclerosis. J Neurol. 1999;246:677–82.
7. Skoretz SA, Flowers HL, Martino R. The incidence of dysphagia following endotracheal intubation: a systematic review. Chest. 2010;137:665–73.
8. Platteaux N, Dirix P, Dejaeger E, Nuyts S. Dysphagia in head and neck cancer patients treated with chemoradiotherapy. Dysphagia. 2010; 25:139–52.
9. Martino R, Silver F, Teasell R, Bayley M, Nicholson G, Streiner DL, et al. The Toronto Bedside Swallowing Screening Test (TOR-BSST©): development and validation of a dysphagia screening tool for patients with stroke. Stroke. 2009;40:555–61.
10. Streiner DL. Diagnosing tests: using and misusing diagnostic and screening tests. J Pers Assess. 2003;81:209–19.
11. Hinchey JA, Shephard T, Furie K, Smith D, Wang D, Tonn S. Formal dysphagia

screening protocols prevent pneumonia. Stroke. 2005;36:1972–6.

12. Lindsay PBP, Bayley MM, Hellings CB, Hill MMM, Woodbury EBM, Phillips SM. Canadian best practice recommendations for stroke care (Updated 2008). CMAJ. 2008;179:E1–93.

13. Duncan PW, Zorowitz R, Bates B, Choi JY, Glasberg JJ, Graham GD, et al. Management of adult stroke rehabilitation care: a clinical practice guideline. Stroke. 2005;36:e100–43.

14. Intercollegiate Stroke Working Party. National clinical guidelines for stroke. London: Royal College of Physicians; 2004.

15. National Stroke Foundation. Clinical guidelines for acute stroke management. Melbourne, Australia: National Stroke Foundation; 2007

16. Martino R, Pron G, Diamant NE. Screening for oropharyngeal dysphagia in stroke: insufficient evidence for guidelines. Dysphagia. 2000;15:19–30.

17. Perry L. Screening swallowing function of patients with acute stroke. Part one: identification, implementation and initial evaluation of a screening tool for use by nurses. J Clin Nurs. 2001;10:463–73.

18. Bours GJ, Speyer R, Lemmens J, Limburg M, de Wit R. Bedside screening tests vs. videofluoroscopy or fibreoptic endoscopic evaluation of swallowing to detect dysphagia in patients with neurological disorders: systematic review. J Adv Nurs. 2009;65:477–93.

19. Lam K, Lam FK, Lau KK, Chan YK, Kan EY, Woo J, et al. Simple clinical tests may predict severe oropharyngeal dysphagia in Parkinson's disease. Mov Disord. 2007;22:640–4.

20. Clave P, Arreola V, Romea M, Medina L, Palomera E, Serra-Prat M. Accuracy of the volume-viscosity swallow test for clinical screening of oropharyngeal dysphagia and aspiration. Clin Nutr. 2008;27:806–15.

21. Nathadwarawala KM, Nicklin J, Wiles CM. A timed test of swallowing capacity for neurological patients. J Neurol Neurosurg Psychiatry. 1992;55:822–5.

22. Suiter DM, Leder SB. Clinical utility of the 3-ounce water swallow test. Dysphagia. 2008;23:244–50.

23. Manor Y, Balas M, Giladi N, Mootanah R, Cohen JT. Anxiety, depression and swallowing disorders in patients with Parkinson's disease. Parkinsonism Relat Disord. 2009;15:453–6.

24. Barker J, Martino R, Reichardt B, Hickey EJ, Ralph-Edwards A. Incidence and impact of dysphagia in patients receiving prolonged endotracheal intubation after cardiac surgery. Can J Surg. 2009;52:119–24.

25. Platteaux N, Dirix P, Dejaeger E, Nuyts S. Dysphagia in head and neck cancer patients treated with chemoradiotherapy. Dysphagia. 2010;25:139–52.

26. Ramsey DJ, Smithard DG, Kalra L. Early assessments of dysphagia and aspiration risk in acute stroke patients. Stroke. 2003;34(5):1252–7.

27. Mann G. MASA: the Mann assessment of swallowing ability. Clifton Park: Singular; 2002.

28. Crary MA, Mann GD, Groher ME. Initial psychometric assessment of a functional oral intake scale for dysphagia in stroke patients. Arch Phys Med Rehabil. 2005;86:1516–20.

29. Martino R, Pron G, Diamant NE. Oropharyngeal dysphagia: surveying practice patterns of the speech-language pathologist. Dysphagia. 2004;19:165–76.

30. McCullough GH, Wertz RT, Rosenbek JC, Dinneen C. Clinicians' preferences and practices in conducting clinical/bedside and videofluoroscopic swallowing examinations in an adult, neurogenic population. Am J Speech Lang Pathol. 1999;8:149–63.

31. Mathers-Schmidt BA, Kurlinski M, Department of Communication S, Disorders WWUBWUSABM-Swe. Dysphagia evaluation practices: inconsistencies in clinical assessment and instrumental examination decision-making. Dysphagia. 2003;18(2):114–25.

32. Wallace KL, Middleton S, Cook IJ. Development and validation of a self-report symptom inventory to assess the severity of oral-pharyngeal dysphagia. Gastroenterology. 2000;118:678–87.

33. Belafsky PC, Mouadeb DA, Rees CJ, Pryor JC, Postma GN, Allen J, et al. Validity and reliability of the eating assessment tool (EAT-10). Ann Otol Rhinol Laryngol. 2008;117:919–24.

34. Cook IJ, Kahrilas PJ. AGA technical review on management of oropharyngeal dysphagia. Gastroenterology. 1999;116:455–78.

35. Andrews J. Amyotrophic lateral sclerosis: clinical management and research update. Curr Neurol Neurosci Rep. 2009;9:59–68.

36. Calcagno P, Ruoppolo G, Grasso MG, De Vincentiis M, Paolucci S. Dysphagia in multiple sclerosis—prevalence and prognostic factors. Acta Neurol Scand. 2002;105:40–3.

37. Gasiorowska A, Fass R. Current approach to dysphagia. Gastroenterol Hepatol. 2009;5:269–79.

38. Mann G, Hankey GJ, Cameron D. Swallowing function after stroke: prognosis and prognostic factors at 6 months [see comments]. Stroke. 1999;30:744–8.

39. Gallagher L. The impact of prescribed medication on swallowing: an overview. Perspect Swallow Swallow Disord (Dysphagia). 2010;19:98–102.

40. Logemann JA. Evaluation and treatment of swallowing disorders. Austin: Pro-Ed; 1998.

41. McCullough GH, Rosenbek JC, Wertz RT, McCoy S, Mann G, McCullough K. Utility of clinical swallowing examination measures for detecting aspiration post-stroke. J Speech Lang Hear Res. 2005;48:1280–93.

42. Hughes TAT, Wiles C. Clinical measurement of swallowing in health and in neurogenic dysphagia. Q J Med. 1996;89:109–16.

43. Lazarus C, Logemann JA, Huang CF, Rademaker AW. Effects of two types of tongue strengthening exercises in young normals. Folia Phoniatr Logop. 2003;55:199–205.

44. Yeates EM, Molfenter SM, Steele CM. Improvements in tongue strength and pressure-generation precision following a tongue-pressure training protocol in older individuals with dysphagia: three case reports. Clin Interv Aging. 2008;3:735–47.

45. Hewitt A, Hind J, Kays S, Nicosia M, Doyle J, Tompkins W, et al. Standardized instrument for lingual pressure measurement. Dysphagia. 2008;23:16–25.

46. Yoshida M, Kikutani T, Tsuga K, Utanohara Y, Hayashi R, Akagawa Y. Decreased tongue pressure reflects symptom of dysphagia. Dysphagia. 2006;21:61–5.

47. McCullough GH, Wertz RT, Rosenbek JC. Sensitivity and specificity of clinical/bedside examination signs for detecting aspiration in adults subsequent to stroke. J Commun Disord. 2001;34:55–72.

48. Utanohara Y, Hayashi R, Yoshikawa M, Yoshida M, Tsuga K, Akagawa Y. Standard values of maximum tongue pressure taken using newly developed disposable tongue pressure measurement device. Dysphagia. 2008;23:286–90.

49. White R, Cotton SM, Hind J, Robbins J, Perry A. A comparison of the reliability and stability of oro-lingual swallowing pressures in patients with head and neck cancer and healthy adults. Dysphagia. 2009;24:137–44.

50. Robbins J, Kays SA, Gangnon RE, Hind JA, Hewitt AL, Gentry LR, et al. The effects of lingual exercise in stroke patients with dysphagia. Arch Phys Med Rehabil. 2007;88:150–8.

51. Volonte MA, Porta M, Comi G. Clinical assessment of dysphagia in early phases of Parkinson's disease. Neurol Sci. 2002;23 Suppl 2:S121–2.

52. Mann G, Hankey GJ. Initial clinical and demographic predictors of swallowing impairment following acute stroke. Dysphagia. 2001;16:208–15.

53. Pace CC, McCullough GH. The association between oral microorgansims and aspiration pneumonia in the institutionalized elderly: review and recommendations. Dysphagia. 2010;25:307–22.

54. Langmore SE, Terpenning MS, Schork A, Chen Y, Murray JT, Lopatin D, et al. Predictors of aspiration pneumonia: how important is dysphagia? Dysphagia. 1998;13:69–81.

55. Groher ME, McKaig TN. Dysphagia and dietary levels in skilled nursing facilities. J Am Geriatr Soc. 1995;43:528–32.

56. Chasen M, Bhargava R. A retrospective study of the role of an occupational therapist in the cancer nutrition rehabilitation program. Support Care Cancer. 2010;18:1589–96.

57. Murphy BA, Dietrich MS, Wells N, Dwyer K, Ridner SH, Silver HJ, et al. Reliability and validity of the Vanderbilt Head and Neck Symptom Survey: a tool to assess symptom burden in patients treated with chemoradiation. Head Neck. 2010;32:26–37.

58. Horner J, Massey EW, Riski JE, Lathrop DL, Chase KN. Aspiration following stroke: clinical correlates and outcome. Neurology. 1988;38:1359–62.

59. Horner J, Massey EW, Brazer SR. Aspiration in bilateral stroke patients. Neurology. 1990;40:1686–8.

60. Daniels SK, Brailey K, Priestly DH, Herrington LR, Weisberg LA, Foundas AL. Aspiration in patients with acute stroke. Arch Phys Med Rehabil. 1998;79:14–9.

61. Leder SB. Videofluoroscopic evaluation of aspiration with visual examination of the gag reflex and velar movement. Dysphagia. 1997;12:21–3.

62. Linden P, Kuhlemeier KV, Patterson C. The probability of correctly predicting subglottic penetration from clinical observations. Dysphagia. 1993;8:170–9.

63. Daniels SK, Ballo LA, Mahoney MC, Foundas AL. Clinical predictors of dysphagia and aspiration risk: outcome measures in acute stroke patients. Arch Phys Med Rehabil. 2000;81:1030–3.

64. Logemann JA, Veis S, Colangelo L. A screening procedure for oropharyngeal dysphagia. Dysphagia. 1999;14:44–51.

65. Davies AE, Kidd D, Stone SP, MacMahon J. Pharyngeal sensation and gag reflex in healthy subjects. Lancet. 1995;345:487–8.

66. Horner J, Buoyer FG, Alberts MJ, Helms MJ. Dysphagia following brain-stem stroke. Arch Neurol. 1991;48:1170–3.

67. Schroeder MF, Daniels SK, McClain M, Corey DM, Foundas AL. Clinical and cognitive predictors of swallowing recovery in stroke. J Rehabil Res Dev. 2006;43:301–10.

68. Daniels SK, Schroeder MF, DeGeorge PC, Corey DM, Foundas AL, Rosenbek JC. Defining and measuring dysphagia following stroke. Am J Speech Lang Pathol. 2009;18:74–81.

69. DePippo KL, Holas MA, Reding MJ. Validation of the 3-oz water swallow test for aspiration following stroke. Arch Neurol. 1992;49:1259–61.

70. Suiter DM, Leder SB, Karas DE. The 3-ounce (90-cc) water swallow challenge: a screening test for children with suspected oropharyngeal dysphagia. Otolaryngol Head Neck Surg. 2009;140:187–90.

71. McCullough GH, Wertz RT, Rosenbek JC, Mills RH, Webb WG, Ross KB. Inter- and intrajudge reliability for videofluoroscopic swallowing evaluation measures. Dysphagia. 2001;16:110–8.

72. Daniels SK, Brailey K, Foundas AL. Lingual discoordination and dysphagia following acute stroke: analyses of lesion localization. Dysphagia. 1999;14:85–92.

73. Groher ME, Crary MA. Dysphagia: clinical management in adults and children. Maryland Heights: Mosby/Elsevier; 2010.

74. Borr C, Hielscher-Fastabend M, Lucking A. Reliability and validity of cervical auscultation. Dysphagia. 2007;22:225–34.

75. Leslie P, Drinnan MJ, Zammit-Maempel I, Coyle JL, Ford GA, Wilson JA. Cervical auscultation synchronized with images from endoscopy swallow evaluations. Dysphagia. 2007;22:290–8.

76. Wang TG, Chang YC, Chen SY, Hsiao TY. Pulse oximetry does not reliably detect aspiration on videofluoroscopic swallowing study. Arch Phys Med Rehabil. 2005;86:730–4.

77. Morgan AT, Omahoney R, Francis H. The use of pulse oximetry as a screening assessment for paediatric neurogenic dysphagia. Dev Neurorehabil. 2008;11:25–38.

Part II

Commonly Used Tests for Evaluation of Deglutitive Disorders

3. Radiographic Evaluation of the Oral/Preparatory and Pharyngeal Phases of Swallowing Including the UES: Comprehensive Modified Barium Swallow Studies

Jeri A. Logemann and Kristin Larsen

Abstract The normal oropharyngeal swallow involves rapid neuromuscular actions to move food or liquid through the mouth and pharynx and into the esophagus in two seconds or less. Evaluation of the normal or abnormal swallow is most often completed using a radiographic videofluoroscopic procedure known as the modified barium swallow (MBS) procedure described in detail in this chapter. The MBS has 3 purposes: 1) To identify the presence and the cause of any aspiration; 2) To identify the presence and cause of any oral or oropharyngeal residue after the swallow; 3) To identify treatment strategies that can improve the patient's swallow. During the MBS various volumes of thin liquids from 1 ml to cup drinking, measured viscosities from thin liquid to nectar, puree, and solid food, voluntary controls including timing and effort of airway closure, increasing muscular effort, etc. and sensory stimulation techniques including boluses of various tastes and carbonation can be introduced as described in the chapter. These procedures are assessed for their effectiveness in improving the oropharyngeal swallow and returning the patient to full oral intake as quickly and safely as possible.

When patients have been suspected by their physicians as having a swallowing disorder, a consultation generally comes to speech-language pathology services in the facility to evaluate the patient. That evaluation constitutes a screening of the patient's swallowing problem. If the patient is alert and awake and generally able to accept something placed in their mouth and attempts to swallow it, then a radiographic study of the oral

R. Shaker et al. (eds.), *Manual of Diagnostic and Therapeutic Techniques for Disorders of Deglutition*, DOI 10.1007/978-1-4614-3779-6_3,
© Springer Science+Business Media New York 2013

cavity, pharynx, larynx, and cervical esophagus is often scheduled. If the patient's ability to follow directions is questioned or if oral function is thought to be impaired, a more detailed assessment at the bedside may be conducted. Typically, however, the major limitation to conducting a radiographic assessment of swallow is the patient's general alertness and acceptance of material in their mouth.

The radiographic examination: The Modified Barium Swallow (MBS). The oropharyngeal swallow is a more rapid and complex physiology than is the esophageal aspect of deglutition and involves three phases. The three phases begin with oral placement, i.e., the manipulation of food in the mouth, as well as reduction of the food to a consistency appropriate for chewing. Typically, if oral preparation is not complete before a swallow attempt, the raw bolus, or bolus that is hard and not reduced to a thickened and softened consistency and mixed with saliva, will result in gagging the patient. Gagging is generally a reflexive response to something in the mouth or pharynx that is too large to be comfortably swallowed. The gag reflex is not a part of the swallow but is a preliminary protection. Oral preparation is the first stage in the oropharyngeal swallow. The oral tongue controls the lateralization of material to the teeth and facilitates chewing. When chewing is complete, the oral tongue will subdivide the material into a size that is capable of being swallowed. The oral tongue collects the sensory information about the material being swallowed; this information is needed to form the appropriate size bolus to be swallowed for its consistency. It will take a variable length of time for this chewing and bolus formation to occur, depending on the patient's dental status and strength in and coordination in buccal and lingual musculature to control the bolus. The tongue is the controlling factor in chewing. If the amount of food in the mouth is too large for the swallow, then a part of the bolus is sequestered into the cheek pouch and held in the mouth for a follow-up swallow, while the main portion of the bolus enters into the oral stage of the swallow. It is becoming clearer that the amount of tongue strength needed is a critical element in facilitating a normal oropharyngeal swallow [1–3]. The oral preparation of the food for swallow is completed when the oral tongue subdivides the bolus to make ready for swallow and holds the bolus on the tongue or on the floor of the mouth in front of a slightly retracted oral tongue.

At this point, the oral stage of swallow begins with an upward–along rolling motion of the oral tongue propelling the bolus back toward the hard and soft palates. If the patient holds the bolus on the floor of the mouth before the swallow and then picks it up and puts it on the tongue to initiate the oral swallow, it is known as a "dipper" swallow [4]. If the bolus is held on the tip of the tongue and the swallow is initiated, it is known as a "tipper" swallow. Dipper swallows occur more often in people over age 60. The reason is unclear.

The pharyngeal stage of swallow is clearly the most complex in its anatomy and physiology, beginning with the actual triggering of the pharyngeal stage. The critical sensory stimulus to elicit the onset of motor control in the pharyngeal stage has not been clearly defined. There are techniques that have been utilized to stimulate that pharyngeal swallow in patients who have trouble eliciting the swallow independently, such as thermal tactile stimulation [5, 6] and carbonated boluses [7], but these are rather gross techniques that are not attempting to directly emulate the neural stimulus needed. When the pharyngeal swallow triggers, a number of pharyngeal events occur in a generally organized fashion, beginning with the superior and anterior movement of the larynx and hyoid bone, the closure of the airway at the levels of the true vocal folds, followed by the entrance to the airway at the arytenoid cartilages and base of epiglottis, and finally, the closure at the epiglottis. The laryngeal and hyoid elevation contribute to narrowing the entrance to the airway. The base of tongue moves backward to meet the anteriorly bulging posterior pharyngeal wall and the medially bulging lateral pharyngeal walls. The pharyngeal walls contract top to bottom sequentially to narrow the pharynx and increase pharyngeal pressure. The upper esophageal sphincter must be opened by a combination of events beginning with relaxation of the cricopharyngeal muscle followed by the pull of the thyroid and hyoid structures. Pharyngeal transit times for the bolus are less than 1 s in normal individuals of all ages. It is prolonged slightly (by a fraction of a second) as the nature of the bolus is thickened. The bolus has passed through the pharynx and the upper esophageal sphincter within a second from its entry into the pharynx.

The definition of the nature of a patient's oropharyngeal dysphagia depends upon careful visualization via radiography. Other techniques have been introduced to also visualize the pharynx but techniques such as videoendoscopy do not enable observation of certain critical aspects of the pharyngeal swallow, such as tongue base posterior movement, levels of airway closure, and/or or upper esophageal sphincter opening. Unfortunately, studies that have compared the results of videoendoscopic and videofluoroscopic studies of the oropharyngeal swallow have asked only limited questions such as, "Is the patient aspirating or not?" Unfortunately, where there is in some manuscripts a correlation between identification of aspiration on videoendoscopy and identification of presence of aspiration on videofluoroscopy, the questions regarding the cause of the aspiration, the timing of the aspiration, and the nature of other specific types of pharyngeal swallow disorders have not been asked. The asking of limited questions can make the two procedures appear equally useful when, in fact, the questions regarding cause and timing of aspiration and other swallow disorders cannot be answered by videoendoscopy [8, 9]. These two manuscripts have clearly shown the elements of the oropharyngeal swallow which are identified using videoendoscopy vs. videofluoroscopy, and this must be kept in mind when selecting one of these two oropharyngeal diagnostic procedures.

Arranging to conduct the MBS. Prior to conducting an MBS, the clinician must determine that the fluoroscopic equipment is capable of visualizing and recording the necessary events. That is the ability to observe the superior and inferior posterior and lateral aspects of the image that normally includes the soft palate superiorly, the tongue base and upper esophageal sphincter inferiorly, the lips anteriorly, and the posterior pharyngeal wall posteriorly. Once the patient has been positioned in the lateral projection to visualize these structures, the clinician must be sure that the fluoroscopic equipment is capable of recording at a minimum of 30 frames per second. Anything less will limit the visualized detail of the oropharyngeal swallow and potentially will miss the identification of some physiologic disorders. For example, aspiration may occur very quickly (in less than a fifteenth of a second in some patients). Similarly, the visualization of a tracheoesophageal fistula in the lower cervical esophagus may not last more than one-fifteenth of a second. These and other disorders may not be identified if the fluoroscope is running slower than 30 frames per second. The MBS is designed not only to define structure but also to define the movement patterns of all of the structures within the oral cavity, pharynx, and upper esophageal sphincter during the swallow.

Generally, before beginning the study, the patient is asked about any allergies to barium or other food substances to be used during the study, prior to conducting the study. If there is a barium allergy, then another radio-opaque substance should be substituted, as desired. The patient may not like the taste of the liquid or other consistencies, but generally the newer barium products are more acceptable to the patient's taste. To obtain the radiographic material, it is generally best to purchase them from Bracco Diagnostics [10], which produces thin liquid barium very similar to water, nectar-thickened barium liquids, honey-thickened liquids, and pureed material. The clinician can select the normal foods they would like to introduce, depending on the patient's swallowing disorder and complaints about foods that are difficult to swallow.

Once the visibility of the image has been defined and the rate of recording has been assured, the protocol for the study should be standardized, at least initially. While the protocol should be standardized, there are variabilities within patients' oropharyngeal swallow that warrant changes in the protocol in order to meet the second major goal of the study, and that is, not only to define the nature of the swallow problem but also to define and introduce treatment as soon as the patient exhibits significant swallowing abnormalities. Such abnormalities include aspiration, its timing and cause, as well as the cause of significant residue anywhere in the mouth and pharynx.

Defining the protocol for the MBS. Over the past 20 years, a number of investigators have defined factors which systematically change the characteristics of the normal oropharyngeal swallow according to age. These variables include the volume of the bolus, the viscosity of the bolus, and the voluntary control exerted over the oropharyngeal swallow. Each of these should be examined systematically during the MBS. Bolus volume is the most critical in making significant changes in oropharyngeal swallow physiology, including the duration of closure of the airway and duration and diameter of opening of the upper esophageal sphincter [11, 12]. Starting with a small volume, 1 mL, enables the clinician to identify any massive aspiration of thin liquids on a small volume, thus restricting the possibility that the patient would aspirate a large amount, yet allowing the clinician to define the etiology of the aspiration for the patient with dysphagia related to a range of diagnoses [13]. Thin liquids are the viscosity of food on which aspiration occurs most often. Rather than dumping larger volumes down the airway, using a 1 mL initial swallow enables a safe look at the patient's basic swallow physiology. It also explains why a patient may have difficulty swallowing saliva which is a small volume (1 or 2 mL) naturally. After swallowing 1–3 swallows of 1 mL, the protocol may expand to 3 mL of liquid of a measuring teaspoon, which is the size of teaspoon that can be carried to the mouth without spillage. Then the study should move to 2–3 swallows of 10 mL, which is a tablespoon volume. Looking at the way in which the swallow systematically changes from 1 to 10 mL volume will explain to the clinician the basic physiology of the patient's swallow of thin liquids. After completing two or three swallows of each of the bolus volumes, the clinician should have the patient take several spontaneous swallows from a cup at the patient's self-selection of volume. Observing the swallows from 1 to 10 mL is important, as there are some visible differences that should occur in the normal swallow, including changing the duration of the laryngeal closure and cricopharyngeal opening or increasing duration as volume increases and increasing the duration of upper esophageal sphincter opening, which should also increase with increasing volume. The upper esophageal sphincter not only opens longer but should open wider as bolus volume increases, such that there is a visible difference between the width of opening on a 1 mL swallow, which is rather small, and the 10 mL volume opening, which should be approximately twice as wide as the 1 mL opening. The efficiency of all of the volumes swallowed should be the same—that is, there should be minimal residue remaining in the pharynx after the swallow as the volume increases. Following two 10 mL swallows out and through the esophagus can serve as a screening of esophageal function.

Changes with age within the normal liquid swallow. After age 60, there are small changes in the normal swallow physiology that should be expected [14, 15]. For example, the efficiency of the swallow is slightly reduced, such that there is a small amount of residue remaining in the pharynx after the swallow in the older person. No significant increase in pharyngeal residue has been seen as the patient moves from ages 60 to 80 or 90 [14, 15].

There are also changes in the frequency of penetration as people age [14, 15]. Penetration is the entry of small amounts of food or liquid into the airway down to a variety of levels but not below the vocal folds [14–16]. Normally, any penetrated material is squeezed from the airway as the swallow progresses or is coughed from the airway after it has entered. Normal healthy individuals have an increasing frequency of liquid penetration as they pass age 60 and an increase in pudding material penetration when they pass age 50 [11]. Generally, in normal healthy individuals there is very infrequent penetration at ages younger than 50 [14–16]. The critical clinical and instrumental diagnostic observation is whether or not the subject clears the penetrated material with a subsequent cough, throat clear, or a swallow.

Another observation occurring quite regularly with aging is an increase in the delay in triggering of the pharyngeal swallow [14, 15]. The pharyngeal swallow typically triggers very quickly with minimal delay in younger individuals but as the individual increases in age, there tends to be a somewhat longer separation between the oral stage of swallow and the pharyngeal stage. This completely fits with the knowledge of changes in reflexive behavior with advancing age. Typically, reflexes become a bit slower as the individual ages and this appears to occur in the trigger of the pharyngeal swallow, which is also a reflexive behavior [14, 15]. These are visible changes in the oropharyngeal swallow with aging. None of them have been found to increase significantly over time so that someone in their 90s has no more frequent penetration than someone in their 60s [16]. There is some variability in healthy elderly individuals who have completely normal oropharyngeal swallow with none of the described changes occurring.

The newest aspect of the radiographic study of the oropharyngeal swallow is the introduction of treatment strategies. If the patient exhibits significant abnormalities in their swallow, including aspiration or excessive residue, then it is important that the clinician select and introduce treatment strategies to improve either or both of these abnormalities after defining their cause. There are several categories of treatment strategies that can be introduced during the study and observed for their effects on the swallow: (1) Change in head, neck, or body posture to direct the bolus differently into the pharynx or esophagus, (2) Altered food consistency and or volume, (3) Introduction of treatment strategies.

Assessment of viscosity effects on oropharyngeal swallow. There are changes in the oropharyngeal swallow as the bolus consistency becomes thicker or more viscous [14]. In general, there is prolonged cricopharyngeal opening as the viscosity of the bolus increases and the duration of airway closure also increases. These changes are usually visible on videofluoroscopy. There are also increases in pressure exerted during the swallow as the bolus becomes more viscous, but they are not visible radiographically.

Introduction of treatment strategies. The identification of the patient's physiologic swallowing disorders and their severity leads to the clinician determining whether or not treatment strategies should introduced. The second major purpose of the MBS is to determine whether there is a way in which the patient is safe to eat or drink at least one consistency of food or liquid by mouth while implementing a treatment strategy that has been verified as improving the efficiency and safety of the swallow physiology during the instrumental examination.

Clinicians typically introduce strategies to improve the swallow in the order of their ease and simplicity for the patient. Generally, postural change is the easiest for patients to use. In general, postural changes result in redirection of food or liquid through the mouth and pharynx during the swallow. They do not require a great deal of extra muscle effort on the patient's part but do require some ability to remember and concentrate on using the posture during each of the swallows. This is difficult for some specific types of patients such as those who have suffered a right CVA or traumatic brain injury [6]. These are four postures most frequently used.

Each of the four postures results in a different effect on the swallow. It is important that clinicians remember that each posture has a different purpose and results in unique physiologic deglutitive change for most patients [17–20]. One posture cannot be used as the only solution to numerous swallowing problems. At times, clinicians overuse a posture like chin down (also known as: chin tuck) or head rotation when, in fact, other postures or combinations may be the best solution. Careful directions of the patient are necessary in ensuring their correct usage. However, postural changes can still be the most effective management procedures to improve the safety and efficiency of the swallow [21].

Postural techniques. The first posture is chin down. Chin down posture has several effects: (1) to push the anterior wall of the pharynx posteriorly so that the tongue base is closer to the posterior pharyngeal wall; (2) to narrow the airway entrance and reduce the aspiration that may slide over the tongue base and into the airway; (3) to slow oral transit such that the bolus, especially of liquid, does not splash as quickly from the mouth into the pharynx; and (4) to widen the valleculae. In some individuals the lowering of the chin drops the tongue base forward, thus widening the valleculae and enabling liquids and other foods to rest in the valleculae before spilling over into the pharynx or before the pharyngeal swallow triggers [17]. This does not occur with every patient but can be quite helpful in some.

The second posture is head rotation. Head rotation is used when there is either a unilateral pharyngeal wall paresis or a unilateral laryngeal paresis. The rotation is done to the damaged side of the larynx or pharynx and closes that side from the path of the bolus. As the patient swallows with head rotation, the bolus moves down the stronger or more normal side of the pharynx or larynx and aspiration is often eliminated. Head rotation can also facilitate opening of the upper esophageal sphincter [17, 18]. Head rotation should always be to the weaker side of the pharynx if there is a difference in the two sides, but whether or not the two sides are different, rotating the head to one side pulls the larynx more away from the posterior pharyngeal wall, thus improving opening of the upper esophageal sphincter [18].

The third posture is lifting the chin up to facilitate emptying of the oral cavity by means of gravity. For patients such as those with motor neuron disease or removal of part or all of the oral tongue, lifting the chin facilitates movement of liquid and thin puree by gravity out of the mouth and into the pharynx. Generally, lifting the chin needs to be combined with a breath hold or supraglottic swallow so that liquid falling from the mouth does not go directly into the airway.

The fourth posture is lying down on the patient's stronger side with a pillow supporting the head but not elevating it or the patient lying down on the back with a pillow maintaining the head in line with the spine, to facilitate reduced aspiration of residue occurring after the swallow. Lying down tends to help the patient maintain normal pharyngeal control during the swallow and enables them to clear residue in two or three repeated swallows so the bolus is cleared without aspiration [19]. If this technique facilitates a safe swallow, then the patient can eat small amounts while lying in the supine or side-lying position. Postural changes have been used since the 1940s and are still being used successfully in some patients. Despite the fact that these procedures have been used for a long time in carefully selected patients does not reduce their effectiveness.

Combining postures. There are times when a single posture will not accomplish the desired clinical goal, but combining postures can achieve a safer or more efficient swallow. For example, combining the chin down and head rotation often gives the best airway closure. Combining chin down posture to narrow the airway entrance and head rotation to the weaker side to direct food down the more efficient side can result in an extremely safe and tight airway closure. Similarly, combining the side lying with chin down may accomplish the same goal.

After a postural technique is prescribed and repeated five to ten times with the patient during X-ray, the patient should be instructed to utilize this posture or postures while taking selected amounts of material by mouth. Then the patient should return for reevaluation radiographically within 1 week. At that time, the patient should be observed while using whatever postures were previously instructed. New directions should not be given until the patient has demonstrated that they are using the postural technique correctly. If they are using it incorrectly, then the patient can be reinstructed in how to use the postural procedure. Some patients can return to safe and efficient swallowing on some diet consistencies, using one or more postural procedures.

Sensory enhancing procedures. Many patients exhibit a sensory disorder in eliciting their pharyngeal stage of swallow. Specifically, they may have difficulty in eliciting the pharyngeal stage of swallow until the bolus has dropped further into the pharynx and, in some cases, into the airway or collected in the pharyngeal spaces including the valleculae and the pyriform sinuses. Techniques which heighten sensation have been shown to facilitate faster airway closure and pharyngeal swallow triggering. These techniques include using a sour bolus [20], a carbonated bolus [7], and using thermal tactile stimulation, (using a size 00 laryngeal mirror to rub the anterior faucial arches on each side for approximately five repetitions and then presenting the patient with small amounts of thin cold liquid) [11]. Doing this during the instrumental evaluation allows observation of the effects of the thermal tactile stimulation in speeding the swallow and potentially eliminating any aspiration that can occur while the swallow is delayed and the bolus remains in the pharynx. Another sensory technique that has been shown to have some effect on the oral and pharyngeal phases is carbonation [7]. Carbonation of the bolus is normally performed by taking an Alka Seltzer or sodium bicarbonate tablet putting it in cold liquid and then giving it to the patient to swallow in half-teaspoon amounts as fast as possible. Very often, swallows of the carbonated material result in a faster triggering of the pharyngeal swallow [7]. Again, these two procedures are appropriate only for patients with a sensory disorder, specifically those with a delay in triggering of the pharyngeal stage of swallow. This disorder occurs frequently in patients who have suffered a stroke, a head injury, or have had surgery to the oropharyngeal region for head and neck cancer [13].

Voluntary control—Swallow maneuvers. The third category of treatment procedures that can be introduced during X-ray to improve the swallow is known as swallow maneuvers [13]. Swallow maneuvers are voluntary techniques designed to effect a specific aspect of the motor control of the pharynx during swallow. There are five such procedures, including (1) the effortful swallow, (2) the supraglottic swallow, (3) the super-supraglottic swallow, (4) the Mendelsohn maneuver, and (5) the tongue holding maneuver. All of these require that a patient be able to follow directions and gain control of the motor mechanism of the swallow. None are painful but all require a slightly slower swallow in process of using each swallow maneuver [13]. They also require greater muscle effort than a normal swallow, so that they can be more difficult for elderly patients and those who are medically fragile or fatigued.

The *effortful swallow* involves squeezing the oral and pharyngeal musculature with greater than normal effort during the swallow. Typically, this maneuver is used when a patient has oral and/or pharyngeal residue after completion of the swallow. The goal is to eliminate or significantly decrease the residue by increasing the pressure used during the swallow [22].

The *supraglottic maneuver* is designed to close the airway at the true vocal folds before and during the swallow. In order to achieve the supraglottic swallow, the patient is instructed to take a breath in, hold their breath in their larynx, not their chest, and continue to hold their breath as they swallow, followed by a light cough to clear any residual material after the swallow. This maneuver is designed for those patients with reduction in airway closure.

The *super-supraglottic swallow maneuver* is designed to close the airway entrance. During this maneuver the patient is instructed to again inhale, hold their breath tightly, and swallow, usually with greater effort, and cough after the swallow. During the MBS, the clinician can observe the gap in the airway entrance. The smaller the gap, the greater the effort used. The difference in the supraglottic and super-supraglottic maneuvers is the degree of effort used to achieve and maintain airway closure at the airway entrance with the super–supraglottic swallow [23]. The increased effort used in achieving the closure typically closes the airway at the entrance with the false vocal folds and arytenoid cartilages. This technique requires more effort than a supraglottic swallow, but does result in a higher level of airway closure. This level of closure is particularly needed in those who have undergone a supraglottic laryngectomy. With a super–supraglottic swallow maneuver, the patient must have good laryngeal lifting following the maneuver in order to clear any residue that may have been left in the larynx or on top of the larynx after the swallow.

The most difficult of the swallow maneuvers is the *Mendelsohn maneuver*, which requires that the patient be able to perceive laryngeal movement during swallow. It is a maneuver more easily done by men than women, probably because of the increased size of the laryngeal cartilage (Adam's apple) in men. The patient is asked to swallow several times and feel kinesthetically whether they can tell if something lifts and lowers in the front of their neck during the swallow. This is explained as the "Adam's apple." Once the patient can feel the elevation of the thyroid, they can be asked to swallow normally and feel the Adam's apple lift as high as it goes and then grab it with their muscles and not let it lower for a few seconds until the swallow is over. The Adam's apple should be grabbed with muscle effort, not with the hand. Patients are instructed to hold their Adam's apple up for several seconds during the swallow and then let go. This results in the prolonged opening of the upper esophageal sphincter as long as the larynx is elevated. Indirect biofeedback can be given as the clinician observes the patient's laryngeal movement and gives them information as to whether they indeed caught their Adam's apple as it elevated and kept it elevated for several extra seconds. Problems in producing the Mendelsohn maneuver typically involve catching the Adam's apple movement too late, thus catching it when it is on its way down and not at its maximum elevated position, or trying to elevate the larynx voluntarily without an actual swallow. Typically, it is easy to observe the laryngeal movement and whether or not it occurs as a part of a swallow, or whether the individual is trying to volitionally lift the larynx, as the larynx tends to jerk as it elevates if voluntary control is being used. Some clinicians have used surface EMG to assist the patient in perceiving laryngeal elevation [24, 25]. The purpose of the Mendelsohn maneuver is to improve upper esophageal sphincter opening by accentuating the laryngeal and hyoid movement, which is the controlling factor for upper sphincter opening in the anterior posterior direction during the swallow [6, 13].

The final swallow maneuver is the *tongue hold maneuver, also known as the Masako maneuver* [26, 27]. The tongue hold maneuver involves the patient holding their tongue gently but firmly between their central incisors such that perhaps a fourth of their oral tongue is extended. Swallowing should be done while holding the tongue in that position. It is difficult to initiate a swallow with the oral tongue in that position and may take an extra second, but in pulling the tongue forward and holding it there, the base of tongue is pulled forward and the posterior pharyngeal wall anterior movement is accentuated. This maneuver is appropriate for the patient with reduced base of tongue or pharyngeal wall movement. The purpose of the tongue hold movement is to strengthen both tongue base posterior movement and anterior pharyngeal movement.

These voluntary maneuvers can be used to exercise the oral, pharyngeal, or laryngeal musculature. Or, the use of the maneuvers can be applied to actual eating. The effortful swallow, the supraglottic swallow, the super–supraglottic swallow, and the Mendelsohn maneuver can all be used to facilitate a more successful or safe swallow and be used in actual nutritional intake. The tongue hold maneuver should not be used during eating as it makes swallowing more awkward and difficult. The effectiveness of each maneuver should be examined on or during the radiographic study.

A fourth mechanism for improving the safety and efficiency of possible oral intake is a *change in diet*. Unfortunately, many patients do not want to eliminate certain kinds of foods such as thin liquids or foods requiring chewing from their diet. Often patients may prefer to take non-oral feeding (tube feeding) to changing or limiting the consistency or volume of their oral diet. Clinicians may identify safest and most efficient diet choices during the radiographic study before and after postural techniques, sensory procedures, and/or swallow maneuvers are evaluated. Because patients tend to dislike diet changes, most clinicians will examine the effectiveness of the other techniques before changing their diet. Typically, patients with problems in airway closure will have difficulty with thin liquids, as will those with a delay in triggering the pharyngeal swallow. Thickening liquids can be evaluated by introducing a liquid diet of nectar-thickened liquids in various volumes from 1 to 3 to 5 and 10 mL, and finally, cup-drinking of nectar-thickened liquids. Generally, nectar-thickened liquids are most acceptable to dysphagic patients [28]. If disorders continue to occur with nectar swallows, a thicker liquid, such as honey, can be introduced. However, there are several studies showing patient dislike for honey and at least one study showing that aspiration pneumonia is likely to occur more often on honey-thickened material [28]. Patient compliance is poor for thickened liquids, especially honey-thickened liquids [28].

Evaluation of exercises procedures. Which of these types of management procedures will be effective in any specific patient will depend somewhat on the patient's characteristics, including age, swallow disorders and severity, their willingness to try the techniques, and other food types [29].

The report. The report of the radiographic study should begin with a description of the patient's oral activity during chewing and bolus shaping prior to initiation of the oral stage of swallow. The report should state in what position the evaluation was completed (lateral and AP), food consistencies and volumes used during the study, as well as behavior and compliance of patient. The oral stage of swallow should be described including oral transit times in relation to normal times reported for various ages [14, 15] and the ability of the patient to chew the bolus if they have reached the cookie consistency and are able to initiate the oral stage of swallow. Any delay in triggering of the pharyngeal swallow should be measured in time (seconds) and then compared with normal data for age [14, 15]. Then, after the pharyngeal swallow has triggered, the elements of the pharyngeal stage should be defined as normal or abnormal. If any interventions are introduced at this point because of aspiration or increased residue, this should be described in terms of their success or failure. The report should indicate when aspiration occurred in terms of pre-, intra-, or post-deglutitive aspiration; this is an important factor in determining treatment and management. Finally, recommendations should be made regarding the patient's ability to maintain an oral diet or need for a non-oral diet or need for a particular food consistency. Finally, the last recommendation presents the need for therapy and the type of therapy needed.

Reports should be sent to the patient's referring physician as soon as possible and any other professional the patient requests. The results are also entered into the patient's chart, so that all others caring for the patients can review the findings. A follow-up phone call to him/her to answer any questions is advised. Use of a check sheet to report the studies is not recommended as such sheets are often difficult to read and interpret, especially by individuals who are not swallowing specialists.

References

1. Lazarus C, Logemann JA, Huang CF, Rademaker AW. Effects of two types of tongue strengthening exercises in young normals. Folia Phoniatr Logop. 2003;55(4):199–205.
2. Robbins J, Gangnon RE, Theis SM, et al. The effects of lingual exercise on swallowing in older adults. J Am Geriatr Soc. 2005;53(9):1483–9.
3. Robbins J, Kays SA, Gangnon RE, et al. The effects of lingual exercise in stroke patients with dysphagia. Arch Phys Med Rehabil. 2007;88(2):150–8.
4. Dodds WJ, Taylor AJ, Stewart ET, Kern MK, Logemann JA, Cook IJ. Tipper and dipper types of oral swallows. AJR Am J Roentgenol. 1989;153(6):1197–9.
5. Lazzara G, Lazarus C, Logemann JA. Impact of thermal stimulation on the triggering of the swallowing reflex. Dysphagia. 1986;1:73–7.
6. Logemann JA. A manual for videofluoroscopic evaluation of swallowing. 2nd ed. Austin: Pro-Ed; 1993.
7. Bülow M, Olsson R, Ekberg O. Videoradiographic analysis of how carbonated thin liquids and thickened liquids affect the physiology of swallowing in subjects with aspiration on thin liquids. Acta Radiol. 2003;44:366–72.
8. Logemann JA, Rademaker AW, Pauloski BR, Ohmae Y, Kahrilas PJ. Normal swallowing physiology as viewed by videofluoroscopy and videoendoscopy. Folia Phoniatr Logop. 1998;50:311–9.
9. Logemann JA, Rademaker AW, Pauloski BR, Ohmae Y, Kahrilas PJ. Interobserver agreement on normal swallowing physiology as viewed by videofluoroscopy and videoendoscopy. Folia Phoniatr Logop. 1999;51:91–8.
10. Bracco Diagnostics. 107 College Road East, Princeton, NJ 08540, USA. http://www.bracco.com (2011). Accessed 17 Feb 2011.
11. Lazarus CL, Logemann JA, Rademaker AW, Kahrilas PJ, Pajak T, Lazar R, et al. Effects of bolus volume, viscosity, and repeated swallows in nonstroke subjects and stroke patients. Arch Phys Med Rehabil. 1993;74(10):1066–70.
12. Kahrilas PJ, Logemann JA. Volume accommodation during swallowing. Dysphagia. 1993;8(3):259–65.
13. Logemann JA. Evaluation and treatment of swallowing disorders. 2nd ed. Austin: Pro-Ed; 1998.

14. Logemann JA, Pauloski BR, Rademaker AW, Kahrilas PJ. Oropharyngeal swallow in younger and older men: videofluoroscopic analysis. J Speech Lang Hear Res. 2002;45(3):434–45.

15. Rademaker AW, Pauloski BR, Colangelo LA, Logemann JA. Age and volume effects on liquid swallowing function in normal women. J Speech Lang Hear Res. 1998;41(2): 275–84.

16. Daggett A, Logemann J, Rademaker A, Pauloski B. Laryngeal penetration during deglutition in normal subjects of various ages. Dysphagia. 2006;21(4):270–4.

17. Welch MV, Logemann JA, Rademaker AW, Kahrilas PJ. Changes in pharyngeal dimensions effected by chin tuck. Arch Phys Med Rehabil. 1993;74(2):178–81.

18. Logemann JA, Kahrilas PJ, Kobara M, Vakil NB. The benefit of head rotation on pharyngoesophageal dysphagia. Arch Phys Med Rehabil. 1989;70(10):767–71.

19. Rasley A, Logemann JA, Kahrilas PJ, Rademaker AW, Pauloski BR, Dodds WJ. Prevention of barium aspiration during videofluoroscopic swallowing studies: value of change in posture. AJR Am J Roentgenol. 1993;160(5):1005–9.

20. Logemann JA, Pauloski BR, Colangelo L, Lazarus C, Fujiu M, Kahrilas PJ. Effects of a sour bolus on oropharyngeal swallowing measures in patients with neurogenic dysphagia. J Speech Hear Res. 1995;38(3):556–63.

21. Takasaki K, Umeki H, Kumagami H, Takahashi H. Influence of head rotation on upper esophageal sphincter pressure evaluated by high-resolution manometry system. Otolaryngol Head Neck Surg. 2010;142(2):214–7.

22. Pouderoux P, Kahrilas PJ. Deglutitive tongue force modulation by volition, volume, and viscosity in humans. Gastroenterology. 1995;108(5):1418–26.

23. Martin BJ, Logemann JA, Shaker R, Dodds WJ. Normal laryngeal valving patterns during three breath-hold maneuvers: a pilot investigation. Dysphagia. 1993;8(1): 11–20.

24. Ding R, Larson CR, Logemann JA, Rademaker AW. Surface electromyographic and electroglottographic studies in normal subjects under two swallow conditions: normal and during the Mendelsohn manuever. Dysphagia. 2002;17(1):1–12.

25. Park JW, Oh JC, Lee HJ, Park SJ, Yoon TS, Kwon BS. Effortful swallowing training coupled with electrical stimulation leads to an increase in hyoid elevation during swallowing. Dysphagia. 2009;24(3):296–301.

26. Fujiu M, Paulosk BR, Logemann JA. Increased postoperative posterior pharyngeal wall movement in patients with anterior oral cancer: preliminary findings and possible implications for treatment. Am J Speech Lang Pathol. 1995;4:24–30.

27. Fujiu M, Logemann JA. Effect of a tongue holding maneuver on posterior pharyngeal wall movement during deglutition. Am J Speech Lang Pathol. 1996;5:23–30.

28. Robbins J, Gensler G, Hind J, Logemann JA, Lindblad AS, Brandt D, et al. Comparison of 2 interventions for liquid aspiration on pneumonia incidence: a randomized trial. Ann Intern Med. 2008;148(7):509–18. Erratum in: Ann Intern Med. 2008;148(9):715.

29. Logemann JA, Rademaker A, Pauloski BR, Kelly A, Stangl-McBreen C, Antinoja J, et al. A randomized study comparing the Shaker exercise with traditional therapy: a preliminary study. Dysphagia. 2009;24(4):403–11.

4. Radiographic Evaluation of the Esophageal Phase of Swallowing

Marc S. Levine

Abstract The barium esophagogram is a valuable diagnostic test for evaluating both structural and functional abnormalities in the esophagus. The study is usually performed as a multiphasic examination that includes upright double-contrast views with high-density barium, prone single-contrast views with low-density barium, and mucosal relief views of the collapsed esophagus. The double-contrast phase optimizes detection of inflammatory or neoplastic diseases, whereas the single-contrast phase optimizes detection of hiatal hernias and lower esophageal rings or strictures. Fluoroscopic examination of the esophagus is also important for assessing motility disorders such as achalasia and diffuse esophageal spasm. The radiologic diagnosis of gastroesophageal reflux disease, other types of esophagitis, benign and malignant esophageal tumors, varices, lower esophageal rings, diverticula, and esophageal motility disorders is considered in this chapter.

Introduction

Barium esophagography is the primary radiologic modality for the evaluation of patients with dysphagia, reflux symptoms, or other clinical findings of esophageal disease. Double-contrast esophagograms are particularly useful for detecting reflux disease and its complications, infectious esophagitis, esophageal carcinoma, and other structural lesions of the esophagus. The fluoroscopic portion of the examination is also useful for assessing esophageal motility and detecting motility disorders such as achalasia and diffuse esophageal spasm. The purpose of this chapter is to review gastroesophageal reflux disease, other types of esophagitis, benign and malignant esophageal tumors, varices, lower esophageal rings, diverticula, and esophageal motility disorders, all of which can be diagnosed on barium esophagography.

R. Shaker et al. (eds.), *Manual of Diagnostic and Therapeutic Techniques for Disorders of Deglutition*, DOI 10.1007/978-1-4614-3779-6_4, © Springer Science+Business Media New York 2013

Technique

Barium studies of the esophagus are usually performed as multiphasic tests that include upright double-contrast views with high-density barium, prone single-contrast views with low-density barium, and mucosal relief views of the collapsed esophagus [1]. The patient first ingests an effervescent agent and then rapidly gulps high-density barium in the upright, left posterior oblique position. The normal distended esophagus has a thin, white contour in profile and a smooth, homogenous appearance en face (Fig. 4.1a). Collapsed or partially collapsed views (i.e., mucosal relief views) show the normal longitudinal folds as thin, straight, delicate structures no more than 1–2 mm in width (Fig. 4.1b). The patient is then placed in a recumbent, right-side down position for double-contrast views of the gastric cardia, which can often be recognized by three or four stellate folds radiating to a central point at the gastroesophageal junction, also known as the cardiac rosette [1].

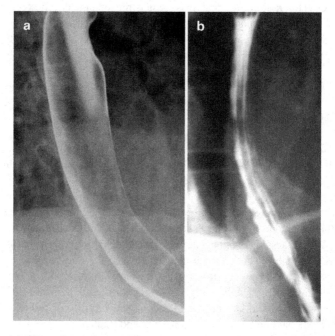

Fig. 4.1. Normal esophagus. Note the normal appearance of the distended (**a**) and collapsed (**b**) esophagus on double-contrast images. The esophagus has a smooth, featureless surface when it is adequately distended.

The patient is then placed in a prone, right anterior oblique position and asked to take discrete swallows of low-density barium to evaluate esophageal motility. The patient next gulps barium to optimally distend the esophagus and better delineate rings, strictures, or hernias that could be missed on upright double-contrast views. Finally, the patient is turned from a supine to a right-lateral position to assess for spontaneous gastroesophageal reflux or reflux provoked by a Valsalva maneuver [1].

A water-siphon test may also be performed to assess for reflux by having the patient swallow several sips of water in a supine, right posterior oblique position. As water passes through the gastroesophageal junction and the lower esophageal sphincter opens, a tiny amount of barium may transiently spurt upwards into the distal esophagus, so-called *physiologic reflux*. When a large volume of barium refluxes into the esophagus, however, this reflux is considered to be pathologic. The water-siphon test has been shown to increase the sensitivity of the barium study for detecting gastroesophageal reflux (though at the cost of a lower specificity) [2].

Gastroesophageal Reflux Disease

The purpose of barium studies in patients with reflux symptoms is not simply to document the presence of a hiatal hernia or reflux but to detect the morphologic sequelae of reflux, including reflux esophagitis, peptic strictures, and Barrett's esophagus. These conditions are discussed separately in the following sections.

Reflux Esophagitis

Double-contrast esophagograms have a sensitivity of almost 90% in detecting reflux esophagitis because of the ability to demonstrate mucosal abnormalities that cannot be visualized on single-contrast studies [2]. The single most common sign of reflux esophagitis on double-contrast esophagograms is a finely nodular or granular appearance with poorly defined radiolucencies that fade peripherally due to edema and inflammation of the mucosa (Fig. 4.2) [3]. This nodularity or granularity almost always extends proximally from the gastroesophageal junction as a continuous area of disease.

52   M.S. Levine

Fig. 4.2. Reflux
esophagitis. There is finely
nodularity or granularity of
the lower third of the
thoracic esophagus due to
edema and inflammation of
the mucosa.

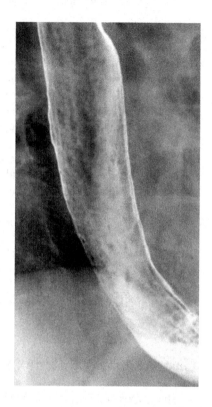

Barium studies may also reveal shallow ulcers and erosions in the distal esophagus. The ulcers can have a punctate, linear, or stellate configuration and are often associated with surrounding halos of edematous mucosa, radiating folds, or sacculation of the adjacent wall (Fig. 4.3) [2]. Other patients may have a solitary ulcer at or near the gastroesophageal junction, often on the posterior wall of the distal esophagus, presumably as a result of prolonged exposure to refluxed acid that pools posteriorly when patients sleep in the supine position [4].

Reflux esophagitis may also be manifested by thickened longitudinal folds due to edema and inflammation extending into the submucosa. However, thickened folds should be recognized as a nonspecific sign of esophagitis from a host of causes. Other patients with chronic reflux esophagitis may have a single enlarged fold that arises at the cardia and extends upward into the distal esophagus as a smooth, polypoid protuberance, also known as an inflammatory esophagogastric polyp [2]. These lesions have no malignant potential, so endoscopy is not warranted when a typical

Fig. 4.3. Reflux esophagitis. This patient has small, shallow ulcers (*arrows*) in the distal esophagus above a hiatal hernia (reproduced with permission from reference [2]).

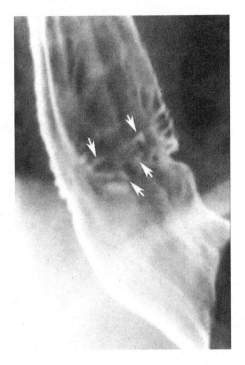

inflammatory esophagogastric polyp is found in the distal esophagus. *If these lesions are unusually large or lobulated and do not have the typical radiographic features of an inflammatory esophagogastric polyp, endoscopic biopsy specimens should be obtained for a definitive diagnosis.*

Scarring and Strictures

Localized scarring from reflux esophagitis may be manifested on barium studies by flattening, puckering, or sacculation of the adjacent esophageal wall, often associated with radiating folds. Further scarring can lead to the development of a circumferential peptic stricture in the distal esophagus [2]. Such strictures typically appear as concentric segments of smooth, tapered narrowing above a hiatal hernia (Fig. 4.4), but asymmetric scarring can lead to asymmetric narrowing with focal sacculation or ballooning of the esophageal wall between areas of fibrosis [2]. Other strictures are manifested by short, ring-like areas of narrowing that can be mistaken for Schatzki rings in patients with dysphagia [2].

Fig. 4.4. Peptic stricture. There is a smooth segment of narrowing (*arrow*) with tapered margins in the distal esophagus above a hiatal hernia due to a reflux-induced (i.e., peptic) stricture.

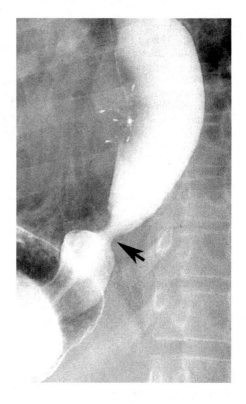

Scarring from reflux esophagitis can also lead to longitudinal shortening of the esophagus and the development of fixed transverse folds, producing a *stepladder* appearance due to pooling of barium between the folds (Fig. 4.5) [5]. This finding should be differentiated from the thin transverse striations (i.e., the *feline esophagus*) seen as a transient phenomenon due to contraction of the longitudinally oriented muscularis mucosae in patients with reflux disease (Fig. 4.6) [6].

Barrett's Esophagus

Double-contrast esophagograms can be used to classify patients with reflux symptoms as being at high, moderate, or low risk for Barrett's esophagus based on specific radiologic criteria [7]. Patients are classified at high risk when barium studies reveal a midesophageal stricture or

Fig. 4.5. Fixed transverse folds in distal esophagus. This patient has a mild peptic stricture (*white arrow*) with pooling of barium between fixed transverse folds (*black arrows*) due to longitudinal scarring and shortening (reproduced with permission from reference [5]).

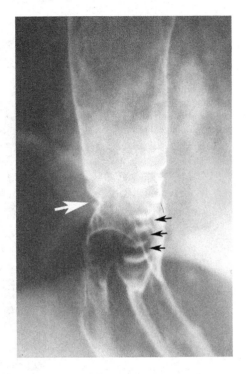

ulcer, usually associated with a hiatal hernia and reflux. A reticular mucosal pattern has also been recognized as a specific radiologic sign of Barrett's esophagus, particularly if adjacent to the distal aspect of a mid *esophageal* stricture (Fig. 4.7) [8]. When these findings are present on barium studies, endoscopy and biopsy should be performed for a definitive diagnosis.

Patients are classified at moderate risk for Barrett's esophagus when barium studies reveal reflux esophagitis or peptic strictures in the distal esophagus. The decision for endoscopy in this group should be based on the age and overall health of the patients (i.e., whether they are reasonable candidates for surveillance). Finally, patients are classified at low risk for Barrett's esophagus when barium studies reveal no structural abnormalities, regardless of the presence or absence of a hiatal hernia or reflux. Most patients are found to be in the low-risk category, and the prevalence of Barrett's esophagus is so small in this group that such individuals can be treated empirically for their reflux symptoms without need for endoscopy [7].

Fig. 4.6. Feline esophagus. There are thin transverse striations due to transient contraction of the muscularis mucosae in a patient with a feline esophagus. These patients almost always have gastroesophageal reflux.

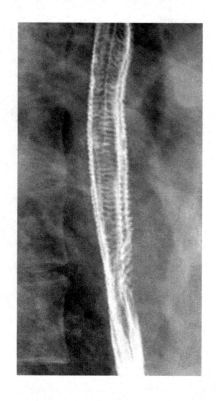

Infectious Esophagitis

Candida Esophagitis

Candida esophagitis usually is manifested on double-contrast barium studies by discrete plaque-like lesions seen as linear or irregular filling defects separated by normal intervening mucosa (Fig. 4.8) [9]. Double-contrast esophagograms have been found to have a sensitivity of 90% in detecting *Candida* esophagitis [10], primarily because of the ability to demonstrate these mucosal plaques. A much more fulminant form of esophageal candidiasis is sometimes encountered in patients with AIDS in whom barium studies reveal a grossly irregular or *shaggy esophagus* caused by innumerable coalescent pseudomembranes and plaques with trapping of barium between these lesions (Fig. 4.9) [9]. When typical findings of *Candida* esophagitis are encountered on double-contrast

Fig. 4.7. Reticular pattern in Barrett's esophagus. There is a mild ring-like stricture (*white arrows*) in the mid esophagus in a patient with Barrett's esophagus. Also note a distinctive reticular pattern extending distally a considerable distance from the stricture (reproduced with permission from reference [8]).

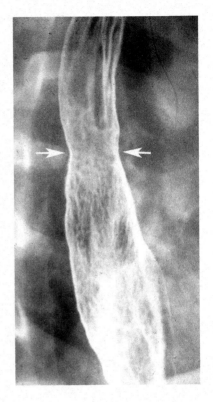

esophagography *in immunocompromised patients, these individuals* can be treated with antifungal agents such as fluconazole without need for endoscopy.

Herpes Esophagitis

The herpes simplex virus is another cause of infectious esophagitis. Herpes esophagitis initially produces small vesicles that subsequently rupture to form discrete, punched-out ulcers on the mucosa. As a result, double-contrast studies may reveal small, superficial ulcers (often surrounded by radiolucent mounds of edema), most commonly in the upper or mid esophagus (Fig. 4.10) [9]. In the appropriate clinical setting, the presence of small, discrete ulcers without plaques should be highly suggestive of herpes esophagitis, as ulceration in candidiasis almost always occurs on a background of diffuse plaque formation.

Fig. 4.8. *Candida* esophagitis. There are multiple discrete plaque-like lesions that have a linear configuration and are separated by normal intervening mucosa.

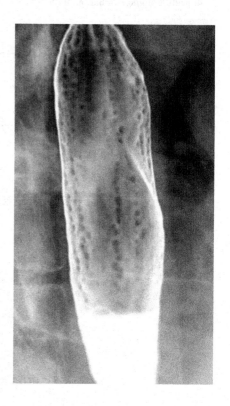

Much less frequently, herpes esophagitis may develop in otherwise healthy patients who have no underlying immunologic problems [11]. Affected individuals usually present with a characteristic flu-like prodrome prior to the sudden onset of severe odynophagia. Barium studies may reveal innumerable tiny ulcers clustered together in the mid esophagus below the left main bronchus [11]. In the appropriate clinical setting, the diagnosis of herpes esophagitis in healthy patients can be suggested on the basis of the radiographic findings without need for endoscopy.

Cytomegalovirus Esophagitis

Cytomegalovirus (CMV) is another cause of infectious esophagitis that occurs primarily in patients with AIDS. CMV esophagitis may be manifested on double-contrast studies by one or more giant, flat ulcers

Fig. 4.9. *Candida* esophagitis with shaggy esophagus. The esophagus has a grossly irregular or shaggy contour due to multiple plaques and pseudomembranes with trapping of barium between these lesions. This fulminant form of *Candida* esophagitis occurs primarily in patients with AIDS.

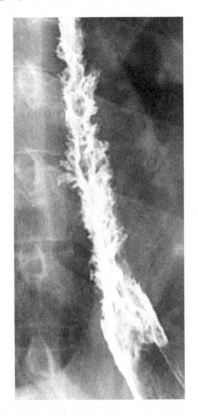

that are several centimeters or more in length [9]. The ulcers may have an ovoid or diamond-shaped configuration and are often surrounded by a thin radiolucent rim of edema (Fig. 4.11). Because herpetic ulcers rarely become this large, the presence of one or more giant ulcers should suggest the possibility of CMV esophagitis in patients with AIDS. However, the differential diagnosis also includes giant HIV ulcers in the esophagus (see next section). Because CMV esophagitis is treated with relatively toxic antiviral agents such as ganciclovir, endoscopy (with biopsy specimens, brushings, and cultures from the esophagus) is required to confirm the presence of CMV infection before treating these patients [9].

Fig. 4.10. Herpes
esophagitis. There are
multiple small, discrete
ulcers (*arrows*) with
surrounding halos of edema
in the mid esophagus due to
herpes esophagitis.

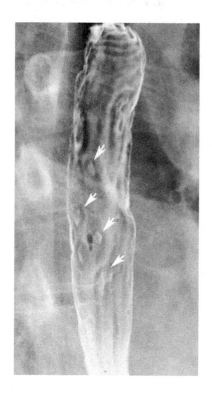

Human Immunodeficiency Virus Esophagitis

Human immunodeficiency virus (HIV) infection of the esophagus
can lead to the development of giant esophageal ulcers indistinguishable
from those caused by CMV esophagitis. Double-contrast esophagograms
typically reveal one or more large ovoid or diamond-shaped ulcers
surrounded by a radiolucent rim of edema (Fig. 4.12), sometimes
associated with a cluster of small satellite ulcers [12]. Occasionally, these
individuals may have associated palatal ulcers or a characteristic
maculopapular rash on the upper body. The diagnosis is established
when endoscopic biopsy specimens, brushings, and cultures reveal no
evidence of CMV esophagitis as the cause of the ulcers. Unlike CMV
ulcers, HIV-related esophageal ulcers usually undergo healing on
treatment with oral steroids [12]. Thus, endoscopy is required in HIV-
positive patients with giant esophageal ulcers to differentiate HIV
esophagitis from CMV esophagitis, so appropriate therapy can be
instituted in these individuals.

Fig. 4.11. CMV esophagitis. This patient with AIDS has a giant, ovoid ulcer in the mid esophagus with a thin surrounding mound of edema (*arrows*). Giant ulcers are characteristic of CMV esophagitis or HIV esophagitis in patients with AIDS (courtesy of Kyunghee C. Cho, M.D., New York, NY).

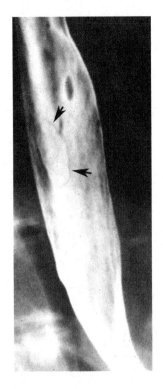

Eosinophilic Esophagitis

Eosinophilic esophagitis (EoE) has been recognized as an increasingly common inflammatory condition of the esophagus, occurring predominantly in young men with long-standing dysphagia and recurrent food impactions, often associated with an atopic history, asthma, or peripheral eosinophilia. The diagnosis of EoE can be confirmed on endoscopic biopsy specimens showing more than 20 eosinophils per high-power field. The etiology is uncertain, but many authors believe EoE develops as an inflammatory response to ingested food allergens in predisposed individuals. As a result, symptomatic patients may have a marked clinical response to treatment with steroids or elemental diets.

The diagnosis of EoE can be suggested on barium studies by the presence of segmental esophageal strictures, sometimes associated with

Fig. 4.12. HIV esophagitis.
A giant, ovoid ulcer is seen
en face in the mid
esophagus with a thin
surrounding mound of
edema (*arrows*). This ulcer
is impossible to
differentiate from the CMV
ulcer in Fig. 4.11
(reproduced with
permission from
reference [12]).

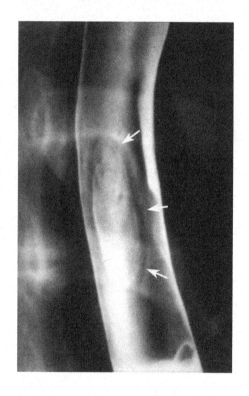

distinctive ring-like indentations, producing a *ringed esophagus*
(Fig. 4.13) [13]. The radiographic diagnosis may also be suggested by
the development of a *small-caliber esophagus* manifested by loss of
caliber of most or all of the thoracic esophagus, which has a mean
diameter of less than 20 mm, a useful threshold for diagnosing EoE on
barium studies (Fig. 4.14) [14].

Drug-Induced Esophagitis

Tetracycline/doxycycline and alendronate sodium are the medications
most commonly responsible for drug-induced esophagitis in the United
States, but other causative agents include potassium chloride, quinidine,
and aspirin or other nonsteroidal anti-inflammatory drugs (NSAIDs).
Affected individuals typically ingest the medication with little or no

Fig. 4.13. Eosinophilic
esophagitis with ringed
esophagus. There is a
smooth, tapered stricture in
the mid esophagus with
distinctive ring-like
indentations (*arrows*) in the
region of the stricture.

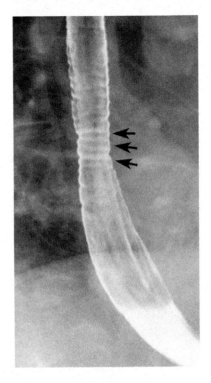

water immediately before going to bed. The capsules or pills usually
become lodged in the mid esophagus where it is compressed by the
adjacent aortic arch or left main bronchus. Prolonged contact of the
esophageal mucosa with these medications presumably causes an irritant
contact esophagitis. Affected individuals may present with severe
odynophagia, but there usually is marked clinical improvement after
withdrawal of the offending agent.

The radiographic findings in drug-induced esophagitis depend on
the nature of the offending medication. Tetracycline and doxycycline
are associated with the development of small, shallow ulcers in the
upper or mid esophagus indistinguishable from those in herpes
esophagitis (Fig. 4.15) [15]. Because of their superficial nature, these
ulcers almost always heal without scarring or strictures. In contrast,

Fig. 4.14. Eosinophilic
esophagitis with small-
caliber esophagus. There is
diffuse loss of caliber of the
entire thoracic esophagus
without a discrete stricture.
Both the ringed esophagus
and small-caliber esophagus
are characteristic of EoE.

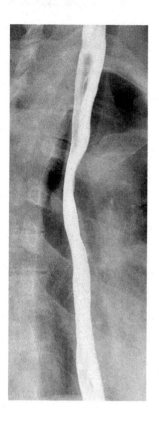

potassium chloride, quinidine, and NSAIDs may cause more severe
esophageal injury, leading to the development of larger ulcers and
possible stricture formation [15]. Alendronate sodium may cause severe
esophagitis with extensive ulceration and strictures that are usually
confined to the distal esophagus [15].

Radiation Esophagitis

A radiation dose of 5,000 cGy or more to the mediastinum may
cause severe injury to the esophagus. Acute radiation esophagitis
usually occurs 2–4 weeks after the initiation of radiation therapy. Most
cases are self-limited, but some patients may have progressive dysphagia
due to the development of radiation strictures 4–8 months after

Fig. 4.15. Drug-induced esophagitis. Several small, discrete ulcers (*arrows*) are present in the mid esophagus due to recent tetracycline ingestion (reproduced with permission from Levine MS. Radiology of the esophagus. Philadelphia, Pa: WB Saunders; 1989).

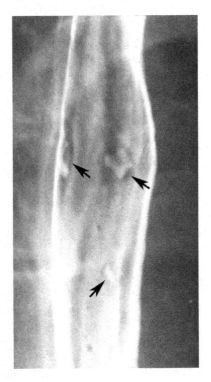

completion of radiation therapy [15]. Such strictures typically appear as smooth, tapered areas of concentric narrowing within a preexisting radiation portal (Fig. 4.16).

Caustic Esophagitis

Ingestion of lye or other caustic agents causes marked esophagitis, eventually leading to stricture formation. Liquid lye causes liquefactive necrosis, resulting in the most severe form of caustic injury to the esophagus [15]. If esophageal perforation is suspected, a radiographic study with water-soluble contrast material may be performed to document the presence of a leak. Such studies may also reveal marked edema, spasm, and ulceration of the affected esophagus [15]. As the esophagitis heals, follow-up barium studies have a major role in determining the

Fig. 4.16. Radiation stricture. There is a smooth, tapered segment of concentric narrowing (*arrows*) in the midthoracic esophagus. This patient had prior mediastinal irradiation.

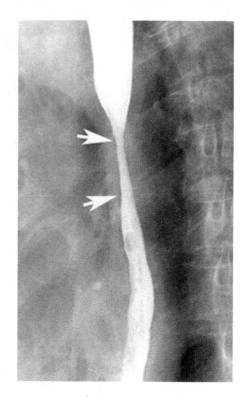

length and severity of developing strictures, which typically involve a long segment of the esophagus (Fig. 4.17). With severe scarring, the esophagus may be reduced to a thin, filiform structure, necessitating esophageal replacement surgery such as a colonic interposition [15].

Other Esophagitides

Alkaline reflux esophagitis is caused by reflux of bile or pancreatic secretions into the esophagus after partial or total gastrectomy [15]. This form of esophagitis is characterized on barium studies by mucosal nodularity or ulceration, or, in severe disease, by distal esophageal

Fig. 4.17. Chronic lye
stricture. This patient has a
long stricture in the thoracic
esophagus from previous
lye ingestion (reproduced
with permission from
reference [15]).

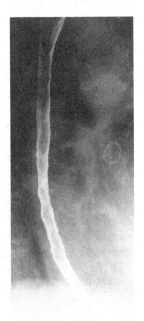

strictures that may progress rapidly in length and severity over a short
period of time [15]. The risk of developing alkaline reflux esophagitis
can be decreased by performing a Roux-en-Y reconstruction to minimize
reflux of alkaline secretions into the esophagus after partial or total
gastrectomy.

Nasogastric intubation is an uncommon cause of esophagitis and
stricture formation in the distal esophagus. It has been postulated that
these strictures result from a severe form of reflux esophagitis caused by
constant reflux of acid around the tube into the distal esophagus [15].
Affected individuals sometimes develop tight esophageal strictures that
progress rapidly in length and severity [15].

Other causes of esophagitis include Crohn's disease, tuberculosis,
graft-versus-host disease, Behcet's disease, and skin disorders involving
the esophagus, such as epidermolysis bullosa dystrophica and benign
mucous membrane pemphigoid [15].

Benign Tumors

Benign tumors of the esophagus comprise only about 20% of all esophageal neoplasms [16]. The vast majority are detected as incidental findings in asymptomatic patients. Squamous papillomas are the most common benign mucosal tumors, appearing on double-contrast studies as smooth or lobulated polyps [16]. Some papillomas may be difficult to differentiate from early esophageal cancers on the basis of the radiographic findings, so endoscopy is required for a definitive diagnosis.

In contrast, leiomyomas are the most common benign submucosal tumors in the esophagus. Affected patients may occasionally present with dysphagia, depending on the size of the tumor and how much it encroaches on the lumen. Leiomyomas usually are manifested on esophagography by smooth submucosal masses, etched in white, that form right angles or slightly obtuse angles with the adjacent esophageal wall (Fig. 4.18) [16]. As a result, these lesions may be indistinguishable from other less common mesenchymal tumors such as fibromas and neurofibromas.

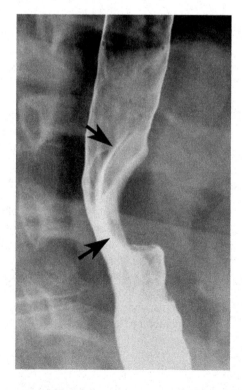

Fig. 4.18. Esophageal leiomyoma. There is a smooth submucosal mass etched in white (*arrows*) in the mid esophagus. Note how the lesion forms obtuse angles with the adjacent esophageal wall.

Fig. 4.19. Fibrovascular polyp. The polyp is seen as a smooth, expansile, sausage-shaped mass (*white arrows*) in the upper thoracic esophagus. A pedicle (*black arrow*) can be identified at the proximal end of the lesion (reproduced with permission from reference [17]).

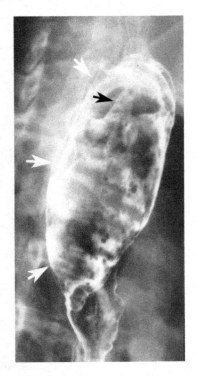

Fibrovascular polyps are rare, benign tumors consisting of fibrovascular and adipose tissue covered by squamous epithelium [16]. Fibrovascular polyps usually arise near the cricopharyngeus, gradually elongating over many years as they are dragged inferiorly by esophageal peristalsis. Rarely, affected individuals may have a spectacular presentation with regurgitation of a mass into the pharynx or mouth or even asphyxia and sudden death if the regurgitated polyp occludes the larynx [16]. Fibrovascular polyps typically appear on barium studies as smooth, expansile, sausage-shaped masses expanding the lumen of the upper esophagus (Fig. 4.19) [17].

Malignant Tumors

Esophageal Carcinoma

Double-contrast esophagography has a sensitivity of greater than 95% in the detection of esophageal cancer [18]. Early esophageal

Fig. 4.20. Superficial spreading carcinoma. There is a focal area of mucosal nodularity in the mid esophagus without a discrete mass. Note how the nodules are poorly defined, merging with one another as a confluent area of disease (reproduced with permission from Levine MS. Radiology of the esophagus. Philadelphia, Pa: WB Saunders; 1989).

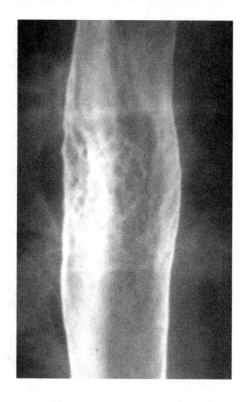

cancers may be manifested on double-contrast studies by plaque-like lesions (often containing flat central ulcers), sessile polyps with a smooth or slightly lobulated contour, or focal irregularity of the esophageal wall [19]. Early adenocarcinomas may also be manifested by a localized area of wall flattening or irregularity within a preexisting peptic stricture [20]. In contrast, superficial spreading carcinoma is characterized by focal nodularity of the mucosa, with poorly defined nodules or plaques that merge together, producing a confluent area of disease (Fig. 4.20) [19, 20].

Advanced esophageal carcinomas usually appear on barium studies as infiltrating, polypoid, ulcerative, or, less commonly, varicoid lesions [20]. Infiltrating carcinomas are manifested by irregular luminal narrowing with mucosal nodularity or ulceration and abrupt, shelf-like proximal and distal margins (Fig. 4.21). Polypoid carcinomas appear as lobulated intraluminal masses, whereas ulcerative carcinomas are seen as giant, meniscoid ulcers surrounded by a thick, irregular rind of tumor

4. Radiographic Evaluation of the Esophageal Phase of Swallowing

Fig. 4.21. Infiltrating
esophageal carcinoma.
There is irregular luminal
narrowing with shelf-like
proximal and distal margins
(*arrows*) in the mid
esophagus due to an
advanced esophageal
carcinoma.

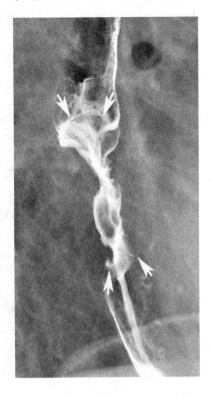

(Fig. 4.22) [20]. Finally, varicoid carcinomas are characterized by submucosal spread of tumor, producing thickened, tortuous defects that mimic the appearance of varices. However, varicoid tumors have a fixed configuration, whereas varices change in size and shape at fluoroscopy. Also, varices rarely cause dysphagia because they are soft and compressible. Thus, it usually is possible to differentiate these conditions on the basis of the clinical and radiographic findings.

Squamous cell carcinomas and adenocarcinomas of the esophagus cannot always be differentiated on barium studies, but squamous cell carcinomas tend to involve the upper or mid esophagus, whereas adenocarcinomas usually are located in the distal esophagus. Unlike squamous carcinomas, adenocarcinomas also have a marked tendency to invade the gastric cardia or fundus, comprising as many as 50% of all malignant tumors at the gastroesophageal junction [20].

Fig. 4.22. Ulcerative carcinoma. A giant meniscoid ulcer (*white arrows*) is seen in the esophagus with a thick, irregular rind of tumor (*black arrows*) surrounding the ulcer. This malignant ulcer can readily be differentiated from the benign CMV and HIV ulcers in Figs. 4.11 and 4.12.

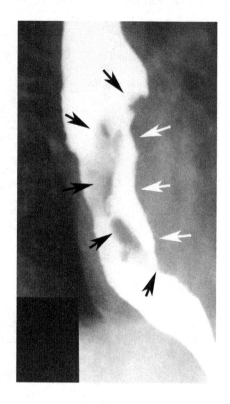

Other Malignant Tumors

Esophageal lymphoma may be manifested on barium studies by submucosal masses, polypoid lesions, enlarged folds, or strictures [21]. Spindle cell carcinoma (formerly known as carcinosarcoma) is another rare tumor characterized by a bulky, polypoid intraluminal mass that expands the lumen of the esophagus without causing obstruction [21]. Other rare malignant tumors involving the esophagus include leiomyosarcoma, malignant melanoma, and Kaposi's sarcoma [21].

Varices

Uphill Varices

Uphill varices usually are caused by portal hypertension with hepatofugal flow through dilated esophageal collaterals to the superior vena cava [22]. Uphill varices may cause marked upper gastrointestinal bleeding. These dilated vascular structures appear on barium studies as serpiginous longitudinal filling defects in the lower thoracic esophagus (Fig. 4.23) and are best seen in the collapsed esophagus with the patient in a prone position, using high-density barium to increase mucosal adherence to the esophageal wall [22]. The differential diagnosis for varices includes varicoid carcinomas and esophagitis with thickened folds.

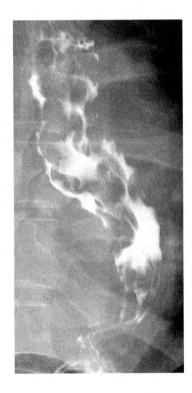

Fig. 4.23. Esophageal varices. Prone single-contrast spot image shows uphill esophageal varices as serpiginous longitudinal defects in the lower esophagus. This patient had portal hypertension.

Downhill Varices

Downhill varices are caused by superior vena cava obstruction with downward flow via dilated esophageal collaterals to the portal venous system and inferior vena cava [22]. Major causes of downhill varices include catheter-related thrombosis of the superior vena cava, bronchogenic carcinoma or other malignant tumors involving the mediastinum, mediastinal irradiation, and substernal goiter [22]. Most patients present with superior vena cava syndrome. The varices typically appear as serpentine longitudinal filling defects which, unlike uphill esophageal varices, are confined to the upper or mid esophagus [22]. Venography, CT, or MR may be performed to confirm the presence of superior vena cava obstruction and determine the underlying cause.

Lower Esophageal Rings

Lower esophageal rings are a frequent finding on esophagography, but only a small percentage cause symptoms. A pathologically narrowed ring, also known as a *Schatzki ring*, causes episodic dysphagia for solids. The pathogenesis is uncertain, but some rings are thought to be caused by scarring from reflux esophagitis.

Lower esophageal rings appear on barium studies as 2–3-mm in height, smooth, symmetric ring-like constrictions at the gas-troesophageal junction, almost always above a hiatal hernia (Fig. 4.24) [23]. The rings can be missed if the distal esophagus is not adequately distended at fluoroscopy, so it is important to obtain prone views during continuous drinking of low-density barium [24]. Conversely, rings can be missed if this region is over distended, causing overlap of the distal esophagus and hernia that obscures the ring [25]. Rings with a maximal diameter greater than 20 mm rarely cause dysphagia, whereas rings with a maximal diameter less than 13 mm almost always cause dysphagia [23]. Esophagography is a sensitive technique for detecting Schatzki rings, sometimes revealing rings that are missed on endoscopy [24].

Fig. 4.24. Schatzki ring.
Prone single-contrast spot
image shows a Schatzki
ring as a smooth,
symmetric, ring-like
constriction (*arrow*) in the
distal esophagus directly
above a hiatal hernia.

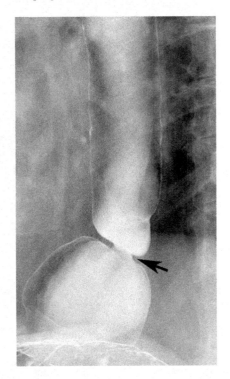

Diverticula

Zenker's Diverticula

Zenker's diverticulum is an acquired mucosal herniation through an
area of weakness in the cricopharyngeal muscle (also known as *Killian's
dehiscence*) just above the cricopharyngeus. The pathogenesis of
Zenker's diverticulum is uncertain, but many patients have cricopharyngeal dysfunction with elevated upper esophageal sphincter
pressures and decreased relaxation of the sphincter during swallowing,
so it has been postulated that cricopharyngeal dysfunction predisposes
to the development of a Zenker's diverticulum.

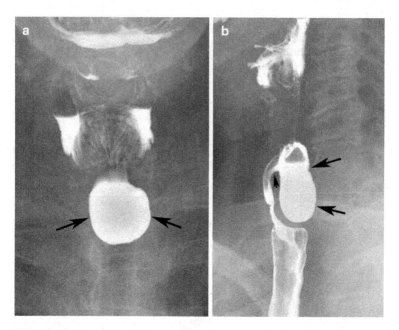

Fig. 4.25. Zenker's diverticulum. (a) A frontal view of the pharynx shows an ovoid midline diverticulum (*arrows*) extending inferior to the piriform sinuses. (b) A lateral view of the pharynx shows the diverticulum (*large arrows*) above an incompletely opened cricopharyngeus indenting the posterior aspect of the pharyngoesophageal junction (*small arrow*). These findings are typical of a Zenker's diverticulum.

When detected on barium studies, Zenker's diverticulum appears on frontal views as a persistent, barium-filled sac in the midline below the tips of the piriform sinuses (Fig. 4.25a). On lateral views during swallowing, the opening of the Zenker's diverticulum above the incompletely opened pharyngoesophageal segment is often surprisingly broad. The sac then courses behind the pharyngoesophageal segment and proximal cervical esophagus (Fig. 4.25b). Barium (or any ingested liquid) within the diverticulum can be regurgitated into the lower hypopharynx during breathing or subsequent swallowing, resulting in overflow aspiration.

Pulsion Diverticula

Pulsion diverticula tend to be located in the distal esophagus and are often associated with esophageal dysmotility [22]. The diverticula appear on barium studies as wide-necked, rounded outpouchings that fail to empty when the esophagus collapses [22]. They usually are discovered as incidental findings in asymptomatic patients. However, a large epiphrenic diverticulum adjacent to the gastroesophageal junction may fill with debris, causing dysphagia, regurgitation, or aspiration [26].

Traction Diverticula

Traction diverticula occur in the mid esophagus and usually are caused by scarring from tuberculosis or histoplasmosis in perihilar lymph nodes [22]. Because traction diverticula contain all layers of the esophageal wall, they maintain their elastic recoil, emptying their contents when the esophagus collapses at fluoroscopy. Traction diverticula often have a triangular or tented appearance resulting from traction on the diverticulum by the fibrotic process in the adjacent mediastinum [22].

Esophageal Intramural Pseudodiverticula

Esophageal intramural pseudodiverticula consist pathologically of dilated excretory ducts of deep mucous glands in the esophagus. The pseudodiverticula appear on barium studies as flask-shaped outpouchings parallel to the long axis of the esophagus (Fig. 4.26) [27]. When viewed en face, these structures can be mistaken for tiny ulcers. When viewed in profile, however, they often appear to be *floating* outside the wall of the esophagus without apparent communication with the lumen [15]. Most pseudodiverticula develop in the distal esophagus in the region of a peptic stricture, likely occurring as a sequela of scarring from reflux esophagitis [27]. Less frequently, pseudodiverticula have a diffuse distribution or are associated with high esophageal strictures (see Fig. 4.26) [27]. When strictures are present, these patients may present with dysphagia, but the pseudodiverticula themselves rarely cause symptoms.

Fig. 4.26. Esophageal intramural pseudodiverticulosis. This patient has a smooth, tapered stricture in the mid esophagus. Multiple pseudodiverticula are also seen in profile as tiny flask-shaped outpouchings (*arrows*) in longitudinal rows parallel to the long axis of the esophagus.

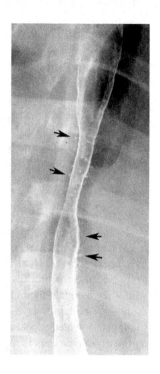

Esophageal Motility Disorders

Achalasia

Primary achalasia is an idiopathic condition involving the myenteric plexus of the esophagus, whereas secondary achalasia is caused by other underlying conditions, most commonly malignant tumor involving the gastroesophageal junction (especially carcinoma of the gastric cardia) [28]. Primary achalasia is characterized by absent primary peristalsis in the esophagus and incomplete opening of the lower esophageal sphincter, manifested on barium studies by tapered, beak-like narrowing of the distal esophagus at or directly adjacent to the gastroesophageal junction (Fig. 4.27) [28]. With advanced disease, the esophagus can become massively dilated and have a tortuous distal configuration, also known as a *sigmoid esophagus*. Because of slow progression of symptoms, affected individuals typically have long-standing dysphagia when they seek medical attention.

Fig. 4.27. Primary achalasia. There is a dilated, aperistaltic esophagus with tapered, beak-like distal narrowing (*arrow*) due to incomplete opening of the lower esophageal sphincter. These findings are characteristic of primary achalasia. Also note retained debris and a standing column of barium in the dilated esophagus. This middle-aged patient had long-standing dysphagia.

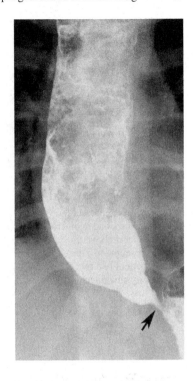

Secondary achalasia is also characterized by absent peristalsis in the esophagus and beak-like distal narrowing [29]. In secondary achalasia, however, the length of the narrowed segment is often greater than that in primary achalasia because of spread of tumor into the distal esophagus (Fig. 4.28) [29]. The narrowed segment can also be asymmetric, nodular, or ulcerated because of tumor infiltrating this region. In some cases, barium studies may reveal other signs of malignancy at the cardia with distortion or obliteration of the normal cardiac rosette [29]. The clinical history is also important, as patients with primary achalasia almost always have long-standing dysphagia, whereas patients with secondary achalasia usually are older individuals (over age 60) with recent onset of dysphagia (less than 6 months) and weight loss [29].

80   M.S. Levine

Fig. 4.28. Secondary
achalasia. There is a dilated,
aperistaltic esophagus with
a longer segment of distal
narrowing (*white arrows*)
than the patient with
primary achalasia in
Fig. 4.27. Also note
irregular narrowing of the
proximal stomach due to a
scirrhous gastric carcinoma
invading the
gastroesophageal junction.
An irregular filling defect
(*black arrows*) is present in
the dilated esophagus due to
impacted food above the
narrowed segment. This
elderly patient had recent
onset of dysphagia and
weight loss.

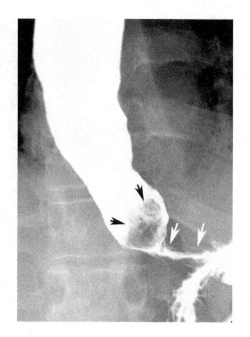

Other Esophageal Motility Disorders

Diffuse esophageal spasm (DES) may be manifested on esophagography by intermittently weakened or absent peristalsis with lumen-obliterating nonperistaltic contractions (NPCs), producing a classic *corkscrew esophagus* (Fig. 4.29) [28]. More commonly, however, these patients have multiple NPCs of mild to moderate severity [30]

Fig. 4.29. Diffuse
esophageal spasm. This
patient has a classic
corkscrew esophagus due to
multiple lumen-obliterating
nonperistaltic contractions
(*arrows*) with trapping of
barium between these
contractions.

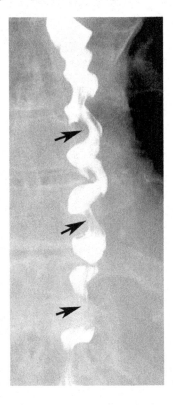

(Fig. 4.30). More than 50% of patients with DES have associated beak-like narrowing of the distal esophagus due to incomplete opening of the lower esophageal sphincter (see Fig. 4.30) [30]. Thus, DES and achalasia may represent opposite ends of a spectrum of interrelated esophageal motility disorders.

Fig. 4.30. Diffuse
esophageal spasm with
lower esophageal sphincter
dysfunction. This patient
has mild to moderate
nonperistaltic contractions
in the esophagus with a
tapered segment of distal
narrowing (*arrow*) due to
incomplete opening of the
lower esophageal sphincter.

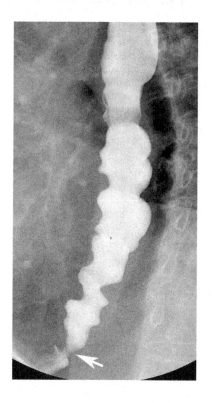

Older patients may have intermittent weakening of peristalsis and multiple NPCs in the distal esophagus in the absence of esophageal symptoms, a relatively common manifestation of aging known as *presbyesophagus* [28].

References

1. Laufer I, Levine MS. Barium studies of the upper gastrointestinal tract. In: Gore RM, Levine MS, editors. Textbook of gastrointestinal radiology. 3rd ed. Philadelphia: WB Saunders; 2008. p. 311–22.
2. Levine MS. Gastroesophageal reflux disease. In: Gore RM, Levine MS, editors. Textbook of gastrointestinal radiology. 3rd ed. Philadelphia: WB Saunders; 2008. p. 337–57.
3. Dibble C, Levine MS, Rubesin SE, Laufer I, Katzka DA. Detection of reflux esophagitis on double-contrast esophagograms and endoscopy using the histologic findings as the gold standard. Abdom Imaging. 2004;29:421–5.

 4. Hu C, Levine MS, Laufer I. Solitary ulcers in reflux esophagitis: radiographic findings. Abdom Imaging. 1997;22:5–7.

 5. Levine MS, Goldstein HM. Fixed transverse folds in the esophagus: a sign of reflux esophagitis. AJR. 1984;143:275–8.

 6. Samadi F, Levine MS, Rubesin SE, Katzka DA, Laufer I. Feline esophagus and gastroesophageal reflux. AJR. 2010;194:972–6.

 7. Gilchrist AM, Levine MS, Carr RF, et al. Barrett's esophagus: diagnosis by double-contrast esophagography. AJR. 1988;150:97–102.

 8. Levine MS, Kressel HY, Caroline DF, Laufer I, Herlinger H, Thompson JJ. Barrett esophagus: reticular pattern of the mucosa. Radiology. 1983;147:663–7.

 9. Levine MS. Infectious esophagitis. In: Gore RM, Levine MS, editors. Textbook of gastrointestinal radiology. 3rd ed. Philadelphia: Elsevier; 2008. p. 359–73.

10. Levine MS, Macones AJ, Laufer I. *Candida* esophagitis: accuracy of radiographic diagnosis. Radiology. 1985;154:581–7.

11. Shortsleeve MJ, Levine MS. Herpes esophagitis in otherwise healthy patients: clinical and radiographic findings. Radiology. 1992;182:859–61.

12. Sor S, Levine MS, Kowalski TE, Laufer I, Rubesin SE, Herlinger H. Giant ulcers of the esophagus in patients with human immunodeficiency virus: clinical, radiographic, and pathologic findings. Radiology. 1995;194:447–51.

13. Zimmerman SL, Levine MS, Rubesin SE, et al. Idiopathic eosinophilic esophagitis in adults: the ringed esophagus. Radiology. 2005;236:159–65.

14. White SB, Levine MS, Rubesin SE, Spencer GS, Katzka DA, Laufer I. The small-caliber esophagus: radiographic sign of idiopathic eosinophilic esophagitis. Radiology. 2010;256:127–34.

15. Levine MS. Other esophagitides. In: Gore RM, Levine MS, editors. Textbook of gastrointestinal radiology. 3rd ed. Philadelphia: WB Saunders; 2008. p. 375–99.

16. Levine MS. Benign tumors of the esophagus. In: Gore RM, Levine MS, editors. Textbook of gastrointestinal radiology. 3rd ed. Philadelphia: WB Saunders; 2008. p. 401–16.

17. Levine MS, Buck JL, Pantongrag-Brown L, Buetow PC, Hallman JR, Sobin LH. Fibrovascular polyps of the esophagus: clinical, radiographic, and pathologic findings in 16 patients. AJR. 1996;166:781–7.

18. Levine MS, Chu P, Furth EE, Rubesin SE, Laufer I, Herlinger H. Carcinoma of the esophagus and esophagogastric junction: sensitivity of radiographic diagnosis. AJR. 1997;168:1423–6.

19. Levine MS, Dillon EC, Saul SH, Laufer I. Early esophageal cancer. AJR. 1986;146: 507–12.

20. Levine MS, Halvorsen RA. Carcinoma of the esophagus. In: Gore RM, Levine MS, editors. Textbook of gastrointestinal radiology. 3rd ed. Philadelphia: WB Saunders; 2008. p. 417–46.

21. Levine MS. Other malignant tumors of the esophagus. In: Gore RM, Levine MS, editors. Textbook of gastrointestinal radiology. 3rd ed. Philadelphia: WB Saunders; 2008. p. 447–64.

22. Levine MS. Miscellaneous abnormalities of the esophagus. In: Gore RM, Levine MS, editors. Textbook of gastrointestinal radiology. 3rd ed. Philadelphia: WB Saunders; 2008. p. 465–93.

23. Schatzki RE. The lower esophageal ring: long term follow-up of symptomatic and asymptomatic rings. AJR. 1963;90:805–10.

24. Levine MS. Abnormalities of the gastroesophageal junction. In: Gore RM, Levine MS, editors. Textbook of gastrointestinal radiology. 3rd ed. Philadelphia: WB Saunders; 2008. p. 495–506.

25. Hsu WC, Levine MS, Rubesin SE. Overlap phenomenon: a potential pitfall in the radiographic detection of lower esophageal rings. AJR. 2003;180:745–7.

26. Fasano NC, Levine MS, Rubesin SE, Redfern RO, Laufer I. Epiphrenic diverticulum: clinical and radiographic findings in 27 patients. Dysphagia. 2003;18:9–15.

27. Levine MS, Moolten DN, Herlinger H, Laufer I. Esophageal intramural pseudodiverticulosis: a reevaluation. AJR. 1986;147:1165–70.

28. Ott DJ. Motility disorders of the esophagus. In: Gore RM, Levine MS, editors. Textbook of gastrointestinal radiology. 3rd ed. Philadelphia: WB Saunders; 2008. p. 323–35.

29. Woodfield CA, Levine MS, Rubesin SE, Langlotz CP, Laufer I. Diagnosis of primary versus secondary achalasia: reassessment of clinical and radiographic criteria. AJR. 2000;175:727–31.

30. Prabhakar AM, Levine MS, Rubesin SE, Laufer I, Katzka DA. Relationship between diffuse esophageal spasm and lower esophageal sphincter dysfunction on barium studies and manometry in 14 patients. AJR. 2004;183:409–13.

5. Fiberoptic Endoscopic Evaluation of Swallowing (FEES)

Susan E. Langmore and Joseph Murray

Abstract The Fiberoptic Endoscopic Evaluation of Swallowing (FEES) is an instrumental assessment of deglutitive function that utilizes a flexible laryngoscope to view pharyngeal and laryngeal structures during swallowing. In this assessment the laryngoscope is placed transnasally and advanced to the pharynx to view structural movements, bolus transit and airway protection. The chapter elucidates the utility and practical application of laryngoscopy to assess swallowing function for the practicing clinician. The chapter includes a description of the procedure and guides the reader in the integration of visual findings that are revealed via the laryngoscope to better identify disordered physiology and further patient management.

Introduction

Flexible laryngoscopy was first used in 1968, allowing medical professionals to view the nasal, pharyngeal and laryngeal structures for purposes of detecting laryngeal pathology and voice function [1]. In 1988, Langmore et al. published the first description of a comprehensive assessment of swallowing using flexible laryngoscopy [2]. This early publication and others [3, 4] described the presentation of food and liquid to patients with the flexible transnasal laryngoscope placed to provide a visualization of events that could be observed during feeding, and the effect of therapeutic intervention. The procedure was purported to have the advantage of being portable, allowing the clinician to assess swallow function at the patient's bedside or clinic and to be without the time constraints or exposure to radiation that hampered the prominent and popular fluoroscopic assessments of oropharyngeal swallowing. Since the inception of the examination, its use has grown considerably and is now used in a variety of settings and in most developed countries

R. Shaker et al. (eds.), *Manual of Diagnostic and Therapeutic Techniques for Disorders of Deglutition*, DOI 10.1007/978-1-4614-3779-6_5, © Springer Science+Business Media New York 2013

throughout the world. It has proved particularly valuable for patients who cannot be transported easily to a fluoroscopy suite, who have laryngeal impairment, or who have need for an extended therapeutic exam. The name given to the particular protocol developed by Langmore and colleagues, fiberoptic endoscopic evaluation of swallowing or FEES, has become a generic signifier for a variety of endoscopic examinations of swallowing described since that time.

Equipment and Technique

The simple analog laryngoscope has changed little since its appearance in medical centers the in the 1960s. Flexible light fibers conduct light from a cold light source and illuminate the pharynx and larynx with a second grouping of light fibers that project the image from the objective lens to the operator's eye. Instrumentation used for the examination has undergone a transformation over the last decade with the advent of small-scale imaging electronics, such as the charge-coupled device (CCD). The image projected from the eyepiece can now be directed to the CCD chip which allows for display of the image on a monitor and recording of the image for review or archival purposes. Analog scopes which were configured to be used with just a light source and were designed to be held up to the operator's eye have begun to be replaced by digital laryngoscopes with CCD imaging chips embedded at the distal tip of the insertion tube (Fig. 5.1).

A wide array of food and liquids can be used for the examination. To maximize visualization of the bolus clinicians may choose foods that reflect light well, such as milk, yogurt, potatoes, or bananas. For foods that do not reflect light well, blue or green dye may be used to assist the endoscopist in discerning food and liquid from surrounding mucosa (Fig. 5.2). Safety concerns related to the use of dye in patients receiving enteral feedings [5] and clinical swallowing examinations have led to a decline in the use of food color in FEES examinations and one study found that there was no benefit for greater visualization of the bolus when using the dye [6]. Nonetheless, many clinicians prefer to dye food or liquid to enhance visualization.

The patient is prepared for the examination with counseling regarding the purpose, risks, benefits and alternatives to the examination. At this time a decision may be made regarding the application of a topical anesthetic and/or vasoconstrictor to the nasal mucosa to make the passage of the scope more comfortable. The effectiveness of topical anesthesia for this purpose is currently unclear with some research indicating a

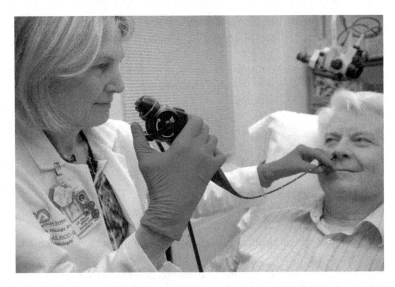

Fig. 5.1. Positioning of patient and endoscopist using a digital "chip in the tip" laryngoscope.

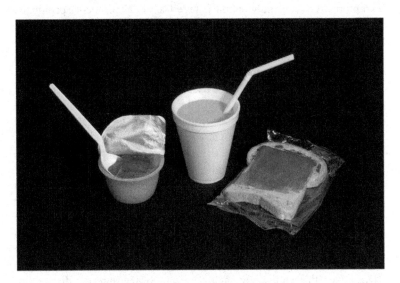

Fig. 5.2. Various food and liquid with blue dye added to enhance visualization of the bolus.

benefit and others indicating that application of these solutions do not have the desired effect of making the exam more comfortable [7] and may even lead to greater discomfort for the patient [8]. Given the equivocal evidence for the use of topical anesthesia, some clinicians will limit their preparation to administration of a vasoconstrictor and lubrication of the insertion portion of the endoscope [9].

Performing the Exam

Once placed transnasally, the endoscope is advanced beyond the nasopharynx to view the mucosal surface structures of the base of tongue, pharynx, and larynx.

Velopharyngeal closure and function should be assessed in patients who present clinically with hypernasality during speech or complaints of nasal regurgitation when eating or drinking. A wide range of congenital, acquired and iatrogenic conditions may contribute to nasopharyngeal incompetence [10]. The acute phase of neurologic diseases such as Miller Fisher Syndrome or Muscular Dystrophy may present with early onset of hypernasality coupled with nasopharyngeal regurgitation [11, 12]. Myesthenia Gravis often presents with hypernasality as an early symptom. A recent publication detailed a FEES protocol specifically designed to elicit VP incompetence and/or pharyngeal weakness [13]. After establishing a baseline swallow, the protocol challenges the patient with repeated swallows of small pieces of bread. A rapid decline in function helps support the diagnosis of myasthenia gravis, after which administration of Tensilon can be used to determine whether the effect of this drug returns the swallow to baseline. Iatrogenic causes such as head and neck surgery, radiation therapy after nasopharyngeal cancer, and uvulopharyngopalatoplasty can also result in nasoregurgitation [14, 15].

During the initial passage of the scope nasopharyngeal closure can be assessed by having the patient alternate between oral plosive and nasal resonant sounds such as/donut/. An estimation of the gap size and location of the gap should be noted. The Golding-Kushner scale is a subjective numeric scoring system used to evaluate relative movement of the velopharyngeal port [16]. Items rated in this scale include right and left lateral pharyngeal wall movement, right and left palate movement and elevation, posterior pharyngeal wall movement, and estimate of gap size. Given that endoscopy cannot absolutely measure the distance of movements, the scale system has some limitations [17]. The clinician should position the scope in the nasopharynx adjacent to the vomer bone

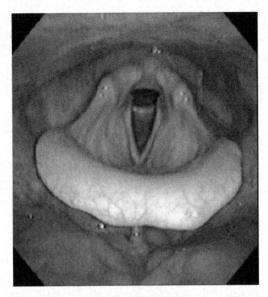

Fig. 5.3. The view typically achieved with the "preswallow position" allows for visualization of portions of the base of tongue, laryngeal structures and subglottic space.

to view velar function. To maximize visualization of the velopharyngeal port it is recommended that the laryngoscope be passed between the inferior and middle turbinates or between the middle and superior turbinates as it enters the nasal cavity rather than along the floor of the nose. This will allow for a greater field of view and a more complete visualization of nasopharyngeal function [18]. The drawback to using this "higher" passage, however, is increasing discomfort for the patient so it should probably be reserved for cases when assessment of VP competence is critical. Following this initial inspection food and liquid can be presented in varying amounts to elicit the finding of nasal regurgitation. The entry point should be noted as well as the volume and consistency of the materials that trigger the event.

For most FEES examinations, the oropharynx, hypopharynx, and larynx are the primary structures of interest. Thus, the endoscopist will need to advance the scope and position it to get an optimal view of these structures before, during, and after the swallow [19]. To attain the preswallow position, the tip of the endoscope is advanced to a position between the soft palate and the tip of the epiglottis where the base of tongue, valleculae, larynx, and both pyriform sinuses are visualized (Fig. 5.3). This "home position" allows for visualization of bolus transit

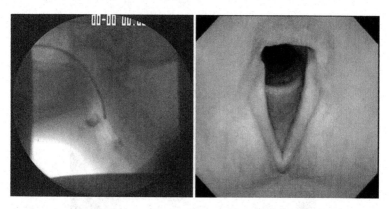

Fig. 5.4. The view achieved with the "postswallow position" allows for closer inspection of the subglottic space.

prior to swallow initiation. Following the swallow, the endoscopist advances the endoscope into the laryngeal vestibule to visualize the larynx, subglottis, and anterior tracheal wall. The postswallow position will allow for the detection of any laryngeal penetration and/or aspiration (Fig. 5.4). Following this close inspection, the endoscope is retracted to the preswallow position to prepare for any subsequent bolus advancement.

During the height of the swallow, the tongue and velum contact the posterior pharyngeal wall and the distal tip of the endoscope will be trapped transiently against the posterior pharyngeal wall by the velum or base of tongue. This causes the light that is projected from the tip of the scope to reflect off of the tissue it is in contact with. This appears as a flash of light that lasts approximately one half of a second in normal subjects [20]. This period of "white-out" occurs during the point of maximal pharyngeal airspace closure and prevents visualization of the bolus during that time. If the pharyngeal airspace is incomplete, an abnormal finding, the view will appear "pink" or the structures will be completely visible. In these patients, the upper esophageal sphincter may even be seen to open.

The 3–5 frames just prior to whiteout and the 3–5 frames immediately following whiteout are critical periods for the endoscopist to visualize. Prior to whiteout, the tongue base and epiglottis advance towards the posterior pharyngeal wall, the lateral pharyngeal walls begin to medialize, and the arytenoids medialize and begin to tilt anteriorly, signaling the onset of the swallow. Immediately after whiteout, the epiglottis is seen to return from its inverted position back to its resting position

Findings from the FEES Exam

While there is no single standardized system for scoring the findings of the FEES exam, efforts have been made to analyze components and stages of swallow function and dysfunction while imaging with a laryngoscope. Integration of these measures and observations allow the examiner to summarize the examination by stating the severity of the problem, the nature of the problem, and the patient's response to therapeutic interventions. In a gross sense, the clinician hopes to characterize the timing, safety, and efficiency of the swallow.

The objective observations begin prior to the presentation of food or liquid with a survey of the anatomic structures of the base of tongue, larynx/pharynx, and assessment of the collection of secretions and the frequency of swallowing. Additionally the clinician may elicit volitional or reflexive motor movements of the base of tongue, pharyngeal and laryngeal structures and also to assess sensory function.

The surface mucosa of the pharynx and larynx should initially be viewed to inspect the structural support for swallowing and barriers to the laryngeal airway. The pharynx and laryngeal structures are configured to collect and contain a bolus as it passively falls out of the oral cavity or is thrust into the pharynx by the tongue. Gravity and/or tongue propusion carries it to the distal pharynx. The clinician should note the overall morphology of the hypopharynx: i.e., the depth of the vallecular space and pyriform sinuses, the availability of these channels, and the height of the aryepiglottic folds to make a determination as to whether these spaces would be able to transiently contain a bolus prior to the initiation of a swallow and would be able to contain residue of material after a swallow without the bolus overflowing into the laryngeal vestibule.

Two recent studies suggest that laryngeal abnormalities are very common in hospitalized patients, especially in those who have been intubated. In a study utilizing FEES to assess swallow function in 99 hospitalized patients, [21], including 67% who had been previously intubated, there was a 79% overall prevalence of laryngopharyngeal abnormalities. Forty-five percent of the patients presented with two or more findings, which included arytenoid edema (33%), granuloma (31%), vocal fold paresis (24%), mucosal lesions (17%), vocal fold bowing (14%), diffuse edema (11%), airway stenosis (3%), and ulcer (6%). Another recent study that assessed 61 patients after extubation, a higher rate of abnormal laryngeal findings were reported, with virtually 100% of patients showing some laryngeal abnormality [22] Edema and erythema were the most common findings, while 39% had either unilateral or bilateral vocal fold immobility. The effect of these abnormalities on swallowing was not reported.

During this initial observation, edema and other mucosal changes as well as intrinsic or extrinsic foreign bodies (e.g., a feeding tube) should be noted as well as their effect on bolus flow. Postsurgical and postradiation anatomical alterations should be noted. The effect of the surgery on the protective barriers should be described. Although one may be concerned that the presence of an endoscope or feeding tube may adversely affect swallowing, two recent studies have found that feeding tubes did not generally impact swallowing [23, 24]. On the other hand, a misplaced tube that has migrated up from the stomach and esophagus and is coiled around the larynx was clearly a detriment.

The finding of secretions in the vestibule should be an immediate visual marker for potential poor performance during the examination. Oropharyngeal secretions are cleared from the hypopharynx by periodic spontaneous swallows. Secretions can accumulate due to a reduction in the frequency of swallowing, a reduction in the effectiveness of the pharyngeal swallow, or a combination of reduced frequency and weakness. The presence of secretions in the laryngeal vestibule has been shown to be highly predictive of aspiration later in the examination [25, 26]. It has also been associated with the development of pneumonia [27, 28].

Spontaneous swallowing may also be considered revealing at the onset of the examination. It is important to note that normal subjects have been reported to swallow approximately three times per minute when a laryngoscope is present in the hypopharynx, much higher than a normal subject without an endoscope placed transnasally [25, 29]. This may be related to increased saliva production resulting from stimulation or irritation to nasal and pharyngeal mucosa. The finding of reduced frequency of swallowing is important to note since, in that same study, neurogenic patients swallowed less than once per minute when compared to their age-matched normal peers [25]. Of note, the patients who aspirated were also found to swallow significantly less frequently than non-aspirating patients.

The finding of secretions in the laryngeal vestibule or trachea and infrequent swallowing (less than once per minute) at the onset of the FEES examination should elicit caution on the part of the clinician, who may want to proceed with great care as the presentation of food and liquid ensues later in the examination (Fig. 5.5).

Observation of Movement of Structures

Tasks designed to specifically assess adequacy of movement of the base of tongue, pharynx, and larynx, can be carried out at this time.

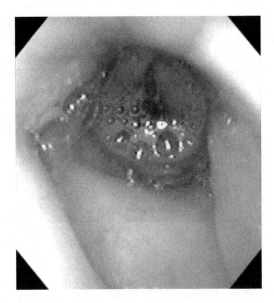

Fig. 5.5. Severely edematous laryngeal/pharyngeal structures with oropharyngeal secretions in the endolarynx.

While the ultimate test of their adequacy occurs during swallowing, endoscopy will not allow for visualization of some of these movements during the height of the swallow.

At a minimum the clinician may wish to have the patient hold their breath or cough to determine if tight laryngeal closure is possible (Fig. 5.6). Phonatory tasks, breath holding, and coughing may reveal unilateral or bilateral laryngeal closure impairments secondary to recurrent laryngeal nerve damage which put the patient at risk of aspiration [30–32]. Both the reflexive and volitional cough requires tight laryngeal closure. This tight closure allows for the buildup and release of subglottic pressure from the tracheal lumen and through the open glottis. If closure of the glottis or supraglottis is impaired as is seen in patients with vocal fold paralysis, a weak or ineffective cough may be observed. The presence of a weakened cough should alert the clinician to the possibility of poor airway clearance in the event of an aspiration event later in the examination [33]. Another task that may be done is to ask the patient to glide up in pitch while phonating "ee." This requires laryngeal elevation which can be visualized endoscopically as a lifting of the arytenoids. The predictive ability of this maneuver for judging adequacy of laryngeal elevation during the swallow, however, has not yet been tested empirically.

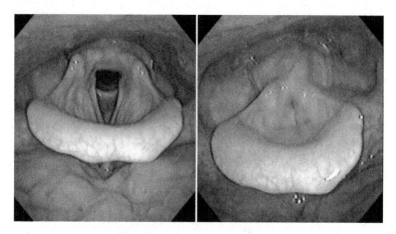

Fig. 5.6. A comparison of the larynx at rest (*left*) and during a valsalva breath hold (*right*).

An impression of pharyngeal muscular contraction can be obtained by observing the "pharyngeal squeeze maneuver" (PSM) which is performed by having the patient sustain a forceful, high pitched /i/ sound and noting the degree of pharyngeal wall movement [34]. A similar fluoroscopic measure was described and validated as a surrogate measure of pharyngeal strength based upon measurements of the pharynx at two points during the swallow. The measure, the "pharyngeal constriction ratio" (PCR) [35] is a measure of the pharyngeal area visible in the lateral radiograph view at the point when a bolus is held in the oral cavity divided by the pharyngeal area at the point of maximum pharyngeal constriction during the swallow. An elevated PCR suggests decreased pharyngeal constriction. A validation of the endoscopic PSM was performed using the PCR as a reference while viewing both events using simultaneous fluoroscopy and endoscopy [36]. In that study patients with an abnormal PSM demonstrated a mean PCR that was significantly higher, indicating a weaker pharynx, ($P < 0.001$) further supporting the validity of the PSM as a surrogate measure of pharyngeal motor integrity.

Assessing Timing of Swallow Onset

Before the field of view is obstructed by the contact of base of tongue or velum against the posterior pharyngeal wall, the bolus can be observed to transit through the pharynx, allowing for an impression of the timeliness or latency of swallow onset. The onset of the pharyngeal swallow is known to be highly variable both within and across subjects [37]. In normal subjects, the bolus is often seen in the valleculae, and occasionally will arrive in the pyriform sinus before the initiation of hyolaryngeal elevation [38, 39]. This pattern of deep bolus advancement gives the endoscopist ample time to observe the initial portion of pharyngeal bolus transit. Before the swallow commences, the operator should be vigilant to position the tip of the endoscope in the preswallow position to view the head of the bolus arriving at the base of tongue. In cases of extreme latency, the tip of the scope should be further advanced to the mid-pharynx to view the containment of bolus in the pyriform sinuses or the entry of the bolus into the laryngeal airway. In 21 patients, Langmore et al. [3] found that specificity compared favorably to the modified barium swallow for identifying swallow latency.

Assessing Aspiration/Penetration

The ability to visualize the mucosal surface of the larynx and trachea with great detail offers great opportunity to the endoscopist for detecting the presence of material in these areas. While the onset of the event of aspiration or penetration may be obscured during at the height of the swallow, the material that remains in the larynx or trachea after the event occurs is easily detected with the laryngoscope. Sensitivity, specificity and inter-rater and intra-rater reliability for penetration and aspiration have been determined to be high [3, 40]. In one study, Leder et al. reported 96% agreement between the two types of evaluations when rating silent aspiration in 56 patients [41]. Leder and Karas also reported 100% agreement between FEES and MBS for penetration and aspiration in a pediatric population [42].

In fact, several studies have shown that detection of aspiration is higher using laryngoscopy than when using fluoroscopy [40, 43–45]. Wu et al. performed both FEES and MBS in 28 patients and reported a 14.3% disagreement between the two examinations for events of penetration and aspiration in which the FEES identified penetration and aspiration in patients when the MBS did not. Similarly, Gerek et al. [44] in a study of 80 subjects using both fluoroscopy and endoscopy reported that FEES offered an advantage for revealing aspiration over fluoroscopy. Perhaps most convincingly, Kelly et al. [43] used a scaled penetration aspiration score [46] to rate simultaneously recorded FEES and VFSS. In this study high inter- and intra-rater reliability was reported but most interesting

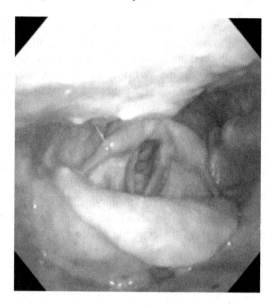

Fig. 5.7. Aspirated material is visible below the glottis.

was that the overall PAS scores were significantly higher for the laryngoscopic view and that the laryngoscopic view revealed aspiration more often than the fluoroscopic view (Fig. 5.7)

Assessing Adequacy of Bolus Clearance

As previously discussed, during the height of the swallow, tissue apposition prevents the clinician from viewing the pharynx or bolus during the height of the swallow. Further, while the endoscope affords a fine visualization of surface mucosa it does not allow for visualization of the oral stage of swallow, movement of submucosal structures, cricopharyngeal opening or striated esophageal transit of the bolus. These limitations hamper the clinician's ability to make determinations regarding adequacy of structural movements by direct observation. Instead, the clinician must rely on visual cues to reveal the underlying cause of the incomplete bolus clearance There is an abundance of literature that can be drawn upon to assist the clinician in this task.

It should be noted that while videofluoroscopy offers superior visualization of swallowing structures deep to the surface, it is still difficult to make determinations regarding the adequacy of the

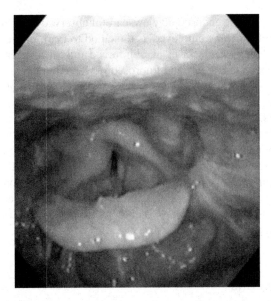

Fig. 5.8. Diffusely retained bolus located in the vallecular space, pyriform sinus, and laryngeal surface of the epiglottis.

movement of those structures. For instance, measurements for laryngeal elevation are highly variable [47] and difficult to assign as being normal or abnormal [48]. There is some evidence to guide the clinician attempting to identify disordered physiology by looking for patterns of bolus retention in the pharynx. A fully efficient swallow will result in little or no retained bolus following a single or secondary clearing swallow. It has long been assumed that when the propulsive components of the swallow become compromised the location of the retained bolus may reveal the physiological deficit. There is now a growing body of literature indicating that pharyngeal pressures may be inferred from observations of retained bolus in the pharynx (Fig. 5.8). For instance, videofluoroscopic swallow studies have demonstrated that when base of tongue retraction is reduced and tongue contact with the posterior pharyngeal wall is weakened, residue remains on the base of tongue and in the valleculae [49]. This finding was reinforced in a study using simultaneous manometry and fluorography [50] which again showed the pairing of reduced pressure at the level of the tongue base and the presence of vallecular residue. In that study reduced pharyngeal shortening and/or reduced laryngeal elevation, were identified to result in pyriform sinus residue. Given that these movements are not directly observable via the endoscopic view, careful observation of the location of the residue can be employed as a method to mark of the locus of a pressure deficit. Pauloski et al. reinforced this in a recent study of simultaneous manometry and fluoroscopy where the clinicians' rating of location of residue had a higher correlation with the region of decreased manometric pressure than did the clinicians' rating of adequacy of movement of structures [51].

Simple measures of swallow efficiency can also be drawn during the FEES examination for the purpose of pre and posttreatment comparisons or to monitor improvements or decline in function over time. For instance, simply counting the number of swallows elicited to clear a premeasured bolus will give the clinician an impression of the efficiency of the swallow. Counting swallows to clear the bolus is easily replicable when the patient is retested at a later date.

Conclusions

The FEES examination allows for the prompt use of portable instrumentation to assess swallowing function in the clinic or at the patient's bedside. The procedure has proven capable of swift identification of ability or disability in swallow function and the prompt implementation of interventions in the form of diet modification, direct interventions or rehabilitation of swallow function. Over the years since its inception, FEES has become a standard assessment practiced in a wide range of settings where these qualities are valued. The procedure has also been used to good effect in research to measure the degree of swallow dysfunction and to test the effect of therapies. While protocols have been published and disseminated [52] further efforts to achieve standardization for scoring and interpretation of the exam are necessary.

References

1. Sawashima M, Hirose H. New laryngoscopic technique by use of fiber optics. J Acoust Soc Am. 1968;43:168–9.
2. Langmore S, Schatz K, Olsen N. Fiberoptic endoscopic examination of swallowing safety: a new procedure. Dysphagia. 1988;2:216–9.
3. Langmore S, Schatz K, Olsen N. Endoscopic and videofluoroscopic evaluations of swallowing and aspiration. Ann Otol Rhinol Laryngol. 1991;100:678–81.

4. Bastian R. Videoendoscopic evaluation of patients with dysphagia: an adjunct to the modified barium swallow. Otolaryngol Head Neck Surg. 1991;104:339–50.
5. FDA Public Health Advisory. FDA Public Health Advisory: Reports of Blue Discoloration and Death in Patients Receiving Enteral Feedings Tinted With The Dye, FD&C Blue No.1. 2003.
6. Leder S, Acton L, Lisitano H, Murray J. Fiberoptic endoscopic evaluation of swallowing (FEES) with and without blue dyed food. Dysphagia. 2005;20:157–62.
7. Nankivell P, Pothier D. Nasal and instrument preparation prior to rigid and flexible nasendoscopy: a systematic review. J Laryngol Otol. 2008;122:1024–8.
8. Frosh A, Jayaraj S, Porter G, Almeyda J. Is local anaesthesia actually beneficial in flexible fibreoptic nasendoscopy? Clin Otolaryngol Allied Sci. 1998;23:259–62.
9. Pothier D, Raghava N, Monteiro P, Awad Z. A randomized controlled trial: is water better than a standard lubricant in nasendoscopy? Clin Otolaryngol Allied Sci. 2006;31:134–7.
10. Rudnick E, Sie K. Velopharyngeal insufficiency: current concepts in diagnosis and management. Curr Opin Otolaryngol Head Neck Surg. 2008;16:530–5.
11. Howell R, Davolos A, Clary M, Frake P, Joshi A, Chaboki H. Miller fisher syndrome presents as an acute voice change to hypernasal speech. Laryngoscope. 2010;120:978–80.
12. Stübgen J. Facioscapulohumeral muscular dystrophy: a radiologic and manometric study of the pharynx and esophagus. Dysphagia. 2008;23:341–7.
13. Warnecke T, Teismann I, Zimmermann J, Oelenberg S, Ringelstein E, Dziewas R. Fiberoptic endoscopic evaluation of swallowing with simultaneous tensilon application. J Neurol. 2008;255:224–30.
14. Tsuneo Y, Minoru S, Yoshihiro K, Takashi N, Ryuichi H, Satoshi E, et al. Functional outcomes and reevaluation of esophageal speech after free jejunal transfer in two hundred thirty-six cases. Ann Plast Surg. 2009;62:54–8.
15. Franklin K, Anttila H, Axelsson S, et al. Effects and side-effects of surgery for snoring and obstructive sleep apnea: a systematic review. Sleep. 2009;32:27–36.
16. Golding-Kushner K, Argamaso R, Cotton R, et al. Standardization for the reporting of nasopharyngoscopy and multiview videofluoroscopy: a report from an International Working Group. Cleft Palate J. 1990;27:337–47.
17. Sie K, Starr J, Bloom D, Cunningham M, de Serres L, Drake A, et al. Multicenter interrater and intrarater reliability in the endoscopic evaluation of velopharyngeal insufficiency. Arch Otolaryngol Head Neck Surg. 2008;134:757–63.
18. Muntz H. Navigation of the nose with flexible fiberoptic endoscopy. Cleft Palate Craniofac J. 1992;29:507–10.
19. Hiss G, Postma N. Fiberoptic endoscopic evaluation of swallowing. Laryngoscope. 2003;113:1386–93.
20. Perlman A, Van Daele D. Simultaneous videoendoscopic and ultrasound measures of swallowing. J Med Speech Lang Pathol. 1993;1:223–32.
21. Postma G, McGuirt W, Butler S, Rees C, Crandall H, Tansavatdi K. Laryngopharyngeal abnormalities in hospitalized patients with dysphagia. Laryngoscope. 2007;117:1720–2.
22. Colton House J, Noordzij J, Burgia B, Langmore S. Laryngeal injury from prolonged intubation; a prospective analysis of contributing factors. Laryngoscope. 2011;121:596–600.

23. Leder S, Suiter D. Effect of nasogastric tubes on incidence of aspiration. Arch Phys Med Rehabil. 2008;89:648–51.

24. Dziewas R, Warnecke T, Hamacher C, Oelenberg S, Teismann I, Kraemer C, et al. Do nasogastric tubes worsen dysphagia in patients with acute stroke? BMC. Neurology. 2008;8:29. http://www.biomedcentral.com/1471-2377/8/28.

25. Murray J, Langmore SE, Ginsberg S, Dostie A. The significance of accumulated oropharyngeal secretions and swallowing frequency in predicting aspiration. Dysphagia. 1996;11:99–103.

26. Donzelli J, Brady S, Wesling M, Craney M. Predictive value of accumulated oropharyngeal secretions for aspiration during video nasal endoscopic evaluation of the swallow. Ann Otol Rhinol Laryngol. 2003;112:469–75.

27. Link D, Willging J, Miller C, Cotton R, Rudolph C. Pediatric laryngoscopic sensory testing during flexible endoscopic evaluation of swallowing: feasible and correlative. Ann Otol Rhinol Laryngol. 2000;109:899–905.

28. Ota K, Saitoh E, Baba M, Sonoda S. The secretion severity rating scale: a potentially useful tool for management of acute-phase fasting stroke patients. J Stroke Cerebrovasc Dis. doi:10.1016/j.jstrokecerebrovasdis.2009.11.015, doi:dx.doi.org.

29. Lear C, Flanagan J, Moorrees C. The frequency of deflutition in man. Arch Oral Biol. 1965;10:83–99.

30. Perie S, Laccourreye O, Bou-Malhab F, Brasnu D. Aspiration in unilateral recurrent laryngeal nerve paralysis after surgery. Am J Otolaryngol. 1998;19:18–23.

31. Bhattacharyya N, Kotz T, Shapiro J. Dysphagia and aspiration with unilateral vocal cord immobility: incidence, characterization, and response to surgical treatment. Ann Otol Rhinol Laryngol. 2002;111:672–9.

32. Nayak V, Bhattacharyya N, Kotz J, Shapiro J. Patterns of swallowing failure following medialization in unilateral vocal fold immobility. Laryngoscope. 2002;112:1840–4.

33. Amin M, Belafsky P. Cough and swallowing dysfunction. Otolaryngol Clin North Am. 2010;43:35–42.

34. Bastian R. The videoendoscopic swallowing study: an alternative and partner to the videofluoroscopic swallowing study. Dysphagia. 1993;8:359–67.

35. Leonard R, Belafsky P, Rees C. Relationship between fluoroscopic and manometric measures of pharyngeal constriction: the pharyngeal constriction ratio. Ann Otol Rhinol Laryngol. 2006;115:897–901.

36. Fuller S, Leonard R, Aminpour S, Belafsky P. Validation of the pharyngeal squeeze maneuver. Otolaryngol Head Neck Surg. 2009;140:391–4.

37. Daniels S, Schroeder M, DeGeorge P, Corey D, Rosebek J. Effect of verbal cue on bolus flow during swallowing. Am J Speech Lang Pathol. 2007;16:140–7.

38. Martin-Harris B, Brodsky M, Michel Y, Lee F, Walters B. Delayed initiation of the pharyngeal swallow: normal variability in adult swallows. J Speech Lang Hear Res. 2007;50:585–94.

39. Stephen J, Taves D, Martin R. Bolus location at the initiation of the pharyngeal stage of swallowing in healthy older adults. Dysphagia. 2005;20:266–72.

40. Wu H, Hsiao Y, Chen C, Chang C, Lee Y. Evaluation of swallowing safety with fiberoptic endoscope: comparison with videofluoroscopic technique. Laryngoscope. 1997;107:396–401.

41. Leder S, Sasaki C, Burrell M. Fiberoptic endoscopic evaluation of dysphagia to identify silent aspiration. Dysphagia. 1998;13:19–21.
42. Leder S, Karas D. Fiberoptic endoscopic evaluation of swallowing in the pediatric population. Laryngoscope. 2000;110:1132–6.
43. Kelly A, Drinnan M, Leslie P. Assessing penetration and aspiration: how do videofluoroscopy and fiberoptic endoscopic evaluation of swallowing compare? Laryngoscope. 2007;117:1723–7.
44. Gerek M, Atala A, Cekin F, Ciyiltepe M, Ozkaptan Y. The effectiveness of fiberoptic endoscopic swallow study and modified barium swallow study techniques in diagnosis of dysphagia. Kulak Burun Bogaz Ihtis Derg. 2005;15:103–11.
45. Tohara H, Nakane A, Murata S, Mikushi S, Ouchi Y, Wakasugi Y, et al. Inter- and intra-rater reliability in fibroptic endoscopic evaluation of swallowing. J Oral Rehabil. 2010;37:884–91.
46. Rosenbek J, Robbins J, Roecker E, Coyle J, Wood J. A penetration-aspiration scale. Dysphagia. 1996;11:93–8.
47. Molfenter S, Steele C. Physiological variability in the deglutition literature: hyoid and laryngeal kinematics. Dysphagia. 2010;26:67–74.
48. Van Daele D, Perlman A, Cassell M. Intrinsic fibre architecture and attachments of the human epiglottis and their contributions to the mechanism of deglutition. J Anat. 1995;186:1–15.
49. Veis S, Logemann J, Colangelo L. Effects of three techniques on maximum posterior movement of tongue base. Dysphagia. 2000;15:142–5.
50. Dejaeger E, Pelemans W, Ponette E, Joosten E. Mechanisms involved in post deglutition retention in the elderly. Dysphagia. 1997;12:63–7.
51. Pauloski B, Rademaker A, Lazarus C, Boeckxstaens G, Kahrilas P, Logemann J. Relationship between manometric and videofluoroscopic measures of swallow function in healthy adults and patients treated for head and neck cancer with various modalities. Dysphagia. 2009;24:196–203.
52. Hey C, Pluschinski P, Stanschus S, Euler HA, Sader RA, Langmore S, et al. A documentation system to save time and ensure proper application of the fiberoptic endoscopic evaluation of swallowing (FEES®). Folia Phoniatr Logop. 2011;63:201–8.

6. Laryngopharyngeal Sensory Testing

Jonathan E. Aviv

Abstract Swallowing can be thought of as the interaction between two distinct, but interrelated phenomena, airway protection and bolus transport. Airway protection requires intact oral, pharyngeal and laryngeal sensory function. Laryngopharyngeal sensory testing specifically assesses a patient's laryngeal and pharyngeal sensation. The sensory testing technique is described in detail with a focus on key technical points. The utility of sensory testing is also described beyond its application in dysphagia to include the evaluation of patients with acid reflux disease, site of lesion testing in the head and neck and in the evaluation of chronic cough, particularly vagal neuralgia and paradoxical vocal fold motion disorder.

Background

Swallowing comprises the interaction between two distinct, but interrelated processes, airway protection and bolus transport [1]. Airway protection depends on normal oral, pharyngeal, and laryngeal sensory function. Flexible Endoscopic Evaluation of Swallowing with Sensory Testing (FEESST) directly assesses a patient's sensory function and predict their ability to protect their airway before administration of food or barium [2, 3].

Patients with swallowing dysfunction may present with a number of other complaints including weight loss, globus sensation, excessive throat mucus, and prandial or post-cibal cough. FEESST has proven beneficial in the initial evaluation of patients with their symptoms. A diagnostic algorithm employed at our center is presented in Fig. 6.1. The algorithm provides a useful framework for which to diagnose and manage patients with swallowing difficulty, depending on the primary presenting complaint.

R. Shaker et al. (eds.), *Manual of Diagnostic and Therapeutic Techniques for Disorders of Deglutition*, DOI 10.1007/978-1-4614-3779-6_6,
© Springer Science+Business Media New York 2013

104   J.E. Aviv

Dysphagia Diagnostic Algorithm

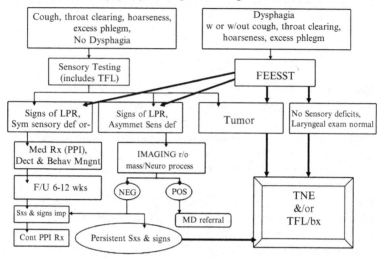

Fig. 6.1. Dysphagia diagnostic algorithm. *Asymmt* asymetry; *Bx* biopsy; *Cont* continue; *Def* deficits; *FEESST* flexible endoscopic evaluation of swallowing with sensory testing; *f/u* follow-up; *Imp* improve; *LPR* laryngopharyngeal reflux; *Med* medical; *Mngnt* management; *r/o* rule out; *Rx* treatment; *Sens* sensory; *TFL* transnasal flexible laryngoscopy; *TNE* transnasal esophagoscopy.

Swallowing dysfunction can be evaluated with two basic approaches, a noninstrument-based approach and an instrument-based approach. Both methods involve administering food to a patient and observing how the patient handles the administered food bolus. The noninstrument-based method is an office or bedside physical examination generally performed as an initial screening exam to gauge the severity of the patient's swallowing complaints. At best, a bedside evaluation of a patient can associate a patient's symptoms with the gravity of their swallowing problem. At worst, a bedside swallowing evaluation can be misleading. Because of the limited nature of the information provided, an instrument-based examination is generally preferred to the bedside evaluation [4, 5].

The two primary means of assessing swallowing ability with an instrument-based approach employ either video fluoroscopy or video endoscopy [6–9]. The primary advantages of the video fluoroscopic swallow study include the ability to evaluate bolus movement through the pharyngoesophageal segment and the capacity to obtain precise and reliable objective measures of swallowing function. Advantages of the endoscopic swallowing evaluation include the absence of radiation exposure and the ability to provide detailed information about pooled saliva, pharyngeal wall movement, mucosal abnormalities, and vocal fold function. In addition FEESST provides information regarding laryngopharyngeal sensation.

Air pulse laryngopharyngeal sensory testing was first described in the early 1990s [10]. The development of the technology was inspired by the swallowing dysfunction endured by head and neck cancer patients following reconstruction of the tongue and pharynx. The desire to provide sensate free tissue reconstruction of the tongue was the original impetus for the development of a method to measure sensation [11]. Laryngopharyngeal sensory testing has evolved to involve the delivery of discrete air pulse stimuli of predetermined pressure to the mucosa innervated by the internal branch of the superior laryngeal nerve (SLN). The sensory challenge evokes the laryngeal adductor reflex (LAR), a brainstem-mediated, fundamental sensory-motor airway protective reflex [12, 13].

The importance of sensation as it relates to swallowing and airway protection in healthy individuals has been previously described [12, 14, 15]. The importance of sensation relative to swallowing in impaired individuals, specifically in patients with swallowing dysfunction after stroke, has suggested that laryngopharyngeal hyposensitivity may be a primary etiology of pneumonia after stroke [16]. Subsequent work showed that stroke patients with dysphagia have laryngopharyngeal sensory deficits and that these deficits may be associated with the development of aspiration pneumonia [17, 18].

Technique

A discrete pulse of air with a bandwidth of 50 ms is delivered to each of the arytenoids to elicit the LAR [13]. The air pulse is delivered from a device called an air pulse sensory stimulator (Vision Sciences Inc, Orangeburg NY) (Fig. 6.2). On one side of the face of the device there is a rheostat that allows the clinician to increase or decrease the strength of the administered air pulse. On the opposite side of the sensory box is a switch and an input for a foot pedal. Manual depression of the switch or depression of the foot pedal attached to the device delivers a 50 ms air pulse. The device is connected via a catheter from the box to a luer lock on the single use disposable endosheath that had been placed on the transnasal flexible laryngoscope that is used to administer the air pulse (Fig. 6.3).

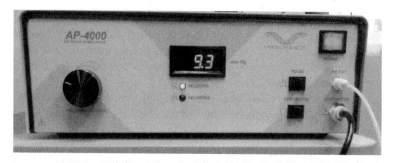

Fig. 6.2. Laryngopharyngeal sensory testing device. On the *left side* of the face of the device is a rheostat which allows the examiner to increase or decrease the strength of the air pulse pressure that is administered. In the *middle* of the device is a digital display which shows the air pulse strength being delivered. The yellow light signifies the device is in standby mode and the green light lights up at the instant a pulse is delivered. The air pulse can be delivered via a foot switch seen on the far *right* of the device, or by manually depressing a switch in either the pulse mode (a 50 ms pulse) or continuous mode, which the examiner can depress for at least 1 s (or 1,000 ms). Also on the *right side* is an air catheter (AIR OUT) which connects the device to a flexible endoscope. At the *top right* of the device face is a green on/off switch.

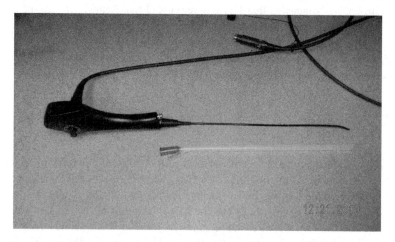

Fig. 6.3. Transnasal flexible laryngoscope with laryngopharyngeal sensory sheath below. Note the ridges at the distal end of the insertion tube of the scope, which is where the blue colored portion of the sensory sheath gets anchored. The luer lock on the proximal portion of the sheath serves to accept the air catheter coming from the sensory device (sensory device not shown).

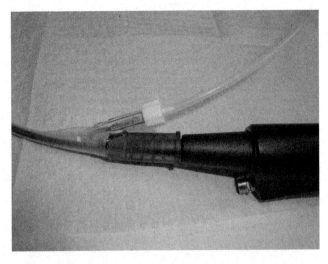

Fig. 6.4. Close up view of air catheter inserted into luer lock of sensory endosheath. The sensory endosheath has already been loaded onto the transnasal flexible laryngoscope and the air catheter from the sensory box is now connected to the luer lock on the sensory endosheath.

The first generation of sensory testing utilized a specialized laryngoscope with a 1.2 mm internal channel. Subsequently a single use disposable endosheath was developed (Medtronic USA, Jacksonville FL) to slide onto most commercially available laryngoscopes. The air catheter is attached to a luer lock on the endosheath and the air pulse can then be administered (Fig. 6.4).

The air catheter should be loaded at 6 o'clock relative to the flexible laryngoscope so that the air pulse emanates inferiorly towards the arytenoid, as opposed to another more superiorly located area in the pharynx, which may deliver the air pulse superiorly towards the nasopharynx (Fig. 6.5). The air pulse is delivered less than 2 mm from the arytenoid and both the right and left sides are tested. If asymmetry is noted, diagnostic imaging of the head and neck is recommended to rule out a mass lesion along the course of the vagus nerve. Stimulation of the SLN not only results in elicitation of the LAR, it also can initiate a swallow, which necessarily results in elevation of the larynx. Elevation of the larynx while the flexible endoscope is stationary at the level of the

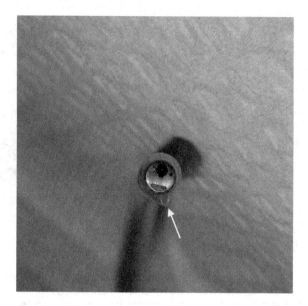

Fig. 6.5. Six o'clock position of air catheter on endoscope. The 1.2 mm catheter tip is shown at the correct 6 o'clock position on the flexible endoscope. It is critical that the examiner make sure that the catheter opening is in this inferiorly based position so the administered air pulse gets directed inferiorly towards the arytenoid, and not in another position which would then direct the air pulse to other areas of the pharynx.

arytenoid can result in inadvertent tracheoscopy. To avoid this, the flexible laryngoscope should be withdrawn towards the oropharynx after the air pulse is administered. The sensory testing is initiated at suprathreshold air pulse pressure values to ascertain the ability to protect the airway. Laryngopharyngeal sensory thresholds are defined as normal if <4.0 mmHg air pulse pressure, moderate if between 4.0 and 6.0 mmHg air pulse pressure, severe if >6.0 mmHg air pulse pressure, and absent if no reaction at a 1 s pulse, which is 20 times as long as the standard 50 ms air pulse width. The referenced URL displays a series of video clips demonstrating laryngopharyngeal sensory testing technique [19].

Indications

Laryngeal sensory testing was initially developed to assess a patient's ability to protect their airway during deglutition, that is, as part of the

FEESST exam [20]. Over the past 20 years, however, primarily due to work with sensory testing performed by gastroenterologists and pulmonologists, it has been shown to be an indicator of acid reflux disease [21, 22], neurogenic cough [23], vagal neuralgia [24], and site of lesion testing [24].

Dysphagia (FEESST)

Laryngopharyngeal sensory testing serves as an additional guide for the clinician managing a patient with dysphagia. The test can help decide whether or not the patient can safely take food by mouth [25].

The relationship between the results of sensory testing and airway safety in dysphagic patients was thoroughly evaluated in a prospective study of 122 patients with dysphagia of numerous etiologies [26]. All patients in the study underwent a FEESST and were divided into two groups, those with an intact and those with an absent LAR (no elicitation of the LAR after continuous air pulse administration). Patients in both groups were administered pureed food and thin liquid and the prevalence of laryngeal penetration and aspiration was determined. Patients with an absent LAR administered pureed food had a prevalence of penetration of 84 % and a prevalence of aspiration of 70 %. Patients with an absent LAR administered thin liquid (water) had a prevalence of penetration of 100 % and a prevalence of aspiration of 93 %. In comparison, patients with an intact LAR administered puree had a prevalence of penetration and aspiration of 9 and 4 % respectively. Patients with an intact LAR administered thin liquid had a prevalence of penetration and aspiration of 34 and 17 % respectively (Fig. 6.6). These results suggest that individuals with an absent LAR are at a significantly increased risk of penetration and aspiration ($p < 0.05$). These findings have significant implications in the determination of diet recommendations.

Cough

Laryngopharyngeal sensory testing is routinely utilized to evaluate the patient with chronic cough. Chronic cough is defined as cough lasting for more than 6 weeks. When a patient has chronic cough with a normal chest X-ray, no active smoking and no current Angiotensin Converting Enzyme (ACE) inhibitor use, workup of the cough should focus on detection and treatment of Upper Airway Cough Syndrome (UACS), formerly known as postnasal drip syndrome (PNDS), non-asthmatic eosinophilic bronchitis (NAEB) and gastroesophageal reflux disease (GERD), alone or in combination [27].

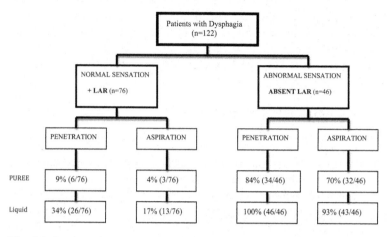

Fig. 6.6. Laryngeal adductor reflex as a predictor of laryngeal penetration and aspiration (effect of laryngeal sensation on swallowing). *LAR* laryngeal adductor reflex.

Once UACS, NAEB, and acid reflux have been ruled out, vagal neuralgia and paradoxical vocal fold motion disorder (PVFMD) should be evaluated as possible etiologies of the cough. An abnormal LAR in the presence of cough suggests a vagal neuropathy and treatment can be initiated appropriately.

Acid Reflux Disease

It has been shown that laryngopharyngeal sensitivity can be reversibly diminished in patients with acid reflux disease [28, 29].

In a study of laryngopharyngeal sensation, acid reflux and pH testing a laryngeal sensory deficit greater than 5 mmHg air pulse pressure (considered a moderate laryngopharyngeal sensory deficit) combined with findings consistent with laryngopharyngeal reflux (LPR) on flexible laryngoscopy, was as sensitive and specific as 24-h pH testing alone in predicting the presence of LPR disease. The addition of a sensory deficit greater than 5.0 mmHg air pulse pressure to flexible laryngoscopy findings increased the diagnostic yield of LPR disease vs. the flexible laryngoscopy findings alone [21] (Table 6.1).

In another study, patients with chronic cough who had positive 24-h pH studies, underwent laryngopharyngeal sensory testing before and after minute infusions of either dilute hydrochloric acid or saline to the

Table 6.1. Reflux finding score (RFS).

Findings	Scoring				
Subglottic edema (pseudosulcus vocalis)		2 if present			4 polyp
Ventricle obliteration		2 if partial			4 if complete
Erythema/hyperemia		2 arytenoids only			4 if complete
Vocal fold edema	1 mild	2 mod		3 severe	4 polyp
Arytenoid/interarytenoid edema	1 mild	2 mod		3 severe	4 obstruction
Posterior commissure hypertrophy	1 mild	2 mod		3 severe	4 obstruction
Granuloma/granulation		2 if present			
Thick endolaryngeal mucus		2 if present			

An RFS > 7 is significant and suggests laryngopharyngeal reflux

hypopharynx. Laryngopharyngeal sensory thresholds in individuals with acid infusions had significantly diminished laryngeal sensory thresholds compared with the saline infusion control group. This data suggests that the sensory integrity of laryngopharynx is significantly impaired following exposure to even small amounts of acid and that patients with chronic cough and pH test-positive GERD have reduced laryngopharyngeal sensitivity compared with healthy controls and this diminished sensation may result in an increased risk of aspiration [22].

Vagal Neuralgia

While the constellation of patient symptoms related to acid reflux disease is vast, the complaint of throat pain, especially unilateral throat pain, is typically not related to peptic injury of the laryngopharynx. Throat pain or pain with phonation is more typical of a neurogenic etiology. Laryngopharyngeal sensory asymmetry may suggest a unilateral vagal afferent neuropathy responsible, at least in part, for their throat pain [24]. Patients with vagal neuropathy may have comorbid LPR at the time of initial presentation. Reflux typically causes a bilateral symmetric sensory deficit [21, 28, 29] and patients will first need to be treated with antacid therapy as well as diet and lifestyle modifications. On follow-up examination at least 6 weeks later, a repeat sensory test is performed in order to "unmask" sensory asymmetry. If asymmetry is present, a vagal etiology of the throat pain is suggested.

Asymmetric sensory deficits may require radiographic imaging (MRI or CT) to rule out a mass along the course of the vagus nerve. Once a negative imaging study is confirmed, the patient may be referred to a physiatrist experienced with head and neck pain or receive a medical regimen including low dose tricyclic antidepressant medications and/or a nerve acquiescing medication such as pregabalin or gabapentin [30].

Paradoxical Vocal Fold Motion Disorder

Another cause of chronic cough that is particularly vexing to diagnose and treat is PVFMD. Described in the early 1980s, PVFMD is a cause of chronic cough often mistaken for asthma, postnasal drip and allergies [31]. Several studies have shown that patients with PVFMD not only have evidence of acid reflux disease but also have laryngeal sensory deficits [23, 32]. Treatment of the acid reflux component with antacids alone is not enough to resolve the cough in these individuals. The patient must also undergo respiratory retraining, which are increased resistance-breathing exercises, typically administered by an SLP. The combination of increased resistance-breathing exercise with antacid therapy resolves the cough in most cases.

Site of Lesion

Symmetry of laryngopharyngeal sensory testing results has been repeatedly emphasized. The most important information that laryngopharyngeal sensory testing provides is an individual's ability to safely protect the airway. The second most important information provided is the presence of sensory asymmetry. If an asymmetry exists, we recommend an imaging study to rule out a mass effect along the course of the vagus nerve (Fig. 6.1).

Summary

Laryngopharyngeal sensory testing allows to precisely assess symmetry and integrity of the afferent loop of laryngopharyngeal sensory functions which, in turn, has implications for management of patients with swallowing disorders and neurologic deficits of the larynx.

References

1. Zamir Z, Ren J, Hogan W, Shaker R. Coordination of deglutitive vocal cord closure and oral-pharyngeal swallowing events in the elderly. Eur J Gastroenterol Hepatol. 1996;8:425–9.
2. Aviv JE, Johnson LF. Flexible endoscopic evaluation of swallowing with sensory testing (FEESST) to diagnose and manage patients with pharyngeal dysphagia. Pract Gastroenterol. 2000;24:52–9.
3. Aviv JE. Sensory discrimination in the larynx and hypopharynx. Otolaryngol Head Neck Surg. 1997;116:331–4.
4. Leder SB, Espinosa JF. Aspiration risk after acute stroke: comparison of clinical examination and fiberoptic endoscopic evaluation of swallowing. Dysphagia. 2002;17(3):214–8.
5. Aviv JE. The bedside swallowing evaluation when endoscopy is an option: what would you choose? Dysphagia. 2002;17:219.
6. Langmore SE, Schatz K, Olsen N. Fiberoptic endoscopic examination of swallowing safety: a new procedure. Dysphagia. 1988;2:216–9.
7. Bastian RW. Videoendoscopic evaluation of patients with dysphagia: an adjunct to modified barium swallow. Otolaryngol Head Neck Surg. 1991;104:339–50.
8. Logemann J. Role of the modified barium swallow in management of patients with dysphagia. Otolaryngol Head Neck Surg. 1997;116:335–8.
9. Logemann JA, Bytell DE. Swallowing disorders in three types of head and neck surgical patients. Cancer. 1979;44:1095–105.
10. Aviv JE, Martin JH, Keen MS, Debell M, Blitzer A. Air-pulse quantification of supraglottic and pharyngeal sensation: a new technique. Ann Otol Rhinol Laryngol. 1993;102:777–80.
11. Urken ML, Weinberg H, Vickery C, Biller HF. The neurofasciocutaneous radial forearm flaps in head and neck reconstruction: a preliminary report. Laryngoscope. 1990;100:161–73.
12. Jafari S, Prince RA, Kim DK, Paydarfar D. Sensory regulation of swallowing and airway protection: a role for the internal superior laryngeal nerve in humans. J Physiol. 2003;550:287–304.
13. Aviv JE, Martin JH, Kim T, Sacco RL, Thomson JE, Diamond B, et al. Laryngopharyngeal sensory discrimination testing and the laryngeal adductor reflex. Ann Otol Rhinol Laryngol. 1999;108:725–30.
14. Addington WR, Stephens RE, Gilliland K, Miller SP. Tartaric acid-induced cough and the superior laryngeal nerve evoked potential. Am J Phys Med Rehabil. 1998;77:523–52.
15. Sulica L, Hembree A, Blitzer A. Sensation and swallowing: endoscopic evaluation of deglutition in the anesthetized larynx. Ann Otol Rhinol Laryngol. 2002;111:291–4.
16. Kidd D, Lawson J, Macmahon J. Aspiration in acute stroke: a clinical study with videofluoroscopy. Q J Med. 1993;86:825–9.
17. Aviv JE, Martin JH, Sacco RL, Diamond B, Zagar D, Keen MS, et al. Supraglottic and pharyngeal sensory abnormalities in stroke patients with dysphagia. Ann Otol Rhinol Laryngol. 1996;105:92–7.

18. Aviv JE. Prospective, randomized outcome study of endoscopy versus modified barium swallow in patients with dysphagia. Laryngoscope. 2000;110:563–74.

19. Laryngopharyngeal sensory testing video clips. http://www.entandallergy.com/vas/gallery/gallery_swallowing_feesst.php

20. Aviv JE, Kim T, Goodhart K, Kaplan S, Thomson J, Diamond B, et al. FEESST: a new bedside endoscopic test of the motor and sensory components of swallowing. Ann Otol Rhinol Laryngol. 1998;107:378–87.

21. Botoman VA, Hanft KL, Breno SM, Vickers D, Astor FC, Caristo IB, et al. Prospective controlled evaluation of pH testing, laryngoscopy and laryngopharyngeal sensory testing (LPST) shows a specific post inter-arytenoid neuropathy in proximal GERD (P-GERD). LPST improves laryngoscopy diagnostic yield in P-GERD. Am J Gastroenterol. 2002;97:S11–2.

22. Phua SY, McGarvey LPA, Ngu MC, Ing AJ. Patients with gastro-oesophageal reflux disease and cough have impaired laryngopharyngeal mechanosensitivity. Thorax. 2005;60:488–91.

23. Cukier-Blaj S, Bewley A, Aviv JE, Murry T. Paradoxical vocal fold motion: a sensory-motor laryngeal disorder. Laryngoscope. 2008;118(2):367–70.

24. Aviv JE, Murry T. Sensory testing alone. In: Aviv JE, Murry T, editors. FEESST: flexible endoscopic evaluation of swallowing with sensory testing. San Diego, CA: Plural Publishing; 2005. p. 57–70.

25. Setzen M, Cohen MA, Mattucci KF, Perlman PW, Ditkoff MK. Laryngopharyngeal sensory deficits as a predictor of aspiration. Otolaryngol Head Neck Surg. 2001;124:622–4.

26. Aviv JE, Spitzer J, Cohen M, Ma G, Belafsky P, Close LG. Laryngeal adductor reflex and pharyngeal squeeze as predictors of laryngeal penetration and aspiration. Laryngoscope. 2002;112:338–41.

27. Irwin RS, Baumann MH, Bolser DC, Boulet LP, Braman SS, Brightling CE, et al. Diagnosis and management of cough executive summary ACCP evidence-based clinical practice guidelines. Chest. 2006;129:1S–23S.

28. Aviv JE, Liu H, Parides M, Kaplan ST, Close LG. Laryngopharyngeal sensory deficits in patients with laryngopharyngeal reflux and dysphagia. Ann Otol Rhinol Laryngol. 2000;109:1000–6.

29. Postma GN, Belafsky PC, Aviv JE, Koufman JA. Laryngopharyngeal reflux testing. Ear Nose Throat J. 2002;81(Suppl):14–8.

30. Dillard JN. Pain pills and other pharmaceuticals. In: Dillard JN, Hirschman LA, editors. The chronic pain solution: the comprehensive, step-by-step guide to choosing the best of alternative and conventional medicine. New York, NY: Bantam Publishing; 2002. p. 171–96.

31. Christopher KL, Wood II RP, Eckert RC, Blager FB, Raney RA, Souhrada JF. Vocal-cord dysfunction presenting as asthma. N Engl J Med. 1983;308:1566–70.

32. Murry T, Branski RC, Yu K, Cukier-Blaj S, Duflo S, Aviv JE. Laryngeal sensory deficits in patients with chronic cough and paradoxical vocal fold movement disorder. Laryngoscope. 2010;120:1576–81.

7. Unsedated Transnasal Esophagoscopy: Endoscopic Evaluation of Esophageal Phase of Deglutition

Gregory N. Postma and Kia Saeian

Abstract   Since 1994 when Shaker first introduced the technique of unsedated transnasal upper endoscopy, technological advances have resulted in the availability of newer "ultrathin" video endoscopes with excellent resolution and a 2 mm working channel that allows for interventions. The technique of unsedated transnasal esophagoscopy which largely avoids the gag reflex thereby allowing for non-sedated examination of the upper G.I. tract is now more widely practiced but has not as of yet received universal acceptance by gastroenterologists. It is more often practiced by otolaryngologists who have more familiarity with nasopharyngeal anatomy. The potential benefits of an unsedated examination including lack of adverse effects from sedation, the cost savings due to lack of work loss and need for a separate visit to an often endoscopy unit make this procedure an attractive option. However, since not all patients tolerate an unsedated examination, attention must be paid to appropriate patient selection. Current applications of the technique and published experience with office-based esophagoscopy, assessment of swallowing disorders, role in head and neck oncology, GERD, dyspepsia and Barrett's esophagus are reviewed. The technique's limitations and potential future applications are also outlined.

Introduction

Since the invention of the distal-lighted, rigid esophagoscope by Chevalier Jackson more than a century ago [1] until the early 1960s, esophagoscopy was predominantly the domain of otolaryngologists. The widespread availability of flexible fiberoptic endoscopy [2, 3] in the last

R. Shaker et al. (eds.), *Manual of Diagnostic and Therapeutic Techniques for Disorders of Deglutition*, DOI 10.1007/978-1-4614-3779-6_7,
© Springer Science+Business Media New York 2013

50 years has not only increased the endoscopic evaluation of the esophagus, but also expanded it to more medical specialties particularly gastroenterologists, and also general and CT surgeons. The vast majority of upper endoscopy and esophagoscopy is now performed with flexible endoscopes (typical diameter 9.6 mm) using a charge-coupled device (CCD) to capture extremely clear images and display them often on high resolution video screens with excellent resolution.

Over time, technological advances led to the production of thinner endoscopes. In 1994, using what now seems a rudimentary 5.3 mm diameter fiberoptic instrument requiring a video convertor device, Shaker introduced the technique of unsedated transnasal esophagogastroduodenoscopy (T-EGD) [4], passed easily through the nose and directed into the esophagus largely avoiding the gag reflex thus allowing patients to avoid sedation. The development of newer "ultrathin" video endoscopes with excellent resolution, brilliant illumination, thinner diameters, and state-of-the-art image quality continue to expand options. These instruments allow for air insufflation and irrigation and provide a 2 mm working channel that can also be used to obtain biopsies and/or to perform other interventions.

When there is no a priori need for examination of the stomach and duodenum, *Transnasal esophagoscopy* (*TNE*) is sufficient and provides an important advance in the care of patients with reflux, dysphagia, head & neck cancer, and esophageal pathology. In part due to established office-based practice patterns and their familiarity with the nose and nasopharynx, otolaryngologists have embraced and further popularized TNE and its diagnostic applications for globus, dysphagia, extraesophageal reflux (EER), and gastroesophageal reflux disease (GERD) [5–7]. The gastroenterology community, however, has not as yet fully embraced the use of this technique in large part due to their endoscopy center-based practice and lack of economic incentive to perform unsedated examinations which may often take just as long if not longer as sedated examination for the physician to perform.

This chapter will describe the technique of TNE, outline its applications in clinical practice, and review published experience with TNE with regard to its utility in diagnosing pathology in the esophagus.

Equipment

Transnasal esophagoscopes are available through multiple vendors (*EE-1580K* (*Insertion diameter: 5.1 mm, working length: 1,050 mm*), *Pentax Precision Instrument Corporation, Montrale, New Jersey*;

Olympus PEF-V (Insertion diameter: 5.3 mm, working length: 620 mm) or GI F-N180In (Insertion diameter:4.9 mm, working length: 1,100 mm), Olympus America Inc., Melville, New York; and Vision Sciences® TNE-2000 with Endosheath (Outer diameter: 4.7×5.4 mm, working length:650 mm), Orangeburg, NY), with even the shortest endoscopes of adequate length to allow a retroflexed view of the gastroesophageal junction (GEJ) and gastric cardia and a diameter small enough to allow comfortable transnasal passage. Additionally, the endoscopes have an air insufflation port and working channel for biopsy and suction. In addition, the TNE2000 has disposable sheaths (TNE 2000) with channel ports that eliminate the need for lengthy cleaning times between patients.

Technique of TNE

Unsedated TNE is an office-based procedure, although some gastroenterologists may perform it in an endoscopy center. The patient may be seated in an ENT examination chair, a standard recliner, or a simple chair. Because of the lack of conscious sedation, cardiopulmonary monitoring and intravenous line placement are unnecessary and pre-procedural preparation is limited to preparation of the patient and particularly one of the nares. A brief sniff test by the patient identifies the more patent nare and that side is topically anesthetized and vasoconstricted. A typical mixture would be 50/50 oxymetazoline (0.05%) and lidocaine (4%). Additional topical anesthetic spray is sometimes used in the oropharynx particularly if a prolonged examination is expected. Care must be taken to avoid excessive application of the spray since this may obscure visualization.

Usually, a lubricating agent (e.g., K-Y Jelly or Xylocaine) is applied to ease passage of the scope. Following this, the TNE endoscope is passed along the floor of the nose in the majority of patients. This places the scope between the nasal floor, nasal septum, and the inferior turbinate. In a few patients with an inferior nasal spur, the endoscope may be passed more superiorly between the septum and the inferior and middle turbinate bones. The scope is deflected inferiorly at the nasopharynx over the soft palate and then the tip of the scope is advanced to medial side of the ipsilateral pyriform sinus, the patient is asked to lean forward, flex the neck fully, and swallow. The experienced endoscopist will note that passage of the endoscope into the esophagus is quite simple and clearly easier than the standard, larger diameter endoscopes, but care must be taken to avoid blind passage and excessive pressure in the pyriform sinus which may result in perforation. At that point, the scope is advanced into the esophageal inlet.

Inside the esophagus, the endoscope is advanced into the stomach. Since the esophagus is collapsed at rest, air insufflation or voluntary swallows by the patient may be necessary to allow for good visualization. Examination of the esophagus and stomach is carried out, with special attention paid to the GEJ. The TNE scope also allows a retroflexed view from the stomach, allowing the endoscopist to perform a complete examination of the GEJ. This is done by flexing the tip fully (210°), while the scope is positioned in the stomach. LES function should be evaluated with the esophagoscope a few centimeters proximal to it, determining if the LES is closed (normal) or open at rest and whether or not it opens and then promptly closes following swallowing.

Using a combination of air insufflation and irrigation, the mucosa of the entire esophagus is examined, while the scope is slowly withdrawn. If mucosal lesions or irregularities are noted, 1.8 mm biopsy forceps are passed through the working channel and multiple biopsies may be obtained. Visualization of the duodenum is feasible with the longer instruments, but slight modifications in technique are required such as deflation of gastric air, foreknowledge that gastric fluid residue will typically pool in the antrum instead of the fundus, and experience with passage into the second portion of the duodenum.

Potential Pitfalls of TNE

Difficult Passage of the Instrument

Difficulty in passing the endoscope through the upper esophageal sphincter (UES) should alert the examiner to the possibility of a hypertonic UES or a Zenker's diverticulum. If the endoscopist finds him or herself in a diverticulum, then suctioning, air insufflation, and gentle rotation of the scope should be used to find the lumen and enter the esophagus. Perforation may occur if the tip of the esophagoscope enters a diverticulum and significant pressure is used.

Dilated Lumen of the Esophagus

The presence of a dilated esophagus or the retention of saliva or swallowed material should alert the endoscopist to the potential for an esophageal motility disorder (e.g., achalasia), stricture or ring, foreign body, diverticula, or mass lesions.

Detection of Esophageal Rings/Strictures

Another potential problem is the difference in ability to recognize subtle esophageal rings/strictures due to the change in perspective using thin instruments by endoscopists familiar with larger diameter instruments. This issue is resolved with experience and care to adequately insufflate.

Excessive Air Distention

A common error is the use of excessive air insufflation during the examination, which can result in abdominal bloating and discomfort for the patient. Air should be gently insufflated to obtain complete visualization of all mucosal surfaces and then suctioned out when possible. The majority of insufflated air is needed when evaluating the LES, and it should be suctioned out at the end of the examination. The awake patient is much more sensitive to gastric distention which in the upright position may also limit diaphragmatic excursion. As a matter of routine, when examining the esophagus on withdrawal, the endoscope should be introduced into the stomach intermittently to suction out excessive air.

Epistaxis

Epistaxis rates ranging from 0.85 to 5% have been noted with the larger diameter (5.3–6.0 mm diameter) endoscopes being associated with higher rates of epistaxis [8, 9]. The patient should be reminded to avoid blowing his/her nose vigorously immediately after the procedure. The cases of epistaxis in our experience resolve with gentle pressure and have not required further intervention.

Vasovagal Episodes

In the largest series reported of 1,100 patients from France, vasovagal events were 0.3% using a 5.3 mm endoscope [8]. Avoiding excessive insufflation minimizes this risk.

Patient Selection

Appropriate patient selection is critical in performing successful TNE. In the same series from France, using 5.9 and 5.3 mm endoscopes, failure rates of 16.7 and 4.7%, respectively, with the different scopes were noted. In addition to the size of the endoscope, female gender, age ≤35 years old, and a junior endoscopist performing the procedure were associated with failure to complete the examination [8]. Patient reassurance and engaging the patient in conversation during the examination can be invaluable in helping guide patients, particularly those with high levels of anxiety, through the procedure.

Examination of GE Junction

Validation Studies of Image Quality and Diagnostic Capability

Since the introduction of TNE, there have been inevitable comparisons to what has been viewed as the "gold standard"-conventional esophagoscopy (CE), which is performed transorally with sedation. Many of these studies have compared the complete upper endoscopy, but some have focused on comparison of esophagoscopy only.

Several studies have compared the two techniques with regard to image quality and diagnostic capability. Older studies generally conclude that TNE is inferior to CE [10, 11]. However, these studies use older generation endoscopes which are generally larger or do not have distal chip technology. Studies utilizing newer small-caliber videoendoscopes have concluded that TNE image quality and diagnostic capability is equivalent to CE [12–17].

One such study compared a prototype 4 mm transnasal videoesophagoscope to a standard 9.8 or 8.6 mm transoral videoendoscope [16]. The study was a prospective trial and examined diagnostic accuracy using CE as the "gold standard." Patients scheduled for CE had TNE performed immediately preceding their scheduled procedure. The diagnostic accuracy of TNE was found to be 100% in 44 patients. The authors also found overall tolerance was similar between the unsedated and sedated examinations.

Barrett's Esophagus

While image quality is important, it is equally, if not more, important to know whether newer techniques of assessment are capable of detecting Barrett's esophagus with similar accuracy to CE. Barrett's esophagus is a tissue diagnosis and requires the endoscopist to obtain biopsy specimens. Two randomized crossover studies have been published addressing this topic [13, 14].

While most cancers in the United States are experiencing a decline in prevalence, esophageal adenocarcinoma is on the rise [18]. BE represents a premalignant condition for adenocarcinoma. TNE is a useful screening examination for BE. In two studies noted earlier, researchers have demonstrated the equivalence of TNE and CE in the diagnosis of BE [13, 14]. Due to its safety, decreased costs, and equivalent findings, TNE may be the screening modality of choice for BE.

In both studies, patients underwent both CE and TNE, with the procedures separated by at least 1 week. The order of the procedures was randomized and endoscopists were blinded as to previous endoscopic results. Biopsies were taken as indicated using 2.2 mm biopsy forceps for CE and 1.8 mm biopsy forceps for TNE.

In the study by Saeian et al., [14] the level of agreement between CE and TNE for detection of dysplasia in biopsy specimens was found to be 91% (κ=0.79) and felt to be in the "excellent" range. Jobe et al. [13] examined several different endpoints including detection of hiatal hernia, esophagitis, and stricture, grading of GEJ abnormalities, and pathologic diagnosis of Barrett's esophagus. In this study, the correlation between CE and TNE was found to vary between 80 and 96% for the different endpoints (κ=0.60–0.84). Interestingly, although both CE and TNE detected Barrett's metaplasia and dysplasia at similar rates, there was only moderate concordance between the two. Each modality detected changes that were "missed" by the other. This likely has to do with inherent sampling error with respect to selected biopsy sites whether a large diameter or ultrathin instrument is used.

Advantages Over Conventional Esophagoscopy

TNE provides a number of advantages over CE. These include improved safety, decreased overall costs, and patient preference.

Safety

The majority of complications during sedated endoscopy are related to sedation. The vast majority of gastroenterologists perform sedated upper gastrointestinal endoscopy. Cardiopulmonary complications account for more than 50% of all adverse events; the majority are aspiration, over-sedation, hypoventilation, and airway obstruction [19]. A 2007 national survey of endoscopists demonstrated that adverse cardiopulmonary events secondary to conscious sedation constitute the majority of endoscopic complications; in fact, 67% of complications and 72% of mortalities were cardiopulmonary related [20].

All sedated patients require vigilance and prompt treatment to avoid potentially catastrophic outcomes. One study, published in 1990, reported that approximately 7% of patients undergoing sedated upper endoscopy desaturated to <80% [21]. Evidence from a database of 21,011 primarily inpatient procedures indicates that serious cardiopulmonary complications and death attributed to conscious sedation during endoscopic procedures are infrequent; they occur at an estimated incidence of 54 and 3 per 10,000 cases, respectively [22]. These rates have likely improved somewhat since this survey was conducted; however, the potential for cardiopulmonary complications continues to exist with sedated endoscopic procedures. In addition, conscious sedation has been associated with paradoxical agitation and anaphylaxis. Use of intravenous access may also be associated with local complications such as phlebitis and hematoma formation. A study comparing sedated patients ($n=154$) and unsedated patients ($n=330$) undergoing upper endoscopy procedures reported that 21% of sedated patients but only 2% of unsedated patients experienced desaturations below 90% [23]. Of special concern is the more extensive examination of the pharynx and epiglottis that has been associated with more pronounced desaturation. One of the most feared complications of esophagoscopy is esophageal perforation. Among the thousands of TNE and TNEGD cases performed, there has been only a single case of esophageal perforation reported, a case performed by a trainee [24].

Cost Savings

TNE is less expensive than CE. The increased direct costs of CE include longer procedure time, recovery room, and recovery time, and the costs associated with the required medications, monitoring, and nursing [25]. The difference in cost has been estimated to be greater than $2,000 per procedure, though prospective cost comparison trials are lacking [26]. Indirect costs are also important. These include loss of work time by both the patient and a caretaker/driver. In contrast, with TNE, most patients are able to return to work or home shortly after the completion of the examination and do not need a caretaker. There are unfortunately no randomized, direct comparison trials that definitively demonstrate the cost saving benefits of unsedated examination.

Patient Preference

Though initial patient anxiety is higher before unsedated TNE, studies have shown a very high patient satisfaction rate, often greater than with CE [9, 24, 25, 27]. Crossover studies have shown that in patients who had both sedated and unsedated exams, the unsedated exam was better tolerated [16]. In one European study, 91% of TNE patients who had previously undergone CE preferred unsedated TNE, but sedation is not necessarily the standard of care for patients undergoing CE in Europe [8]. In our experience in the US population, patient education and patient selection is of paramount importance and we have learned that it is not safe to assume that a patient automatically would prefer not to take a day off from work for a procedure.

Role of TNE in Clinical Practice

The role of TNE continues to evolve in both the diagnostic and therapeutic realms particularly due to the high yield of pathology found on unsedated TNE examinations when performed in an otolaryngology practice with rates of pathologic findings approaching 50% [9, 28].

Indications for TNE can be divided into three major categories: esophageal, extraesophageal, and procedure-related. Esophageal indications include dysphagia, refractory or long-standing gastro-esophageal reflux, evaluation of a radiologic abnormality on barium swallow, and screening for Barrett's metaplasia. Extra esophageal indications include globus pharyngeus, panendoscopy with biopsy for head and neck cancer, follow-up examinations of head and neck cancer patients, chronic cough, and moderate-to-severe EER.

TNE, Transnasal-EGD, and Conventional EGD

The majority of otolaryngologists performing TNE do not attempt to visualize the entire stomach or even enter the duodenum. This begs the question of whether or not an esophagoscopy alone is sufficient for otolaryngology patients and whether a complete esophagastro-duodenoscopy (EGD) would be more appropriate. This question was addressed in a study by Wildi et al. [37] in which 175 patients underwent EGD and the findings were stratified according to their symptoms. Their study demonstrated that patients *without* daily dyspeptic symptoms, abdominal pain, nausea, or a history of gastric or duodenal ulcers were unlikely to have pathology identified in the stomach or duodenum. Therefore, isolated esophagoscopy is sufficient in routine otolaryngology patients.

TNE in Head and Neck Oncology

Panendoscopy is part of the standard evaluation of individuals with head and neck squamous cell carcinoma (HNSCCa). Often, these patients possess co-morbidities that increase the risk of general anesthesia. In-office TNE allows for an examination of the aerodigestive tract without the morbidity of anesthesia. Biopsies can also be obtained; studies have reported a very high congruence rate for biopsies using TNE compared with standard (operating room-based) panendoscopy [29].

TNE may also play a role in the follow-up of patients with treated head and neck cancer. Studies from Taiwan and North America have shown a high incidence of esophageal abnormalities after the treatment of the head and neck primary [30, 31].

Farwell et al. prospectively performed TNE on 100 patients at least 3 months after treatment for HNSCCa [32]. The findings on esophagoscopy included peptic esophagitis (63%), stricture (23%), candidiasis (9%), Barrett's (8%), gastritis (4%), and carcinoma (4%). Only 13% had a normal esophagoscopy. This work and others strongly suggest that esophageal pathology is extremely common in patients treated for head and neck cancer and that the severity of dysphagia symptoms is *not* predictive of a normal endoscopy, and the decision to perform screening esophagoscopy in this population must not be based on patient symptoms alone. These findings support routine esophageal screening after head and neck cancer treatment.

TNE-Assisted Procedures

A wide variety of procedures may be performed using TNE. These include biopsies of the laryngopharynx and esophagus, esophageal, neopharyngeal, and nasopharyngeal stricture balloon dilation, secondary tracheo-esophageal puncture [33–35], the delivery of flexible lasers, and insertion of wireless pH monitoring devices [36].

The role of TNE and evaluation of esophageal motility remains to be proven. Because the patient is awake, the pharyngeal phase of swallowing can also be evaluated for the presence or absence of aspiration and pharyngeal residue. Traditionally, endoscopic evaluation of esophageal motility has been discredited in part because of the role of sedation and its effects on motility. In the absence of the need for sedation, TNE has been used to evaluate dysphagia. This assessment may be enhanced by feeding the patient food-colored applesauce with the TNE in place with normal motility involving esophageal transit in less than 13 s. While this technique for evaluation of dysphagia remains to be validated, it is an intriguing application of TNE.

Conclusions

The safety, tolerability, and accuracy of TNE are now well established. Controlled studies have demonstrated its equivalence to CE in a variety of different measures, including its ability to offer a comprehensive examination and assessment of the esophagus. Combined with its relative cost benefits and safety profile, TNE has become an important part of the armamentarium for diagnosis and management of patients with dysphagia, extraesophageal/gastroesophageal reflux disease, and head and neck cancer.

References

1. Jackson C. The life of Chevalier Jackson: an autobiography. New York: The Macmillan; 1938. p. 229.
2. Burnett W. An evaluation of the gastroduodenal fibrescope. Gut. 1962;3:361–5.
3. Lopresti P, et al. Clinical experience with a glass-fiber gastroscope. Am J Dig Dis. 1962;7:95–101.

4. Shaker R. Unsedated trans-nasal pharyngoesophagogastroduodenoscopy (T-EGD): technique. Gastrointest Endosc. 1994;40(3):346–8.

5. Aviv JE, et al. Office-based esophagoscopy: a preliminary report. Otolaryngol Head Neck Surg. 2001;125(3):170–5.

6. Belafsky PC, et al. Transnasal esophagoscopy. Otolaryngol Head Neck Surg. 2001;125(6):588–9.

7. Kumar VV, Amin MR. Evaluation of middle and distal esophageal diverticuli with transnasal esophagoscopy. Ann Otol Rhinol Laryngol. 2005;114(4):276–8.

8. Dumortier J, et al. Unsedated transnasal EGD in daily practice: results with 1100 consecutive patients. Gastrointest Endosc. 2003;57(2):198–204.

9. Postma GN, et al. Transnasal esophagoscopy: revisited (over 700 consecutive cases). Laryngoscope. 2005;115(2):321–3.

10. Birkner B, et al. A prospective randomized comparison of unsedated ultrathin versus standard esophagogastroduodenoscopy in routine outpatient gastroenterology practice: does it work better through the nose? Endoscopy. 2003;35(8):647–51.

11. Dean R, et al. A comparative study of unsedated transnasal esophagogastroduodenoscopy and conventional EGD. Gastrointest Endosc. 1996;44(4):422–4.

12. Catanzaro A, et al. Prospective evaluation of 4-mm diameter endoscopes for esophagoscopy in sedated and unsedated patients. Gastrointest Endosc. 2003; 57(3):300–4.

13. Jobe BA, et al. Office-based unsedated small-caliber endoscopy is equivalent to conventional sedated endoscopy in screening and surveillance for Barrett's esophagus: a randomized and blinded comparison. Am J Gastroenterol. 2006;101(12):2693–703.

14. Saeian K, et al. Unsedated transnasal endoscopy accurately detects Barrett's metaplasia and dysplasia. Gastrointest Endosc. 2002;56(4):472–8.

15. Sorbi D, et al. Unsedated small-caliber esophagogastroduodenoscopy (EGD) versus conventional EGD: a comparative study. Gastroenterology. 1999;117(6):1301–7.

16. Thota PN, et al. A randomized prospective trial comparing unsedated esophagoscopy via transnasal and transoral routes using a 4-mm video endoscope with conventional endoscopy with sedation. Endoscopy. 2005;37(6):559–65.

17. Trevisani L, et al. Unsedated ultrathin upper endoscopy is better than conventional endoscopy in routine outpatient gastroenterology practice: a randomized trial. World J Gastroenterol. 2007;13(6):906–11.

18. Conio M, et al. Long-term endoscopic surveillance of patients with Barrett's esophagus. Incidence of dysplasia and adenocarcinoma: a prospective study. Am J Gastroenterol. 2003;98(9):1931–9.

19. Waring JP, et al. Guidelines for conscious sedation and monitoring during gastrointestinal endoscopy. Gastrointest Endosc. 2003;58(3):317–22.

20. Sharma VK, et al. A national study of cardiopulmonary unplanned events after GI endoscopy. Gastrointest Endosc. 2007;66(1):27–34.

21. Hart R, Classen M. Complications of diagnostic gastrointestinal endoscopy. Endoscopy. 1990;22(5):229–33.

22. Arrowsmith J, et al. Results from the American Society for Gastrointestinal Endoscopy/ US Food and Drug Administration Collaborative Study on complication rates and drug use during gastrointestinal endoscopy. Gastrointest Endosc. 1991;37:421–7.

23. Banks MR, Kumar PJ, Mulcahy HE. Pulse oximetry saturation levels during routine unsedated diagnostic upper gastrointestinal endoscopy. Scand J Gastroenterol. 2001; 36(1):105–9.

24. Zaman A, et al. A randomized trial of peroral versus transnasal unsedated endoscopy using an ultrathin videoendoscope. Gastrointest Endosc. 1999;49(3 Pt 1):279–84.

25. Garcia RT, et al. Unsedated ultrathin EGD is well accepted when compared with conventional sedated EGD: a multicenter randomized trial. Gastroenterology. 2003; 125(6):1606–12.

26. Watts TL, Shahidzadeh R, Chaudhary A, et al. Cost savings of unsedated transnasal esophagoscopy. Paper presented at: 87th Annual Meeting of the American Broncho-Esophageal Association; April 26–27, 2007; San Diego, CA.

27. Mulcahy HE, et al. A prospective controlled trial of an ultrathin versus a conventional endoscope in unsedated upper gastrointestinal endoscopy. Endoscopy. 2001; 33(4): 311–6.

28. Andrus JG, Dolan RW, Anderson TD. Transnasal esophagoscopy: a high-yield diagnostic tool. Laryngoscope. 2005;115(6):993–6.

29. Postma GN, et al. The role of transnasal esophagoscopy in head and neck oncology. Laryngoscope. 2002;112(12):2242–3.

30. Su YY, Fang FM, et al. Detection of metachronuous esophageal squamous carcinoma in patients with head and neck cancer with use of transnasal esophagoscopy. Head Neck. 2010;32(6):780–5.

31. Wang CP, Lee YC, et al. Unsedated transnasal esophagogastroduodenoscopy for the evaluation of dysphagia following treatment for previous head neck cancer. Oral Oncol. 2009;45(7):615–20.

32. Farwell DG, Rees CJ, et al. Esophageal pathology in patients after treatment for head and neck cancer. Otolaryngol Head Neck Surg. 2010;143(3):375–8.

33. Bach KK, Postma GN, Koufman JA. In-office tracheoesophageal puncture using transnasal esophagoscopy. Laryngoscope. 2003;113(1):173–6.

34. Vaghela HM, Moir AA. Hydrostatic balloon dilatation of pharyngeal stricture under local anaesthetic. J Laryngol Otol. 2006;120(1):56–8.

35. Doctor VS. In-office unsedated tracheoesophageal puncture. Curr Opin Otolaryngol Head Neck Surg. 2007;15(6):405–8.

36. Belafsky PC, et al. Wireless pH testing as an adjunct to unsedated transnasal esophagoscopy: the safety and efficacy of transnasal telemetry capsule placement. Otolaryngol Head Neck Surg. 2004;131(1):26–8.

37. Wildi SM, Glenn TF, et al. Is Esophagoscopy alone sufficient for patients with reflux symptoms? Gastrointest Endosc. 2004;59(3):349–54.

8. Manometry of the UES Including High-Resolution Manometry

Benson T. Massey

Abstract Manometry of the upper esophageal sphincter and pharynx is used for the measure of the contractile activity of these structures at rest, during deglutition, and in response to various stimuli. The anatomic asymmetry, movement, and fast responses of these structures challenge the performance characteristics of most manometric systems. The advent of solid-state high-resolution manometry addresses the limitations of earlier systems. However, currently available commercial systems continue to have limitations in performance, cost, and durability. The field is further limited by the lack of consensus in the field regarding specific definitions for manometric phenomena, as well as the absence of universally applicable and available normative data sets.

Introduction

Manometry of the upper esophageal sphincter (UES) and pharynx is a technique used to assess the anatomy and function of these structures via inferential interpretation of intraluminal pressure patterns. Clinically, the goal is to confirm normal function or detect disordered function, so as to guide clinical management. The working assumption is that the recorded pressure signatures reflect the "natural" (i.e., un-instrumented) activity of the adjacent musculature. To the extent that these assumptions are valid, intraluminal manometry is a useful technique. However, there are situations where the interplay between study conditions and manometer technical limitations renders such assumptions erroneous. The manometrist who is not cognizant of these situations is at risk to make incorrect interpretations and diagnoses.

R. Shaker et al. (eds.), *Manual of Diagnostic and Therapeutic Techniques for Disorders of Deglutition*, DOI 10.1007/978-1-4614-3779-6_8, © Springer Science+Business Media New York 2013

The indications for manometry of the pharynx and UES are as follows:

1. Locate the UES relative to other structures. Typically, in clinical practice, this is performed to locate the borders of the UES relative to the nasal sill reference point, to allow placement of other recording devices (e.g., pH sensors) at a defined location relative to the UES. However, the relative intraluminal position of the UES relative to other structures (e.g., lower esophageal sphincter, lips, and velum) can also be recorded.
2. Record the basal tonic activity of the UES during inter-deglutitive intervals.
3. Determine the completeness of inhibition of UES tone (both degree and duration) during deglutition. Determine the timing of this inhibition relative to the timing of pharyngeal contractions (or other deglutitive motor phenomena). Assess the magnitude of pharyngeal contraction and UES after-contraction during deglutition.
4. Measure the intrabolus pressure, to assess for abnormal bolus transport dynamics. A series of such measurements, over a range of bolus volumes, can allow recognition of abnormal distensibility of a structure.
5. Identify the response of the UES to sensory stimuli and changes in cortical activity.
6. Assess the effect (beneficial or adverse) of therapeutic interventions on the function of the pharynx and UES.

Challenges for Manometric Recording and Interpretation

Multiple challenges must be recognized and overcome for manometric recordings of the pharynx and UES to have acceptable fidelity and correct interpretations. Many of these challenges are not present for manometric recordings in the smooth muscle portion of the esophagus, so that assumptions used for interpretation in this distal region are not appropriate in the more proximal segment.

Unlike the tubular esophagus, the anatomy in the region of the UES and pharynx exhibits striking radial asymmetry. Depending upon the manometric sensor orientation, the wall adjacent to it has considerable variation in muscle content, including complete absence of any contractile element. There is correspondingly extreme variation in magnitude of pressures recorded around the circumference of the lumen. Striking changes in axial pressure are also present, depending upon the location of the sensor within the UES high pressure zone and the pharynx. Hence, determination of whether a recorded pressure is abnormally high or low depends upon precise knowledge about the location of that sensor. There is also functional laterality at the UES, which is composed of what can be considered a left and a right cricopharyngeus muscle, each with separate innervation. Thus, there is the potential for a unilateral defect in function.

In addition, the location of the UES is not stationary. Its position relative to a point sensor can shift with changes in neck position. Even when the neck is held stationary, the UES has an orad movement that can exceed 2 cm during deglutition [1]. This means that a point sensor positioned at the location of the maximal pressure in the UES at rest is almost certainly going to be displaced into the lower pressure region of the cervical esophagus during deglutition. The manometric signal will have the spurious appearance of UES relaxation. This displacement can last up to 1 s, which is over twice the actual duration of inhibition of the cricopharyngeus muscle on electromyography [2]. Thus, impaired relaxation of the UES following that axial movement can be missed (Fig. 8.1). While this problem can be overcome to some extent by placing a pressure sensor at the location of maximal UES orad excursion during deglutition, accurate recording remains hampered because the UES movement varies somewhat from swallow-to-swallow. Thus, without concurrent imaging from another modality, such as videofluoroscopy, one cannot reliably determine whether a single point sensor is located in the region of the UES during its movement. Accounting for UES movement during pressure recordings requires use of a perfused sleeve device or use of multiple, closed-spaced point sensors (with "e-sleeve" software incorporated into high-resolution manometric software).

Compared to the smooth muscle region of the esophagus, the UES and pharynx exhibit more rapid and extreme pressure changes. Recording these changes requires a correspondingly greater fidelity of the manometric apparatus. Pressure transients up to 600 mmHg and pressure wave velocities of up to 25 cm/s can be observed in some regions of the pharynx [3]. To achieve a 98% accuracy when recording these phenomena, the manometry system must have a flat frequency response of 48 Hz [4]. This cannot be achieved with perfused manometry systems.

The UES between swallows has a highly variable "resting" pressure that depends upon the rate of firing of its motor neurons, which are located in the nucleus ambiguus. The firing rate of these at any given

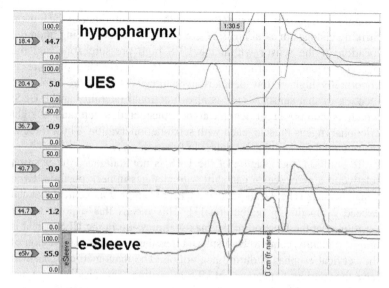

Fig. 8.1. Line tracing from a solid-state, high-resolution manometry study in a patient with impaired deglutitive UES relaxation. The transducer labeled UES is positioned at the midpoint of the UES high pressure zone at rest, with the transducer labeled hypopharynx located 2 cm proximally. Note that with deglutition, UES channel appears to record a complete UES relaxation. However, the UES moves orad to the more proximal channel, which shows impaired relaxation. The e-sleeve channel seen at the *bottom* of the figure also shows the impaired UES relaxation.

moment is influenced by input from multiple afferent sensory pathways and higher cortical centers. It is therefore impossible to determine whether a given pressure in the UES is abnormally high or low without knowledge of the ongoing external factors modifying that pressure. Basal UES pressure increases with emotional stress, speech, and crying [5–7]. This author has observed pressures in excess of 200 mmHg sustained for over a minute after aspiration-induced coughing. The stimulus of movement of the manometry catheter within the UES can cause a pressure increase, and the recorded pressure is higher with larger diameter catheters [8]. The duration of UES relaxation increases with larger swallowed bolus volumes [9].

Not all pressure phenomena in the pharynx and UES reflect the underlying motor activity of these structures. The cricopharyngeus muscles have intrinsic elastic properties and exhibit a tonic resistance to stretch [10]. Even when the muscles are paralyzed, a manometry catheter distending the lumen of the UES can record a "resting" pressure of up to

25 mmHg [11]. This is another reason for larger diameter catheters to record larger basal pressures in the UES on pull-through studies. Catheters whose cross-sectional dimensions conform more closely to the slit-like anatomy of the UES record lower pressures overall and less radial variation in the recorded pressure [12, 13].

The action of muscles extrinsic to the pharynx and UES can alter the recorded intraluminal pressure. For example, contraction of the thyrohyoid muscles (or its analog in other species) acts to pull upon the UES, and this can produce a fall in the recorded UES pressure even when the muscle itself is not relaxing [14]. Turning the head also alters the pressures recorded in the UES [15, 16].

From a fluid mechanics perspective, intraluminal pressures can be considered to exist within two pressure domains [17]. Within the first, the manometer has circumferentially contiguous contact with the wall of the lumen and no bolus lies between these structures. In this situation, the recorded "contact" pressures will be directly proportionate to the forces generated by contractile activity of the muscle in the adjacent wall. In the second, the manometer resides freely with the bolus fluid, without contacting the adjacent wall. In this situation, the recorded "intrabolus" pressures do not directly reflect the contractile activity of the muscle in the adjacent wall. Intrabolus pressure also is affected by such factors as the diameter and length of the lumen through which the bolus passes, as well as the downstream pressure in the lumen receiving the bolus.

During deglutition, most of the interval of UES relaxation overlaps the interval of UES opening and bolus flow. Hence, the manometer is largely recording an intrabolus pressure during the period of UES relaxation. For small bolus volumes, this intrabolus pressure remains relatively low, and the recorded pressure signature suggests a "complete" UES relaxation. However, with larger bolus volumes, and pathologic processes that impede bolus transit, this intrabolus pressure can become significantly elevated. The result can be an apparent abnormal UES deglutitive relaxation response in terms of absolute nadir pressure and/or duration of low pressure. This almost certainly explains the reports of abnormal deglutitive relaxation of the UES in esophageal achalasia [18, 19], a condition associated with high downstream pressures due to esophageal retention of fluid. Treatment to relieve this distension restores the UES residual pressures to normal [20].

An assumption of intraluminal manometry is that the contact and intrabolus pressures recorded are negligibly affected by the presence of the catheter. There are several conditions in which this assumption is violated sufficiently to affect the pressure recordings. As mentioned previously, the size of the manometric catheter affects the recorded UES pressure. If the lumen is sufficiently narrowed by a pathologic process, the additional luminal narrowing by the presence of the catheter is no longer negligible and considerably higher intrabolus pressures may be recorded. Manometry catheters are relatively incompressible. While manometry catheters are relatively flexible, they still must exhibit some resistance to radial deformity and almost complete resistance to axial deformity to facilitate catheter passage. These physical properties mean that if the catheter does not "hang freely" within the lumen, it is possible for forces generated at remote sites to be transmitted through the shaft of the catheter to the region of interest. In this situation, the recorded pressure does not necessarily reflect either the contact pressure or the intrabolus pressure that would have otherwise been observed at that location. For this phenomenon to occur, the movement of the catheter must be constrained at two separate points. The catheter usually has one constraint proximally, as it is secured to prevent dislodgement. There can also be transient proximal fixation during deglutition due to elevation and contraction of the velum, when the catheter is passed through the nasopharynx. Changes in the lumen angulation, diameter, and distensibility may produce a second fixation site for the catheter. This may explain why extreme neck deflection alters the pressures recorded at the UES [21].

Use of manometry for clinical inference requires some knowledge of whether or not the recorded pressures during different phenomena fall within the normal range. Unfortunately, data sets for normal values are extremely limited for the currently available manometric systems. For example, one of the largest reported data sets for normal values only included subjects under the age of 50 [22]. Yet multiple studies have indicated that pressures recorded in the region of the UES are related to age [23, 24] and most of the patients seen clinically fall outside this age range evaluated in this study. Because of differences in catheter dimensions and recording fidelity, normal values for different measured parameters may vary among systems. Different studies have used different definitions of events. For example the duration of deglutitive UES relaxation may be defined as the interval of relatively stable low pressure, the interval between when the pressure falls below and then rises above 50% of the resting pressure, and complex computationally derived intervals. Determination of the start and end points of pressure-related phenomena can be difficult, due to the inherent instability of pressure baselines. This introduces an element of subjectivity into the measurement, resulting at worst in biased readings and at best in difficulty comparing values reported in different studies. Use of defined algorithms for automated data point identification can overcome some of this subjectivity. However, the need for a human input to exclude events with artifacts from analysis again introduces some subjectivity into the process.

Adding to the above difficulties is a lack of consensus over what constitutes an abnormal value for any parameter. Given some inherent variation in recorded pressure phenomena from swallow-to-swallow, data from multiple swallows are usually recorded for each subject. For a parameter such as nadir UES pressure, this could be reported as the average value, the range of values, or the highest value. Any of these could be compared to the range of average values for each subject in the data set or the range of average values for all swallows among all subjects in the data set. Given that, by statistical definition, about 5% of values in normal subjects will fall outside the 95% of normalcy, one cannot be certain that a value in this 5% range in any particular patient represents a true pathologic state rather than the extreme end of normal variation in function. There is no agreement as to whether abnormal deglutitive UES relaxation should be defined by the presence of abnormalities on (1) any swallow, (2) all swallows, or (3) the majority of swallows. Until these issues regarding the determination of normalcy are addressed by additional investigation or consensus within authoritative bodies in the field, clinical manometry of the UES and pharynx will remain a fairly qualitative and subjective exercise.

Finally, the available manometric systems each have particular limitations in their actual operation that either introduce artifact into the pressure recordings or affect the recording conditions for the study. These will be discussed in the next section.

Performance Characteristics of Different Manometric Systems

Perfused Point Sensors

Perfused point sensors have long been used for manometric recording within the esophageal body. The catheters for these manometric systems are relatively cheap and extremely durable. This is less the case with the perfusion pump apparatus, where pressure leaks or retained air in the system seriously degrades the recording fidelity. Even at its best, a perfused point sensor does not have an adequate frequency response to record dynamic pressure phenomena in the region of the UES and pharynx. Perfused manometry systems have their pressure transducers located externally to the subject. If the sidehole from which the perfusing fluid enters the lumen is not at the level of the external transducer, there will be a hydrostatic pressure offset that will affect the baseline pressure recordings. Thus, studies need to be performed with the sideholes at the level of the external transducer or pressure readings need to be recorded relative to a pressure other than atmospheric pressure, such as intra-esophageal or intra-pharyngeal pressure. The stimulus of the water perfusate within the pharynx may activate reflex responses in the UES, alter the natural swallowing rate, and predispose certain patients to aspiration.

Point sensors can record the axial UES pressure profile at any given moment by recording pressure changes, while the sensor is pulled through the length of the sphincter high pressure zone. However, without knowing the radial orientation of the sensor, this information is relatively meaningless. Attempts at recording basal sphincter pressure changes over time by placing the sensor at the location of maximal pressure on a pull-through are going to be affected by any movement of the sphincter relative to the sensor, including those associated with head and neck movement and deglutition. The result is that spurious relaxations of the UES may be recorded. Given these limitations, the main use for single point sensors would be for locating the upper and lower borders of the UES (e.g., relative to the nares), so as to guide placement of other intraluminal sensors, such as pH probes, at fixed locations relative to the UES.

Solid-State Point Sensors

Solid-state point sensors avoid many of the limitations of perfused point sensors by having an adequate frequency response and no stimulation from perfusate. They are also easily referenced to atmospheric pressure regardless of subject position. Unidirectional point sensors still suffer from uncertain radial orientation within the lumen. This can be overcome to some extent by the use of solid-state sensors that obtain circumferentially averaged pressure information. Of course, such sensors lose any ability to provide information on the radial variation in pressure within the lumen. Solid-state point sensors are like their perfused counterpoints in being unable to record UES pressure meaningfully during its movement.

Solid-state manometric point sensors tend to be expensive and fragile. In addition, the pressures are affected by the ambient temperature. Thus, calibration of these sensors needs to be performed at body temperature or the manometric system needs to incorporate software to adjust for thermal drift in the recordings. A large problem for these sensors with prolonged recordings is a drift in the baseline that is in addition to temperature effects. The genesis of this drift is unclear, but may be related to fluid absorption in the catheter around the pressure transducer or transducer deformation by adherent debris. At any rate, in this author's experience, the resulting drift can be considerable and is not necessarily linear throughout the course of the manometric study, which makes algorithmic correction schemes suboptimal.

Perfused Sleeve Sensors

The concept of the perfused sleeve sensor is that it records the highest intraluminal pressure seen anywhere along its length. The sensor is positioned across a sphincter so that during any axial movement of the sphincter it remains adjacent to the sleeve sensor. Hence, any observed fall in pressure results from a relaxation rather than displacement of the sphincter. Perfused sleeve sensors have a unidirectional radial recording of pressure. Special sleeve sensors with flattened cross sections have been developed that allow consistent anterior–posterior orientation (the direction of maximal pressure) within the UES [25]. Sleeve sensors require point sensors at either end to identify the location of the UES high pressure zone and allow placement so that the proximal end of the sleeve remains above the location of the most orad excursion of the UES during deglutition.

The perfused sleeve is useful for tracking the "resting" pressure of the UES for prolonged periods. Its frequency response for recording sphincter relaxations, during either deglutition or in response to other stimuli, is acceptable, and the device can identify failed deglutitive relaxation of the UES. However, once the pharyngeal contraction reaches the proximal end of the sleeve, that contraction will produce the highest pressure occurring over the length of sleeve and be recorded, instead of the pressure within the UES at that point. As a consequence, the perfused sleeve tends to under-record the duration of UES relaxation.

Limitations in frequency response for recording phasic pressure increases are even worse than those for perfused point sensors. While relatively cheap, perfused sleeve sensors suffer the same risk of technical artifacts, reference pressure difficulties, and stimulation by the perfusate of perfused point sensors. An artifact unique to the perfused sleeve sensor can occur if the opening of the UES is relatively stenosed and/or doesn't relax with deglutition. In this situation, the brisk orad movement of the UES can drive fluid back up the sleeve, producing a pressure spike that gives the appearance of an exaggerated contraction of the sphincter.

Solid-State High-Resolution Manometry

Within the past decade, advances in computer processing capability, combined with development of solid-state catheters incorporating multiple closely spaced sensors, have allowed the concept of high-resolution manometry to become a practical reality for recording in the region of the pharynx and UES. The catheters have point sensors that record average pressures around the circumference of the catheter. However, multiple sensors (up to 36) are present and sufficiently closely spaced (usually 1 cm apart) that the UES is always over at least one sensor during axial movements. Hence, failure of relaxation will not be missed. An additional advantage of having so many sensors available is that concurrent recordings from the esophageal body and lower esophageal sphincter can be obtained. In this author's experience a substantial portion of patients with abnormalities in deglutitive UES function have additional manometric abnormalities identified distally [26].

Data from each sensor can be displayed as a line tracing. The close spacing of the data allows for algorithms for interpolating and displaying estimated pressures between actual sensor data, giving the appearance of continuous pressure information along the entire length of the luminal axis at any given point. This interpolated pressure data is then depicted on a computer display in "contour plots," wherein the horizontal axis depicts time, the vertical axis depicts axial distance along the lumen, and pressure information for any point on the length-time continuum is represented on a color scale (Fig. 8.2a, b). This representation of the manometric data has proven to be highly intuitive and easier for novices in the field to master. The large number of sensors available means that positioning of any one sensor relative to a structure, such as the UES, does not have to be precise. Measurements of UES location tone and relaxation are performed post-hoc. Some commercially available systems have software with an "e-sleeve" feature: what this does is take the pressure data from several adjacent sensors (typically positioned over the locations of the sphincter during rest and excursion) and display on a channel at any instant the

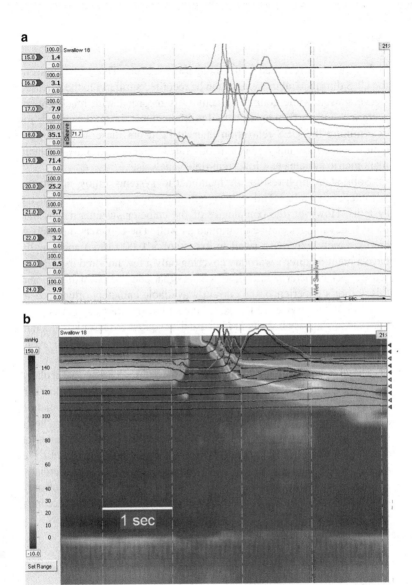

Fig. 8.2. (**a**) Solid-state high-resolution manometry of the UES and pharynx. Line tracings represent pressure records from ten adjacent circumferentially sensitive pressure transduces spaced 1 cm apart. The sensor located 19 cm from the nares is located close to the maximum basal UES pressure. During deglutitive UES relaxation, the UES is displaced proximally, giving an incorrect appearance on that channel of a relaxation in excess of 0.6 s. The e-sleeve, displaying the highest pressure seen over multiple channels, provides a more realistic inhibition of about 0.3 s. (**b**) Identical swallow to that depicted in (**a**). However, individual line tracings are superimposed over a contour plot that represents pressure on a color scale (seen at *left*) and generates interpolated data points between adjacent channels. Following UES relaxation, a pressure wave exceeding 200 mmHg moves down through the pharynx and UES.

highest pressure recorded from among these sensors. Thus, relaxations of the UES during axial movement can be recorded similarly to the perfused sleeve sensor, while contractile activity is recorded with much greater accuracy. Other computational algorithms have been developed for determining the UES relaxation interval [22], but these are somewhat complex and have not yet been incorporated into commercially available manometric systems to allow "real-time" analysis.

Solid-state high-resolution manometric systems enjoy all of the advantages that other solid-state systems have over perfusion manometry systems. However, the complexity of the catheter systems means that their disadvantages can be multiplied as well. The catheters themselves are extremely expensive (well in excess of $10,000 U.S.) and usually have a manufacturer's warranty covering only a few hundred uses. More sensors per catheter means more sensors that can fail prematurely, and this author's experience, the currently available catheters often need to be sent out for service well ahead of the end of the warranty period. For this reason, the busy manometry lab usually requires at least two catheters (ideally on about 100 prior uses apart in their duty cycles) to avoid downtime and schedule disruption.

The baseline drift during prolonged recordings can be particularly bothersome with high-resolution systems, particularly because the drift can be highly variable from channel-to-channel, throwing off the interpolation software considerably over the course of a study. Because the catheter sensors are circumferentially indiscriminate, artifacts from constraints of catheter movement (where one side of the catheter pushes against the adjacent wall) are less easily identified as such. Some commercially available manometric systems have default sampling frequencies of only about 30/s, which may be inadequate in some situations for accurate recording of pressure transients in the region of the pharynx and UES.

Manometry Combined with Other Instrumentation

Many studies have employed manometry of the UES and pharynx in concert with recordings of other phenomena. These include endoscopy/laryngoscopy, intraluminal pH/impedance, electromyography of different muscles, and videofluoroscopy. Concurrent recordings allow correlation of manometrically identified events with other phenomena, such as the timing of UES relaxation relative to vocal cord adduction, the relationship between UES relaxation and opening, and the response of the UES to gastroesophageal reflux. When isolated point sensors are used, concurrent videofluoroscopy is essential to be certain that the sensor seemingly recording deglutitive UES relaxation is actually within the sphincter at that moment. These other recording modalities are discussed elsewhere within the text.

Manometry of the UES and pharynx can also be combined with instrumentation to evoke different reflex responses. For instance, air injected into the esophageal body can elicit the UES belch response, while balloon distension in the esophageal body can provoke UES contraction. Slow infusion of water into the hypopharynx can be used to assess the threshold for reflexive swallow and associated UES responses [27].

Protocol for Performance and Interpretation of Manometry of the Pharynx and UES

The following description of the manometric examination is based upon the use of solid-state high-resolution manometry, since that is the modality that is currently provided by most equipment venders. The general principles apply to the use of other techniques, although perfusion manometry has additional requirements, such as avoiding ongoing perfusion of recording channels located in the pharynx to avoid excessive triggering of swallowing and potential aspiration. Depending upon the operation of the particular manometry lab, some components of the following protocol will be performed by the manometry nurse or technician, while other aspects will be performed by the clinician responsible for final analysis and interpretation of the manometry study.

Pre-procedure Preparation

At the start of the day's manometry lab session, the equipment should be turned on and verified to be in working order. There is nothing worse than to have the patient intubated for the procedure, only to discover that the study must then be canceled because of equipment malfunction! Calibration protocols should be performed. The manometric catheter should be documented to have undergone appropriate disinfection, cleaning, and storage since its last use. All ancillary equipment to conduct the study should be available and within easy reach during the procedure. This should include tape, topical anesthetic, decongestant spray, cotton swabs for applying the anesthetic, lubricating jelly, tissues or paper towels, soft-tipped syringes with water, emesis basin, exam gloves, and examining gown to cover the patient's clothing. The cart, chair, or table upon which the patient will be studied should be cleaned and have clean linens.

When the patient is brought into the examining room, their identity and procedure should be confirmed. Identifying data should be entered into the manometric system database and checked for accuracy. The indication for the procedure should be confirmed with the patient, as well as information about which clinicians should receive reports about the findings from the study. The patient should be queried about medication allergies; prior difficulties with epistaxis or nasal deformity; previous manometric studies and any difficulties with these; and time of last food or liquid intake. Ideally, patients will have gone at least 4 h without any substantial oral intake, other than sips of liquids for medications, to reduce the risk of gagging up their last meal during the intubation. If this is the patient's first manometry study, the procedure should be explained to the patient, with emphasis upon what the patient will experience during the study. Any remaining questions or concerns should be solicited and addressed. The patient should be assessed for their ability to position themselves appropriately on examining cart, obvious nasal deviation, their cognitive ability to follow instructions during the procedure, and overt signs of extreme anxiety about the test. The patient should be asked to place the examining gown over their clothing and to loosen or remove any restrictive clothing around the neck or face.

Intubation of the Patient

Allow the patient to sit on the exam cart. Pinch each nostril shut with a finger and have the patient sniff deeply through the other; the side with the best airflow should be selected for the initial intubation attempt. If the upper nasal passages show signs of congestion, administer a topical short-acting decongestant. Unless contra-indicated, apply a topical anesthetic to the nasal passage, using an agent such as a lidocaine gel. This author's preferred technique is to apply this with a long cotton swab, starting at the entrance to the nares and then working slowly and gently backwards with additional gel on the swab until contact is made with the back wall of the nasopharynx. The ability to slightly tap the swab against the back of the nasopharynx without a response from the patient is a good sign of adequate topical anesthesia. Advancing the swab in this

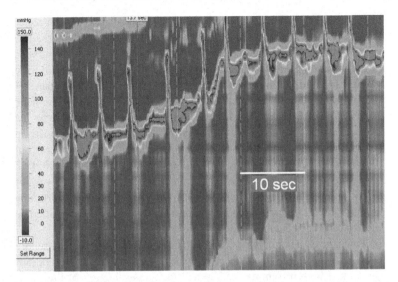

Fig. 8.3. Contour plot showing pressure data during patient intubation with a solid-state high-resolution manometry catheter. The patient is swallowing repeatedly about every 5 s. Very early in the study, the high pressure region of the UES with superimposed swallow-related pressure changes is easily identified, confirming correct intubation of the catheter tip in the esophagus. The UES pressure band moves to the *top* of the screen as the catheter is advanced into the esophagus.

way allows detection of any altered anatomy that may prevent passage of the catheter. Some practitioners prefer a brief nasal spray with a mixture of 1% lidocaine and a decongestant.

Lubricate the catheter with additional anesthetic or other gel and advance the catheter along the path previously taken by the swab. Once the catheter tip contacts the back wall of the nasopharynx, the patient should tuck the chin down as far as possible. Apply additional pressure to have the catheter tip turn and advance it about another 5–10 cm until a slight resistance indicates that the catheter is abutting the top of the UES or pyriform recess. At this point have the patient take a dry swallow while simultaneously advancing the catheter. The goal is to advance the catheter tip into the proximal esophagus during the orad excursion and relaxation of the UES. It is helpful during this process to observe the monitor, since successful passage has a characteristic appearance (Fig. 8.3).

Some patients with oropharyngeal dysphagia may have difficulty in advancing the catheter past the UES during dry swallows. For some patients, having them swallow sips of water while passing the catheter can help, but this should not be tried if the patient is already observed to be having difficulty handling their oral secretions. Another alternative, for patients who are felt to be contracting the UES during deglutition, is to try advancing the catheter between swallows, again observing the monitor for evidence of successful esophageal intubation. Some patients cover the esophageal inlet with the epiglottis despite appropriate neck flexion. The catheter tip may then deflect back into the hypopharynx. At other times the catheter tip will deflect backwards out of the pyriform recess. These situations cannot be identified during blind intubation, but their presence is suggested by repeated failed attempts at intubation. In such situations, the only reasonable recourse is to use endoscopy or videofluoroscopy to guide the catheter in the right direction. Endoscopy in this situation has an advantage because the endoscope tip can often be used to push the catheter in the proper direction.

Once the catheter tip has passed into the esophagus it should normally be advanced until the tip is identified to be in the stomach on the monitor, since most high-resolution studies will include evaluation of the lower esophageal sphincter and esophageal body. The catheter is then secured to the nose with tape, and the position of the catheter is noted on the manometry software. Depending on the height of the patient and the manometric catheter, the catheter may need to be repositioned more proximally later, to assure that an adequate number of recording channels are located in the region of the pharynx and UES. Enter any change in position on the manometry software.

Performing the Manometry Study

Before starting the data collection portion of the manometry study, give the patient a few minutes to rest and recover from the intubation experience. Often the stimulus of intubation, especially if it has been difficult, stimulates saliva production and increases the spontaneous swallow rate. Do not start the data collection until the spontaneous swallow rate falls to about once per minute. For esophageal body assessment, the patient is usually given 5 mL water swallows while recumbent. These can also be used for assessing UES relaxation and pharyngeal contraction. For more complete and reliable analysis of the UES and pharynx, have the patient take several dry swallows as well while recumbent, then have them change to a sitting position, and repeat the 5 mL water and dry swallows. Changing positions is important because some subjects become anxious while trying recumbent swallows or position their necks at extremes of flexion or extension; these may alter the manometric appearance of the swallow. The addition of dry swallows is important, especially in patients with cervical dysphagia for solids, because some patients are found to have abnormal UES relaxation with dry swallows while relaxation with wet swallows remains relatively unaffected [28]. During the study, make note of when the subject is talking, moving, crying, or otherwise visibly agitated, as these will affect the pressure seen in the UES between swallows.

Manometric Data Scoring and Interpretation

The following parameters are usually scored and interpreted from the manometric data obtained at the pharynx and UES: (1) location of top of UES, (2) length of UES, (3) basal UES pressure, (4) percent of wet and dry swallows showing UES relaxation response, (5) nadir pressure during UES relaxation, (6) duration of UES relaxation, (7) amplitude of pharyngeal contraction, and (8) coordination of UES relaxation with pharyngeal contraction. Additional parameters that could be assessed include propagation velocity of the pharyngeal pressure wave, and intrabolus pressure within the pharynx and UES (although this latter makes assumptions about whether the pressure at a given point is actually intrabolus, unless the manometry is performed concurrently with videofluoroscopy or impedance).

The location of the top of the UES relative to the nares depends on the subject's body habitus. The length of the UES can vary somewhat during the course of the study and can vary with the level of UES activation also. Typical values are in the range of 2–4 cm. The clinical meaning of higher or lower values is uncertain. Equally uncertain is the meaning of "resting" UES pressure, given its extreme variability from minute to minute. A major limitation of most commercial manometric analysis software is that it forces a recording of "baseline" UES pressure right at the start of the study, at a time when most patients may still be agitated by the intubation process. Almost invariably, towards the end of the study, when the patient is acclimated to the presence of the catheter and routine of the study, lower pressures are observed. Given these considerations, my practice is to position the e-sleeve over the UES high pressure zone and take several readings throughout the length of the study, trying to score periods as far from swallows, coughs, gags, talking, and movement as possible and recording values at end expiration. I then report these as a range, rather than a mean, since this conveys the (usually great) range of variability in the basal UES pressure so recorded. The upper range is usually <100–150 mmHg when recorded in this fashion. Values higher than this, when seen only early in the study, likely reflect intolerance of the study by the subject and are discounted. The clinical significance when pressures are elevated above the usual range during periods without obvious provocative stimulation is uncertain. Some patients with persistently elevated pressures above 150 mmHg or transient elevations in excess of 300–500 mmHg in this author's experience have been found to have myotonic or myopathic changes upon direct EMG recordings of the cricopharyngeus muscles. These elevated pressures may be a marker for underlying pathology, rather than a cause for symptoms; however, sensitivity and specificity of such elevated pressures for any disorder is completely unknown.

Analysis of UES pressure changes during deglutition requires the use of either an e-sleeve or a careful determination of which pressure sensor is adjacent to the UES when it completes its orad movement. While it is possible to score pressure changes at the sensor located closest to the midpoint of the UES high pressure zone at rest, this sensor is almost invariably recording from the esophageal body during most of the swallow. As discussed previously, the apparent interval of UES inhibition from this sensor (usually 0.6–1.0 s) is almost twice the duration of UES deglutitive inhibition detected on EMG recordings from the cricopharyngeus muscles [2], and is actually the interval of the deglutitive excursion of the UES. Using the e-sleeve, nadir pressures at the UES during dry and 5 mL water swallows are usually below 10–15 mmHg. Determination of the duration of UES deglutitive inhibition in clinical practice currently requires a somewhat subjective assessment of the times of onset and offset of this inhibition. Using the e-sleeve, typical values for such inhibition durations are 200–400 ms for dry swallows and 300–500 ms for 5 mL water swallows. The clinical implications of a subject having a minority of swallows with parameters outside these ranges are unclear. It should be remembered that not all elevated deglutitive residual pressures reflect abnormal UES relaxation. The causes for elevated residual pressures are listed in Table 8.1.

Deglutition related contraction pressures in the hypopharynx are typically in excess of 200 mmHg on high-resolution solid-state manometry. Pressures <100 mmHg raise the possibility of pharyngeal weakness, although the lack of circumferential discrimination of the

Table 8.1. Causes for elevated deglutitive nadir UES pressure.

Impaired deglutitive UES relaxation
Impaired anterior traction on the UES
Reduced distensibility of the pharyngoesophageal segment
Elevated downstream pressure in the esophageal lumen
Unrecognized swallow of a larger or more viscous bolus
Extreme angulation of neck during swallow
Calibration drift in baseline pressure

transducers makes it impossible to determine whether the abnormality is unilateral or bilateral. Hypopharyngeal contractions with onset either before the start or after the termination of the period of UES inhibition indicated some disruption in the coordination of muscle contractions at the level of the central pattern generator for swallowing.

As stated previously, when using manometry alone, identifying a pressure as being from the intrabolus region is somewhat presumptive. In the region of the UES and pharynx this is usually identified clinically as a lower amplitude pressure "ramp" preceding the major upstroke of the post-deglutitive contraction of the pharynx and UES. In this region, for 5 mL water swallows, the value is usually <10–15 mmHg [9, 22]. Higher values indicate abnormal downstream resistance to bolus flow. Dramatic increases in intrabolus pressure with larger bolus volumes indicate impaired distensibility of the pharyngoesophageal segment, as can be seen with cricopharyngeal bars [29] and Zenker's diverticula [30].

Conclusions

Manometric assessment of the pharynx and UES remains a challenging procedure to perform and interpret properly. It requires a detailed understanding of normal and disordered anatomy and physiology of the structures involved. The manometrist must remain aware of the limitations of the manometric apparatus being used and how its presence affects the function of the structures being studied. With these caveats in mind, manometry remains a useful, but not sufficient, tool for assessing some aspects of the structure and physiology of the pharynx and UES and aids in the diagnosis of disorders affecting these structures.

References

1. Kahrilas PJ, Dodds WJ, Dent J, Logemann JA, Shaker R. Upper esophageal sphincter function during deglutition. Gastroenterology. 1988;95(1):52–62.
2. Ertekin C, Aydogdu I. Electromyography of human cricopharyngeal muscle of the upper esophageal sphincter. Muscle Nerve. 2002;26:729–39.
3. Dodds WJ, Hogan WJ, Lydon SB, Stewart ET, Stef JJ, Arndorfer RC. Quantitation of pharyngeal motor function in normal human subjects. J Appl Physiol. 1975; 39(4):692–6.
4. Orlowski J, Dodds WJ, Linehan JH, Dent J, Hogan WJ, Arndorfer RC. Requirements for accurate manometric recording of pharyngeal and esophageal peristaltic pressure waves. Invest Radiol. 1982;17(6):567–72.
5. Cook IJ, Dent J, Collins SM. Upper esophageal sphincter tone and reactivity to stress in patients with a history of globus sensation. Dig Dis Sci. 1989;34(5):672–6.
6. Omari T, Snel A, Barnett C, Davidson G, Haslam R, Dent J. Measurement of upper esophageal sphincter tone and relaxation during swallowing in premature infants. Am J Physiol. 1999;277(4 Pt 1):G862–6.
7. Cook IJ, Dent J, Shannon S, Collins SM. Measurement of upper esophageal sphincter pressure. Effect of acute emotional stress. Gastroenterology. 1987;93(3):526–32.
8. Lydon SB, Dodds WJ, Hogan WJ, Arndorfer RC. The effect of manometric assembly diameter on intraluminal esophageal pressure recording. Am J Dig Dis. 1975; 20(10):968–70.
9. Cook IJ, Dodds WJ, Dantas RO, et al. Opening mechanisms of the human upper esophageal sphincter. Am J Physiol. 1989;257(5 Pt 1):G748–59.
10. Medda BK, Lang IM, Dodds WJ, et al. Correlation of electrical and contractile activities of the cricopharyngeus muscle in the cat. Am J Physiol. 1997;273(2 Pt 1):G470–9.
11. de Leon A, Thörn SE, Wattwil M. High-resolution solid-state manometry of the upper and lower esophageal sphincters during anesthesia induction: a comparison between obese and non-obese patients. Anesth Analg. 2010;111(1):149–53.
12. Dire C, Shi G, Manka M, Kahrilas PJ. Manometric characteristics of the upper esophageal sphincter recorded with a microsleeve. Am J Gastroenterol. 2001; 96(5):1383–9.
13. Bardan E, Kern M, Torrico S, Arndorfer RC, Massey BT, Shaker R. Radial asymmetry of the upper oesophageal sphincter pressure profile: fact or artefact. Neurogastroenterol Motil. 2006;18(6):418–24.
14. Asoh R, Goyal RK. Manometry and electromyography of the upper esophageal sphincter in the opossum. Gastroenterology. 1978;74(3):514–20.
15. Logemann JA, Kahrilas PJ, Kobara M, Vakil N. The benefit of head rotation on pharyngoesophageal dysphagia. Arch Phys Med Rehabil. 1989;70(10):767–71.
16. Takasaki K, Umeki H, Kumagami H, Takahashi H. Influence of head rotation on upper esophageal sphincter pressure evaluated by high-resolution manometry system. Otolaryngol Head Neck Surg. 2010;142(2):214–7.
17. Brasseur JG, Dodds WJ. Interpretation of intraluminal manometric measurements in terms of swallowing mechanics. Dysphagia. 1991;6(2):100–19.

18. Dudnick RS, Castell JA, Castell DO. Abnormal upper esophageal sphincter function in achalasia. Am J Gastroenterol. 1992;87(12):1712–5.

19. DeVault KR. Incomplete upper esophageal sphincter relaxation: association with achalasia but not other esophageal motility disorders. Dysphagia. 1997;12(3):157–60.

20. Yoneyama F, Miyachi M, Nimura Y. Manometric findings of the upper esophageal sphincter in esophageal achalasia. World J Surg. 1998;22(10):1043–6.

21. Castell JA, Castell DO, Schultz AR, Georgeson S. Effect of head position on the dynamics of the upper esophageal sphincter and pharynx. Dysphagia. 1993;8(1):1–6.

22. Ghosh SK, Pandolfino JE, Zhang Q, Jarosz A, Kahrilas PJ. Deglutitive upper esophageal sphincter relaxation: a study of 75 volunteer subjects using solid-state high-resolution manometry. Am J Physiol Gastrointest Liver Physiol. 2006;291(3):525–31.

23. Shaker R, Ren J, Podvrsan B, et al. Effect of aging and bolus variables on pharyngeal and upper esophageal sphincter motor function. Am J Physiol. 1993;264(3 Pt 1): G427–32.

24. van Herwaarden MA, Katz PO, Gideon RM, et al. Are manometric parameters of the upper esophageal sphincter and pharynx affected by age and gender? Dysphagia. 2003;18(3):211–7.

25. Kahrilas PJ, Dent J, Dodds WJ, Hogan WJ, Arndorfer RC. A method for continuous monitoring of upper esophageal sphincter pressure. Dig Dis Sci. 1987;32(2):121–8.

26. Knuff DA, Hogan WJ, Shaker R, Massey BT. Esophageal motor disturbances are common in patients with UES dysfunction. Dysphagia. 2006;21:314.

27. Dua K, Surapaneni SN, Kuribayashi S, Hafeezullah M, Shaker R. Protective role of aerodigestive reflexes against aspiration: study on subjects with impaired and preserved reflexes. Gastroenterology. 2011;140(7):1927–33.

28. Knuff DA, Kounev VJ, Lawal A, Hogan WJ, Shaker R, Massey BT. Abnormal UES deglutitive function is improved with water swallows compared to that seen with dry swallows. Dysphagia. 2006;21:297.

29. Dantas RO, Cook IJ, Dodds WJ, Kern MK, Lang IM, Brasseur JG. Biomechanics of cricopharyngeal bars. Gastroenterology. 1990;99(5):1269–74.

30. Cook IJ, Gabb M, Panagopoulos V, et al. Pharyngeal (Zenker's) diverticulum is a disorder of upper esophageal sphincter opening. Gastroenterology. 1992;103(4): 1229–35.

9. Manometric Assessment of the Esophagus

Jeffrey L. Conklin

Abstract   The methods for manometric evaluation of esophageal motor function have become much more sophisticated in the last decade. The advent of high-resolution manometry allows us for the first time to view esophageal motor function as a complete spatial and temporal continuum from the pharynx to the stomach. It makes the study more comfortable for the patient, more easily and reliably done by the nurse or technician, and more easily interpreted by the clinician. This chapter provides an introduction to high-resolution manometry, identifies what manometry measures, explains manometry equipment and describes how esophageal manometry is done. It reveals the color topographic patterns seen with normal and abnormal esophageal motor function.

Introduction

The manometric methods for recording, displaying, and analyzing esophageal motor function grew rapidly in the last decade. Rudimentary manometry equipment was first developed in the nineteenth century, but the first reliable, high fidelity manometry systems were pioneered by Dodds and Arndorfer in the mid-1970s [1]. These systems consisted of side-hole catheters perfused by a low-compliance pneumo-hydraulic pump. Manometry could be used to study esophageal motor function in the clinical setting for the first time. Shortly thereafter, catheters with solid-state sensors were introduced. Both types of catheter measured pressure at five to eight points along their length, with 3–5 cm intervals between sensing sites. These configurations left large gaps in recorded pressure data giving an incomplete view of esophageal motor function. This was the state-of-the-art until the early 1990s when Clouse and Staiano gave birth to high-resolution manometry, which dramatically

R. Shaker et al. (eds.), *Manual of Diagnostic and Therapeutic Techniques for Disorders of Deglutition*, DOI 10.1007/978-1-4614-3779-6_9,
© Springer Science+Business Media New York 2013

increased the number of sensors along the catheter and shortened the interval between sensors to 1 cm [2, 3]. They used computer algorithms to interpolate pressures between recording sites, and plot the pressure data as pressure contour or topographic plots. Esophageal motor function could be viewed, for the first time, as a complete spatial and temporal continuum from the pharynx to the stomach. This display of high-resolution pressure data, initially called high-resolution manometry, has recently been named high-resolution pressure topography (HRPT).

What Processes Does Esophageal Manometry Elucidate?

The esophagus and its sphincters transport what is swallowed from the pharynx to the stomach, guard against the reflux of damaging gastric contents into the esophagus and airways, and clear the esophagus, should reflux occur. Successful completion of these functions depends upon the integration of complex neuromuscular processes in the central nervous system, myenteric plexus, and muscular components of the esophagus. Esophageal manometry allows clinicians to observe the functional outcomes of these neuromuscular processes when normal or disordered. In many cases, the diagnosis of specific esophageal motor abnormalities can be made.

The esophagus is a roughly 20 cm long muscular tube that is closed at its upper and lower ends by sphincters. The upper esophageal sphincter (UES) partitions the pharynx from the esophagus, and is seen manometrically as a zone of high pressure at the cephalad extent of the esophagus. Its muscular components include the cricopharyngeus muscle, portions of the inferior constrictors, and the proximal esophagus [4]. These are striated muscles that are controlled by the CNS. It is an unusual sphincter because its anterior aspect is the cricoid cartilage, which is not deformable, and its posterior component is primarily the cricopharyngeus muscle, which inserts laterally on the cricoid. This gives the UES a slit-like appearance at rest, when the cricopharyngeus is tonically contracted. This configuration produces an asymmetrical pressure profile, with pressures recorded laterally being lower than anterior and posterior pressures. This means that pressures measured by directional pressure sensors, like the water-perfused side-hole catheters, vary as a function of the sensors radial orientation within the sphincter.

As pharyngeal peristalsis approaches, the UES opens to allow bolus passage into the esophagus. Opening of the UES results from traction on the cricoid cartilage by contraction of the infrahyoid and suprahyoid muscles elevating the hyolaryngeal complex, relaxation of the cricopharyngeus and pressure within the swallowed bolus. Sphincter closure coincides with arrival of the pharyngeal peristaltic pressure wave. This complex neuromuscular process is seen manometrically as a rapid drop in UES pressure to approximate intraesophageal pressure followed by an increase in pressure that overshoots resting UES pressure, and a gradual return to resting pressure.

The body of the esophagus is comprised of inner circular and outer longitudinal muscle layers named according to the orientation of their muscle cells. The top 5 % of the esophagus is striated muscle that has a somatic innervation [5]. Peristalsis here results from patterned activation of brainstem neurons that sequentially innervate the striated esophageal musculature. The musculature of the middle 35–40 % is a mixture of striated and smooth muscle known as the transition zone. The bottom 50–60 % of the esophagus is smooth muscle. Sandwiched between the muscle layers is a flat plexus of neurons called the myenteric plexus. It gets neural inputs from the CNS, and supplies the smooth muscle with its terminal motor innervation [6]. Peristalsis in the smooth muscle esophagus is controlled by complicated interactions of the CNS, myenteric plexus, and smooth muscle [7, 8]. Even with these striking regional differences in neuromuscular control mechanisms, the esophagus normally moves a swallowed bolus along its length without interruption. Esophageal peristalsis is a ring of circular muscle contraction that begins with arrival of pharyngeal peristalsis at the UES, and propagates down the esophagus to the esophagogastric junction (EGJ). Esophageal peristalsis is seen manometrically as a wave of increased pressure that sweeps along the esophagus (Figs. 9.1 and 9.2). The amplitude of peristalsis normally decreases along the transition zone and increases once again in the smooth muscle segment. A small, simultaneous rise in intraluminal pressure typically precedes the peristaltic pressure wave. It is pressure in the bolus that is being propelled along the esophagus. The esophagus also shortens by 2.0–2.5 cm in response to swallowing. This shortening results from contraction of the longitudinal musculature. Esophageal shortening, and restoration of the original length at the end of peristalsis are frequently observed with HRPT.

The lower esophageal sphincter (LES) is a specialized muscle at the EGJ, which is composed of two muscular components: the "clasp" and "sling" fibers [9]. The clasp fibers are circularly oriented smooth muscle

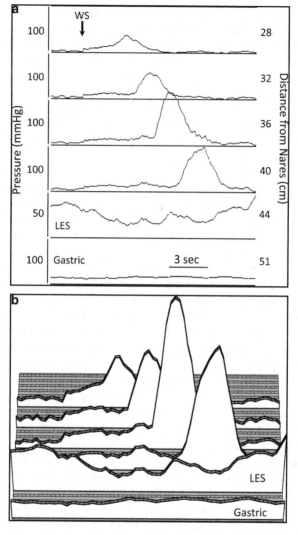

Fig. 9.1. Conversion from low-resolution manometry to high-resolution pressure topography (HRPT). Conventional, low-resolution manometry systems record pressures from sensors that are spaced at relatively long intervals, usually 3–5 cm. This recording (**a**) was acquired by a high-resolution manometry system, but is displayed in the line mode and from only 6 of 36 sensors to mimic a conventional manometry recording. Pressure data are presented as line plots stacked one on top of another, giving a 2-dimensional display. The data can be presented in a 3-dimensional space by stacking the pressure tracings from front to back instead of one on top of the other (**b**). Adding pressure data from all 36 sensors allows simultaneous recording from the pharynx to proximal stomach, and gives much more spatially detailed information about esophageal motor function

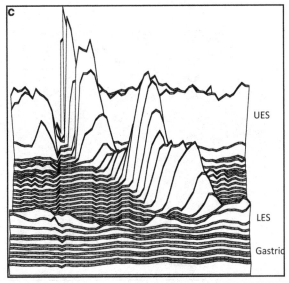

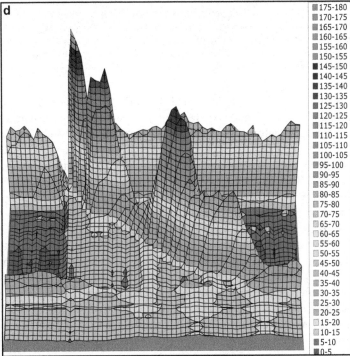

Fig. 9.1. (continued) (**c**). In fact, this image begins to have the appearance of a landscape with mountains, valleys, and plains. Colors can be assigned to different pressures (**d**). If (**d**) is rotated or tilted forward so we look down upon it, the 3-dimensional image is collapsed into the 2-dimensional HRPT.

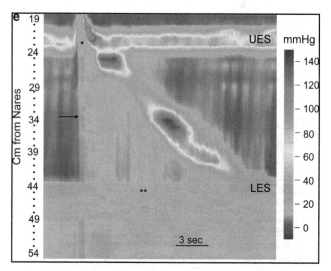

Fig. 9.1. (continued) (**e**). The color bar on the *right* indicates the relationship of color to pressure, and probe location relative to the nares is on the *right*. The *single asterisk* indicates opening of the UES and the *double asterisk* opening of the LES. Pressure in the bolus as it is pushed along the esophagus is indicated by the *lighter blue* color pointed out by the *arrow*.

cells that form a semicircle around the anterior, posterior, and lesser curvature aspects of the EGJ. The sling is a long band of smooth muscle that runs obliquely on the anterior stomach, curves around the EGJ adjacent to the gastric greater curve and ends on the posterior stomach. Esophageal manometry identifies a 2–4 cm wide zone of higher pressure at the EGJ (Figs. 9.2 and 9.3). Resting pressure at the EGJ is a composite of contraction generated by the clasp and sling fibers, and the diaphragm, which normally flanks the LES. The component of resting pressure at the EGJ contributed by the LES depends upon tonic contraction of the sphincter muscles. This results from cellular properties intrinsic to the sphincter muscle and activity of its excitatory and inhibitory innervations [7, 10, 11]. Pressure contributed by the diaphragm is seen as a cyclical rise and fall of pressure produced by diaphragmatic contraction and relaxation during respiration [12, 13] (Fig. 9.3). Because these structures are not symmetrically arranged around the EGJ, the LES pressure profile is not symmetrical. The recorded pressure depends to some extent upon the type of catheter used: circumferential sensors average the pressure around the entire pressure profile, while point sensors give the pressure over a small arc of the pressure profile.

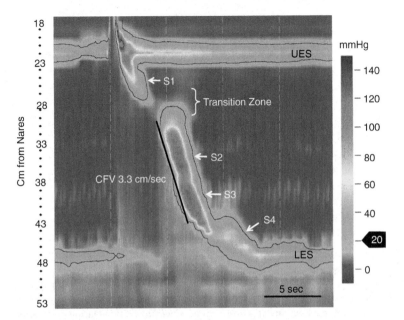

Fig. 9.2. HRPT of normal pharyngeal, esophageal, and LES motor function. The HRPT extends from the pharynx (18–20 cm) to the stomach (49–53 cm). Esophageal peristalsis is composed of four overlapping contractile segments (S1–S4). S1 is generated by contraction of the striated muscle esophagus. Peristalsis in the smooth muscle esophagus is represented by S2 and S3. S4 is the LES contracting at the end of peristalsis and descending to its resting position at the level of the crural diaphragm. The *black line* outlining some parts of the image is the 20 mmHg isobaric contour line. It can be used to estimate the velocity of peristalsis in the smooth muscle esophagus, the contractile front velocity (CFV). The CFV is the slope of a line connecting the 20 mmHg isobaric contour line at the proximal and distal extents of the smooth muscle esophagus, S2 and S3.

Shortly after swallowing is initiated the tonically contracted LES relaxes. Vagal efferent neurons in the dorsal motor nucleus of the vagus are activated with swallowing [14, 15]. They terminate on myenteric neurons that in turn innervate the LES. Nitric oxide made in inhibitory myenteric neurons activates cellular processes in the LES muscle that cause its relaxation [16, 17]. This is recorded manometrically as a 5–10 s drop in LES pressure (Figs. 9.1, 9.2, and 9.5). The sphincter remains relaxed until the peristaltic contraction arrives. With arrival of the peristaltic pressure wave the LES contracts vigorously and then settles back to its resting pressure.

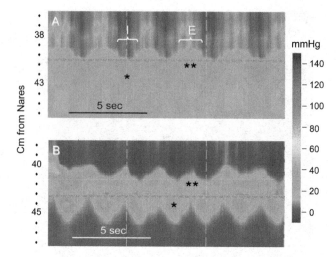

Fig. 9.3. The esophagogastric junction at rest. Pressures produced at the normal EGJ are shown in (**a**). Under normal circumstances, pressure at the EGJ is a composite of tonic LES contraction (*double asterisk*) and cyclical crural diaphragm contraction with inspiration (*single asterisk*). During inspiration (I) pressure decreases in the thoracic cavity, and during expiration (E) it increases. The opposite is true in the abdominal cavity. The point at which pressure across the EGJ during inspiration becomes negative relative to intraabdominal pressure is called the respiratory or pressure inversion point (PIP). The location of the PIP is the location of the *dashed line*, and it indicates the level of the diaphragm. Spatial separation of the diaphragm from the LES (**b**) indicates the presence of a hiatal hernia. This hernia is small.

Manometry Equipment

In the last decade manometric techniques have made monumental strides. The advent of HRPT allowed a much more spatially detailed view of esophageal motor function. All manometry setups consist of two hardware components. The first are pressure sensors/transducers, which sense pressure within the esophageal lumen and convert it to an electrical signal. This component may be a water-perfused, side-hole catheter coupled to volume-displacement transducers, or solid-state pressure sensing devices [18]. Perfused systems use a polyvinyl catheter with channels running along its length. Each channel ends in a small lateral opening facing out at a different level equidistant from its neighbor. This allows pressure to be measured simultaneously at regular intervals along the catheter. A low-compliance pneumo-hydraulic pump slowly injects bubble-free water into the channels. Volume-displacement transducers convert pressure in each channel to an electrical signal. The recorded pressure rises when contraction of the esophageal wall impedes the flow of water through the side-hole. Generally, the amplitude and timing of pressure increases reflect the force and timing of the circular muscle contraction. Factors other than the force of contraction may influence pressure measurements and fidelity of pressure recording. These include compliance of the recording system, diameter of the side-hole, and the perfusion rate [18, 19]. Artifacts may also occur if debris blocks the side-hole or perfusion channel, or if there are air bubbles in the tubing. Water-perfused manometry catheters have the great advantages of being inexpensive and very durable. A major disadvantage is that their frequency-response characteristics are slow, so that they do not faithfully record contractile events in striated muscle structures. In addition, the geometry of these catheters makes accurate recording of pressures in concentrically asymmetrical structures unreliable. The best example of this is the UES, which has a slit-like shape. This means that pressures recorded by a directional sensor like a side-hole will be higher in the anterior–posterior axis of the UES than laterally.

The other commonly used sensing device is a linear array of solid-state pressure transducers spaced at regular intervals along a catheter. These sensors are better able to record motor activity in the pharynx and UES because their faster frequency-response characteristics more faithfully record the rapid striated muscular events in these regions. Many of the confounding factors that may confuse the data obtained with the perfused catheter are not encountered with solid-state devices. They are also less cumbersome to use and require less technical expertise. These devices have the disadvantages of being more fragile and more expensive.

Both water-perfused and solid-state high-resolution manometry catheters are commercially available. They have from 22 to 36 sensors spaced at intervals of as little as 1 cm along the catheter length.

The second component of any manometry system is a recording device that can amplify, store, and display those electrical signals. Today this is typically a computer equipped with analogue to digital converters and software that allows the analysis of pressure data and its display on a video monitor.

Indications for Esophageal Manometry

The indications for esophageal manometry are relatively limited. Its primary indication is in the evaluation of dysphagia not caused by pathological processes like esophagitis, esophageal ulcers or strictures, and esophageal cancers that are elucidated by endoscopy and/or radiological studies. Manometry can also be used to evaluate atypical or noncardiac chest pain, but only after cardiac disease, the esophageal disorders listed above, musculoskeletal pain syndromes and anxiety disorders have been excluded. Primary disorders of esophageal motor dysfunction that are unambiguously associated with chest pain, like achalasia and esophageal spasm, are uncommon. Nevertheless, esophageal manometry remains the standard method for diagnosing achalasia, because it is more sensitive than radiographic studies for this purpose. Hypertensive peristalsis, also known as nutcracker esophagus, is also associated with chest pain and dysphagia, but its relationship to symptoms is less clear. Esophageal manometry is often used, as well, to determine involvement of the esophagus by collagen vascular diseases or generalized GI motor disorders.

Esophageal manometry is the most precise method to identify the upper border of the LES for accurate pH probe placement [20]. It is relatively widely used prior to Nissen fundoplication and bariatric surgery, particularly when the patient complains of esophageal symptoms. The surgical approach may be modified or abandoned when peristalsis in the smooth muscle esophagus is weak or absent. HRPT in particular has found utility in the evaluation of chest pain or dysphagia following surgical antireflux and bariatric procedures. It easily identifies incomplete LES relaxation, elevated intrabolus pressures (IBPs), and/or peristaltic dysfunction when the fundoplication or Lap band is too tight. It also identifies abnormal pressurization of the gastric pouch and occasional disordered motor function in the jejunal limb of a gastric bypass. HRPT is also invaluable in the evaluation of patients who remain symptomatic after Heller myotomy: it easily identifies an incomplete myotomy.

Performance of Esophageal Manometry

Patient Preparation

The patient should not eat or drink for at least 6 h prior to the procedure, and even longer if achalasia is expected. The exception to this is the taking of medications need for the patient's well-being. In general, they should avoid medications that influence esophageal motor function, including caffeine, calcium channel blockers, phosphodiesterase inhibitors, organic nitrates, prokinetic agents, loperimide, opiate antagonists or agonists, adrenergic antagonists and agonists, and anticholinergic agents like tricyclic antidepressants. Again, exception must be made for medications required for patient well-being. Using sedation to ease the intubation process should be avoided if at all possible. If the catheter is placed at the time of endoscopy, it is best to use a very short acting agent like propofol alone for sedation. If sedation is used it must be included as part of the manometry report. Local anesthesia with intranasal 2 % viscous lidocaine helps the patient tolerate the procedure, but is not universally used. It can be introduced by squirting the viscous lidocaine into the nares and having the patient sniff, or with the gel on a cotton swab that is placed in the nasopharynx. Its use should also be documented. HRPT has made the use of swallow and respiration detectors a thing of the past.

Equipment Preparation

As with any procedure in which the GI tract is intubated great pains must be taken to assure that the catheter and other equipment have been cleaned and maintained according to instructions of the manufacturer and local infection control agencies. The recording equipment should be calibrated according to manufacturer's instruction prior to probe placement. The catheter type and configuration should be documented in the manometry report.

Performance of the Procedure

The use of high-resolution manometry systems has greatly simplified and shortened the duration of esophageal manometry testing. Detailed descriptions of how esophageal manometry should be performed with older and increasingly less used low-resolution manometry catheters and systems are described in detail elsewhere [21] and will not be covered here.

These days the manometry catheter is almost universally passed after local anesthesia to the nasopharynx. The catheter is then passed into the nasopharynx and down the esophagus. Having the patient sip and swallow water during the intubation process facilitates catheter placement: as long as the patient is swallowing they cannot gag. Most high-resolution manometry catheters have a sensing segment long enough to span from the pharynx to the stomach (Figs. 9.1 and 9.2). This makes it quite easy for the operator to position the catheter so that it simultaneously records pressure for the pharynx, UES, esophagus, LES, and proximal stomach. High-pressure zones produced by the UES and LES, and cyclical pressure changes produced by diaphragmatic contraction and relaxation are easily identified (Figs. 9.1 and 9.2). Once in position, the catheter does not have to be moved to complete the study, as in the older "pull-through" method. After the catheter is positioned the patient is placed supine or at most sitting up 30°. When a water-perfused catheter is used, it is important to keep the patient supine with the external pressure transducers positioned at the same level as the mid-thorax. This is to avoid artifactual pressures generated in a column of water.

After the catheter is placed and the patient positioned, some time should be allowed for the patient to accommodate to the catheter. Repetitive or involuntary swallowing and gagging, which are frequent at the beginning of the study, usually resolve as accommodation occurs. High resting UES pressure and high amplitude contraction of the striated muscle of the esophagus are often seen at the beginning of the study. They are not a pathological process, but a response to irritation by the catheter. Both diminish as the patient accommodates to the catheter. Once the patient is comfortable, they are asked not to swallow for 30 s so baseline UES and LES resting pressures can be measured. Next water swallows are given to evaluate the motor functions of the UES, esophagus, and LES. Swallows of 3–5 cc given at intervals of no less than 20–30 s are used for this purpose. This timing gives the relaxed LES time to recover its resting pressure, and avoids deglutitive inhibition; that is, swallow induced inhibition of a first peristaltic contraction by a second swallow occurring during propagation of the first swallow. When doing impedance manometry or standard high-resolution manometry it is possible to "challenge" the esophagus with a viscous bolus. The viscous bolus material is commercially available or may be approximated by applesauce. This approach can be useful in patients with dysphagia who have a normal manometry with wet swallow because it uncovers esophageal motor dysfunction not identified with liquid swallows [22, 23]. After evaluating esophageal motor function, the high-resolution manometry catheter can be pulled back and positioned to assess pharyngeal motor function [24, 25]. Having the patient say ka-ka-ka locates where velopharyngeal closure occurs, partitioning the nasopharynx from the mesopharynx. Water swallows can then be used to observe pharyngeal peristalsis and UES opening. The high spatial and temporal fidelity of modern HRM catheters makes reliable assessment of pharyngeal motor function possible for the first time.

Principles of High-Resolution Pressure Topography

The advent of HRPT has truly changed the way we think about the evaluation of esophageal motor function. This came about largely due to two technological developments. First, the miniaturization of solid-state pressure sensors allowed the incorporation of many closely spaced sensors along the length of the catheter. These catheters have as many as 36 pressure sensors spaced at 1 cm intervals along the catheter length, yielding a 35 cm sensing segment This increases the spatial resolution of esophageal manometry dramatically, by allowing simultaneous recording of pressure at short intervals from the pharynx to proximal stomach. The second breakthrough was the development of sophisticated computer algorithms that convert all of this pressure information into pressure topography plots that depict pressures as colors, with each pressure being assigned a unique color. Pressure is interpolated between sensors to display a continuous high-resolution color topography plot that allows us to view esophageal motor events as a spatial-temporal continuum. Almost everyone is familiar with this type of presentation in the form of color weather radar, which expresses intensity of rain as color variation. HRPT also allows us for the first time to see normal and abnormal motor function as patterns. What normal esophageal motor function looks like with HRPT and how we translate from low-resolution line plots of pressure to the topographic color contour are depicted in Fig. 9.1.

In many instances, abnormalities of esophageal motor function can be recognized as a particular pattern seen in the high-resolution color topography plot [25–27]. Once these patterns are learned detailed numerical analysis of the HRPT is often not needed to make the diagnosis. A number of new analytical tools and techniques are being developed to quantify the large amount of data found in the HRPT, and to standardize its use. The most detailed of these methods is called the Chicago Classification [28]. It is an algorithmic scheme for diagnosing esophageal motor abnormalities. It is still an evolving method.

Evaluation of the LES and Esophagogastric Junction

HRPT simplifies evaluation of the structural and functional characteristics at the EGJ. Some of the methodology for evaluating esophageal function presented here utilizes the Chicago Classification as it existed when this document was written. There are likely to be some future modifications as the classification system is still evolving. After the catheter is properly positioned across the EGJ, the station pull-through maneuver is not needed to characterize the resting properties of the EGJ. The high-pressure zone encountered at the EGJ is a composite of pressures generated by the LES and crural diaphragm (CD) [12, 13, 29, 30]. During respiratory expiration the CD relaxes so that EGJ pressure is primarily, but not exclusively, that of the resting LES [31]. With inspiration the CD contracts and the EGJ pressure becomes a composite of CD and LES contraction. This is easily seen in the HRPT as a cyclical variation in pressure at the EGJ (Fig. 9.3). Because diaphragmatic and LES contraction are distinguishable, the spatial relationship of one to the other can be discerned. It becomes a relatively easy task to identify and quantify hiatal hernias. When no hernia is present the pressure profiles of the LES and diaphragm are coincident. With a hiatal hernia their pressure profiles diverge: LES pressure is shifted cephalad to the diaphragm (Figs. 9.3 and 9.4). Identifying what is called the respiratory or pressure inversion point (PIP) facilitates sizing of hiatal hernias [25, 26, 32]. During inspiration, pressure drops in the chest and increases in the abdomen. The PIP is the location at or near the EGJ where this switch occurs, indicating a change in location from the abdominal cavity to the thoracic cavity. It approximates the location of the diaphragm. The morphology of the EGJ has been subclassified into three subtypes based upon its pressure profile. Type I is normal with no separation of the LES (Fig. 9.3a) and CD, type II has a separation of ≤2 cm (Fig. 9.2b), and type III (Fig. 9.4) has a separation of >2 cm. Type III is further subdivided into type IIIa, in which the PIP is just above the CD, and type IIIb, in which it is above the LES [32].

One of the primary purposes of esophageal manometry is to evaluate adequacy of swallow-induced LES relaxation. Unfortunately, no consensus was ever reached on how this should be done with conventional manometry. This is probably because several confounding factors complicate the task. Foremost among these is the significant esophageal shortening that accompanies swallowing [33, 34]. As shortening occurs, the point-like pressure sensor on a conventional manometry catheter may drop out of the high-pressure zone into the stomach. This artifact mimics LES relaxation.

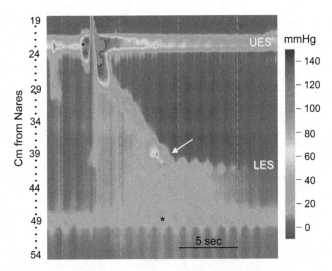

Fig. 9.4. Large hiatal hernia. Here we see a 7–8 cm hiatal hernia. Diaphragmatic contraction is indicated by the *asterisk* and is positioned 49 cm from the nares. The LES is in the range of 40 cm from the incisors. It is relatively common to see the LES location only for a short period after arrival of the peristaltic wave. Notice that arrival of the peristaltic pressure wave at the EGJ is seen in the color contour as an obtuse angle (*arrow*). This is a useful way to identify a profoundly hypotensive LES.

Close spacing of pressure sensors along the HRM catheter makes it easy to identify and track LES location, even when significant esophageal shortening occurs. The other major artifact making accurate measurement of relaxed LES pressure difficult is diaphragmatic contraction during LES relaxation. Two software algorithms have been devised to obviate these confounders and evaluate adequacy of LES relaxation. The routinely reported measure of LES relaxation is the residual pressure. Both algorithms determine pressure within the relaxation window, a window that straddles the high-pressure zone and stretches from opening of the UES to arrival of the peristaltic contraction at the LES (Fig. 9.5). The first is the 3-s nadir (3SN), which finds the continuous 3-s interval during LES relaxation that has the lowest mean pressure relative to intragastric pressure. The second is called the 4 s integrated relaxation pressure (IRP) [35]. It is the lowest average pressure over four continuous or discontinuous seconds within the relaxation window. The IRP is probably a marginally better measure than 3SN because it is influenced less by diaphragmatic contraction if the subject is breathing rapidly. An IRP of less than 15 mmHg is used as normal because it is the best value for differentiating achalasia from normal or other esophageal disorders [35].

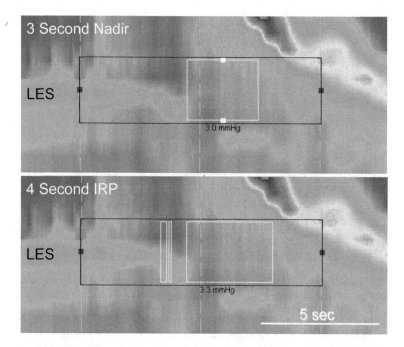

Fig. 9.5. Measurement of residual LES pressure. Two software algorithms are used to determine the adequacy of LES relaxation. Both determine pressure within the deglutitive relaxation window, a window that straddles the high-pressure zone and stretches from opening of the UES to restoration of the LES to its resting position (*black boxes*). This is the spatial and temporal domain within which LES relaxation is evaluated. The eSleeve™ is used to set the spatial extent of the window, 6 cm by default. This assures that esophageal shortening does not take the LES out of the measurement window. The first algorithm is the 3-s nadir (3SN). It identifies the continuous 3-s interval during LES relaxation that has the lowest mean pressure relative to intragastric pressure (*white box*). The second is called the 4 s integrated relaxation pressure (IRP). It is the lowest average pressure over four continuous or discontinuous seconds within the relaxation window (*white boxes*).

Evaluation of Esophageal Body Function

Esophageal peristalsis is seen in the HRPT as an overlapping series of contractions in segments termed S1–S4 along the length of the esophagus (Fig. 9.2) [2, 36]. The first contractile segment (S1) passes from the lower border of the UES to a pressure trough at about the level of the aortic arch called the transition zone. S1 corresponds functionally with peristaltic contraction of the striated muscle esophagus. The smooth muscle esophagus is divided into S2 and S3. The last segment (S4) is a region over which the peristaltic pressure wave slows. The genesis of S4 is complex. During peristalsis longitudinal muscle contraction shortens the esophagus, essentially producing a physiological hiatal hernia. It remains shortened as the peristaltic pressure wave arrives in the distal esophagus, producing the radiographic phrenic ampulla. S4 is contraction of the LES at the end of peristalsis, emptying of the phrenic ampulla and restoration of the LES to its resting position near the crural diaphragm [37].

One of the great advantages of HPRT is that it allows determination of isobaric contours (Figs. 9.2, 9.6, and 9.7). An isobaric contour that defines 20 or 30 mmHg can be used to determine the velocity of peristalsis in the smooth muscle esophagus. Thirty mmHg was initially chosen because it is the pressure that reliably differentiates IBP from luminal closure pressure, thereby delineating luminal closure by the peristaltic contraction [38]. It is also the peristaltic pressure that predicts bolus clearance [39].

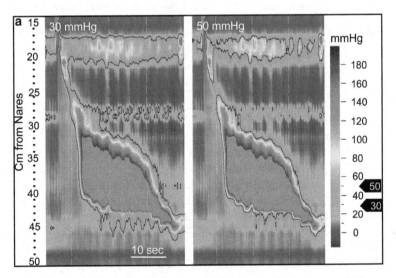

Fig. 9.6. Isobaric contours can be used to distinguish esophageal spasm (**a**) from an elevated intrabolus pressure caused by pressurization of the bolus ahead of the peristaltic contraction against some outlet obstruction (**b**). In (**a**) 30 and 50 mmHg isobaric contour lines are applied to a rapidly propagating contraction that is indicative of esophageal spasm, CFV of 8.3 cm s^{-1}. In this case, the 30 and 50 mmHg isobaric contour lines at the wave front are parallel indicating that the CFV will be calculated as close to the same in both cases. In (**b**) 30 and 50 mmHg

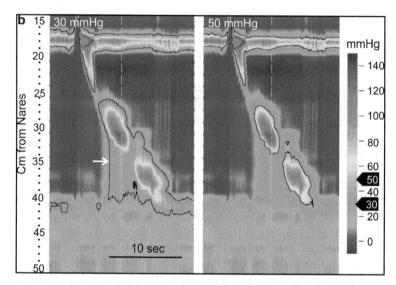

Fig. 9.6. (continued) isobaric contour lines are applied to a peristaltic contraction pressurizing the bolus ahead of it. The straight vertical portion of the 30 mmHg contour line (*arrow*) delimits a high intrabolus pressure. Note that pressures in the bolus are isobaric. Using the 30 mmHg isocontour will give an artifactually rapid CFV. In this case, adjusting the isobaric contour line to 50 mmHg gives the true CFV.

The velocity of peristalsis in the smooth muscle esophagus can be determined by calculating the slope of a line connecting the 20 or 30 mmHg contour line at the cephalad extent of S2 to the 20 or 30 mmHg contour at the distal extent of S3. This is called the contractile front velocity (CFV). The upper limit of normal, defined as the 95th percentile of the mean in normal individuals, is 4.5 cm/s [40]. Spastic contraction is defined as a CFV >8.0 cm/s, essentially simultaneous contraction (Fig. 9.6).

The IBP is a rise in pressure in the region between the advancing peristaltic contraction and the EGJ (Figs. 9.1e and 9.6b). Small increases in IBP are routinely seen with normal esophageal motor function. IBPs greater than 15 mmHg are considered abnormal, and are usually a sign of esophageal outlet obstruction. An elevated IBP with preserved peristalsis may be caused by a fundoplication, peptic stricture, eosinophilic esophagitis, or early achalasia. The validity of CFV breaks down as a measure of wave front velocity when the pressure inside the bolus being propelled down the esophagus is greater than 30 mmHg (Fig. 9.6). In this situation, the CFV is artificially rapid because it is calculated from the leading edge of the IBP. Recognizing the pattern of

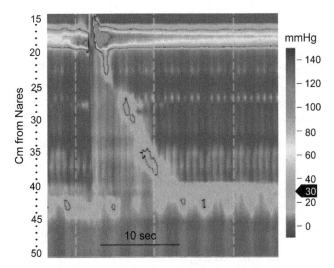

Fig. 9.7. Using isobaric contour lines to identify hypotensive or failed peristalsis. In this panel 30 mmHg isobaric contour lines are applied to the peristaltic sequence. There are gaps in the contour lines where pressure is below 30 mmHg. A gap of >3 cm in the 30 mmHg contour indicates hypotensive peristalsis.

elevated IBP, or increasing the magnitude of the isobaric contour line, 50 mmHg has been suggested, can compensate for the artifact.

Historically a peristaltic pressure below 30 mmHg was used to define ineffective hypotensive peristalsis because below this pressure bolus transit does not reliably occur [39]. Isobaric contour lines can be used to evaluate the integrity of peristalsis in the smooth muscle esophagus (Fig. 9.7). Hypotensive peristalsis is defined as peristaltic pressure wave with no pressure above 30 mmHg or a ≥3 cm gap in the 30 mmHg isobaric contour. Bolus transit is also impaired when there is a 2 cm gap in the 20 mmHg contour [40].

The intensity of smooth muscle contraction is evaluated with a software algorithm that calculates the *distal contractile integral* (DCI). It is the integral of pressure, duration, and length of contraction in the smooth muscle esophagus, segments S2 and S3 [27, 41]. It is expressed as mmHg s^{-1} cm^{-1}. Peristaltic sequences with a DCI of >5,000 mmHg s^{-1} cm^{-1} are considered abnormal and are termed hypertensive peristalsis [27, 41]. This is akin to what was called nutcracker esophagus from conventional manometry. The hypertensive segment may involve S2, S3, or both. Hypertensive contraction, >180 mmHg, isolated to the LES may also occur when the peristaltic pressure wave reaches the LES.

Table 9.1. Classification of individual smooth muscle esophageal responses to wet swallows by high-resolution pressure topography.

Normal (Fig. 9.2)
  <3 cm defect in the 30 mmHg isobaric contour distal to the TZ, CFV
  <8 cm^{-1}, IBP <15 mmHg, and DCI <5,000 mmHg s^{-1} cm^{-1}
Hypotensive peristalsis (Fig. 9.7)
  Normal CFV with >3 cm defect in the 30 mmHg isobaric contour of the
  wavefront distal to the TZ
Absent peristalsis
  No propagating contractile wavefront and minimal (<3 cm) contractile
  activity, or esophageal pressurization
Hypertensive peristalsis
  Normal CFV with a DCI >5,000 mmHg s^{-1} cm^{-1}
Spasm (Fig. 9.6a)
  Rapidly propagated (CFV >8 cm s^{-1})
Elevated intrabolus pressure (Fig. 9.6b)
  IBP >15 mmHg compartmentalized between the EGJ and the peristaltic
  wavefront
Panesophageal pressurization (Fig. 9.8)
  No peristaltic pressure wave with esophageal pressurization from the UES to
  the EGJ of >30 mmHg IBP

Transition zone (TZ); contractile front velocity (CFV); distal contractile integral (DCI);
intrabolus pressure (IBP); upper esophageal sphincter (UES).
Modified from Pandolfino et al. [28]. The most recent iteration of the Cicago
classification was recently published [43].

These tools are used in the new Chicago classification of smooth muscle esophageal motor disorders (Tables 9.1 and 9.2) [28]. In Table 9.1 are the tools used to evaluate single peristaltic sequences and in Table 9.2 the clinical diagnoses arising from these descriptions. While this classification system appears detailed and somewhat cumbersome, it remains a work in progress and is likely to change as more correlations between the HRPT and pathological processes are observed. In fact, a great deal of diagnostic information can be gleaned by recognizing the topographical patterns of normal and disordered esophageal function without using any numerical evaluation [26].

Pharyngeal and UES Motor Function

HRPT allows reliable manometric evaluation of pharyngeal and UES motor function for the first time (Fig. 9.8a) [24]. At the end of the study the catheter can be drawn back so that pressures are recorded from the nasopharynx to the upper esophagus. Typically the catheter is positioned

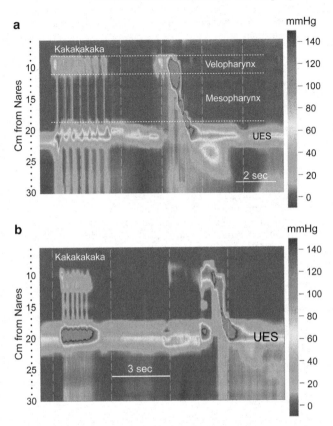

Fig. 9.8. Pharyngeal motor function. The pharyngeal response to vocalization and swallowing is seen in (**a**). Saying "kakakaka" produces velopharyngeal contraction that partitions the nasopharynx from the mesopharynx. With swallowing velopharyngeal contraction occurs just before the UES opens. Then pharyngeal peristalsis sweeps very rapidly to the UES. Pharyngeal pressure approximates that of the upper esophagus while the UES is open during pharyngeal peristalsis. This pressure is pharyngeal intrabolus pressure. When pharyngeal intrabolus pressure is elevated it suggests functional obstruction at the pharyngoesophageal junction (**b**). In this case the cause was an obstructing cricopharyngeal bar.

so that the distal sensor is 40 cm from the nares. Vocalization by saying kakakakaka identifies the location and function of the velopharynx, where the velum closes against the posterior pharyngeal wall, and the mesopharynx, the pharynx between the velopharynx and UES. With a swallow, there is velopharyngeal closure followed very shortly by UES opening and then mesopharyngeal peristalsis. Normally, pressure in

Table 9.2. Motility disorders of the smooth muscle esophagus according to The Chicago classification.

Disorders with normal EGJ relaxation (mean IRP <15 mmHg) and normal IBP
Absent peristalsis
    100 % wet swallows with absent peristalsis
Hypotensive peristalsis (Fig. 9.7)
    More than 30 % of swallows with hypotensive or absent peristalsis
Hypertensive peristalsis
    Normal CFV, mean DCI >5,000 and <8,000 mmHg s^{-1} cm^{-1} or LES after
    contraction >180 mmHg
Spastic nutcracker
    Normal CFV, mean DCI >8,000 mmHg s^{-1} cm^{-1}
Distal esophageal spasm
    CFV >8 cm s^{-1} with >20 % of wet swallows
        Segmental spasm limited to S2 or S3
        Diffuse spasm involving both S2 and S3 (Fig. 9.6a)
Disorders with impaired EGJ relaxation (IRP >15 mmHg) and/or elevated IBP
(mean >15 mmHg)
Achalasia (Fig. 9.9)
    All types have mean IRP >15 mmHg and absent peristalsis
        Type I—little or no panesophageal pressurization
        Type II—panesophageal pressurization
        Type III—esophageal spasm
Functional EGJ obstruction (Fig. 9.6b)
    Normal CFV, max-IBP >15 mmHg with >30 % of swallows
    compartmentalized
    Between the peristaltic wave and the EGJ

Transition zone (TZ); contractile front velocity (CFV); distal contractile integral (DCI); intrabolus pressure (IBP); integrated relaxation pressure (IRP); esophagogastric junction (EGJ).

Modified from Pandolfino et al. [28]. The most current iteration of the Chicago classification was recently published [43].

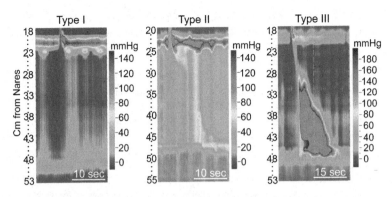

Fig. 9.9. Subclassification of achalasia. Classically achalasia is defined as failed or compromised LES relaxation and failure of peristalsis in the smooth muscle esophagus. Achalasia is now classified as three types, all of which have failed or compromised LES relaxation [42]. Type I is characterized by little or no pressure activity in the esophagus. This type is associated with more esophageal dilatation and only a modest response to therapy, with myotomy being the most successful. Type II has panesophageal pressurization, and is responsive to any of the standard therapies. Type III has spastic esophageal contractions, and is poorly responsive to therapy.

mesopharynx, pharyngeal IBP, approximates that of the proximal esophagus while the UES is open. If pharyngeal IBP is elevated it suggests obstruction at the pharyngoesophageal junction [25, 26]. This is typically seen with an obstructing cricopharyngeal bar (Fig. 9.8b). Weak or failed mesopharyngeal peristalsis suggests a neuromuscular disease. We are only at the beginning of our understanding of the pharyngeal HRPT. More detailed analytical tools will be developed for this region in the future.

References

1. Steff JJ, Dodds WJ, Hogan WJ, Linehan JH, Stewart ET. Intraluminal esophageal manometry: an analysis of variables affecting recording fidelity of peristaltic pressures. Gastroenterology. 1974;67:221–30.
2. Clouse R, Staiano A. Topography of the esophageal peristaltic pressure wave. Am J Physiol. 1991;261:G677–84.
3. Clouse R, Staiano A. Topography of normal and high-amplitude esophageal peristalsis. Am J Physiol. 1993;265:G1098–107.
4. Kahrilas PJ, Dodds WJ, Dent J, Logemann JA, Shaker R. Upper esophageal sphincter function during deglutition. Gastroenterology. 1988;95:52–62.

5. Roman C. Nervous control of esophageal peristalsis. J Physiol. 1966;58:79–108.

6. Christensen J, Robison BA. Anatomy of the myenteric plexus of the opossum esophagus. Gastroenterology. 1982;83:1033–42.

7. Conklin JL, Christensen J. Motor functions of the esophagus. In: Johnson LR, Christensen J, Alpers D, Jacobsen ED, Walsh J, editors. Physiology of the gastrointestinal tract (Chapter 4). 3rd ed. New York: Raven Press; 1994. p. 33–40.

8. Doty RW. Neural organization of deglutition. In: Code CF, editor. Handbook of physiology, section 6. Alimentary canal, vol. 4. Washington: American Physiological Society; 1968. p. 1861–902.

9. Lieberman-Meffert D, Allgower M, Schmid P, Blum AL. Muscular equivalent of the lower esophageal sphincter. Gastroenterology. 1979;76:31–8.

10. Goyal RK, Rattan S. Genesis of basal sphincter pressure: effect of tetrodotoxin on lower esophageal sphincter pressure in opossum in vivo. Gastroenterology. 1976;71:62–77.

11. Holloway RH, Blank EL, Takashashi I, Dodds WJ, Dent J, Sarna SK. Electrical control activity of the lower esophageal sphincter in unanesthetized opossums. Am J Physiol. 1987;252:G511–21.

12. Mittal RK, Rochester DF, McCallum RW. Sphincteric action of the diaphragm during a relaxed lower esophageal sphincter in humans. Am J Physiol. 1989;256:G139–44.

13. Boyle JT, Altschuler SM, Nixon TE, Tuchman DN, Pack AI, Cohen S. Role of the diaphragm in the genesis of lower esophageal sphincter pressure in the cat. Gastroenterology. 1985;88:723–30.

14. Rossiter CD, Norman WP, Jain M, Hornby PJ, Benjamin S, Gillis RA. Control of the lower esophageal sphincter pressure by two sites in the dorsal motor nucleus of the vagus. Am J Physiol. 1990;256:G899–906.

15. Paterson WG, Anderson MA, Anand N. Pharmacological characterization of lower esophageal sphincter relaxation induced by swallowing, vagal efferent nerve stimulation, and esophageal distension. Can J Physiol Pharmacol. 1992;70:1011–5.

16. Murray J, Du C, Ledlow A, Bates JN, Conklin JL. Nitric oxide: mediator of nonadrenergic noncholinergic responses of opossum esophageal muscle. Am J Physiol. 1991;261:G401–6.

17. Tøttrup A, Svane D, Forman A. Nitric oxide mediating NANC inhibition in opossum lower esophageal sphincter. Am J Physiol. 1991;260:G385–9.

18. Arndorfer RC, Steff JJ, Dodds WJ, Linehan JH, Hogan WJ. Improved infusion system for intraluminal esophageal manometry. Gastroenterology. 1977;73:23–7.

19. Dodds WJ, Steff JJ, Hogan WJ. Factors determining pressure measurement accuracy by intraluminal esophageal manometry. Gastroenterology. 1976;70:117–20.

20. Marples MJ, Mughal M, Bancewicz J. Can an esophageal pH electrode be accurately positioned without manometry? In: Siewert JR, Holscher AH, editors. Diseases of the esophagus. New York: Springer; 1987. p. 789–91.

21. Murray JA, Clouse RE, Conklin JL. Components of the standard oesophageal manometry. Neurogastroenterol Motil. 2003;15:591–606.

22. Blonski W, Hila A, Jain V, Freeman J, Vela M, Castell DO. Impedance manometry with viscous test solution increases detection of esophageal function defects compared to liquid swallows. Scand J Gastroenterol. 2007;42:917–22.

23. Basseri B, Pimentel M, Shaye OA, Low K, Soffer EE, Conklin JL. Apple sauce improves detection of esophageal motor dysfunction during high-resolution manometry evaluation of dysphagia. Dig Dis Sci. 2010;56:1723–8.

24. Takasaki K, Umeki H, Enatsu K, Tanaka F, Sakihama N, Kumagami H, Takahashi H. Investigation of pharyngeal swallowing function using high-resolution manometry. Laryngoscope. 2008;118:1729–32.

25. Fox MR, Bredenoord AJ. Oesophageal high-resolution manometry: moving from research into clinical practice. Gut. 2008;57:405–23.

26. Conklin JL, Pimentel M, Soffer EE. A color atlas of high-resolution manometry. New York: Springer Science and Business Media, LLC; 2009.

27. Pandolfino JE, Ghosh SK, Rice J, Clarke JO, Kwiatek MA, Kahrilas PJ. Classifying esophageal motility by pressure topography characteristics: a study of 400 patients and 75 controls. Am J Gastroenterol. 2008;103:27–37.

28. Pandolfino JE, Fox MR, Bredenoord AJ, Kahrilas PJ. High-resolution manometry in clinical practice: utilizing pressure topography to classify oesophageal motility abnormalities. Neurogastroenterol Motil. 2009;21:796–806.

29. Mittal RK, Rochester DF, McCallum RW. Effect of the diaphragmatic contraction on lower oesophageal sphincter pressure in man. Gut. 1987;28:1564–15648.

30. Mittal RK. The crural diaphragm, an external lower esophageal sphincter: a definitive study. Gastroenterology. 1993;105:1565–7.

31. Klein WA, Parkman HP, Dempsey DT, Fisher RS. Sphincterlike thoracoabdominal high pressure zone after esophagogastrectomy. Gastroenterology. 1993;105:1362–9.

32. Pandolfino JE, Kim H, Ghosh SK, Clarke JO, Zhang Q, Kahrilas PJ. High-resolution manometry of the OGJ: an analysis of crural diaphragm function in GORD. Am J Gastroenterol. 2007;102:1056–63.

33. Dodds WJ, Stewart ET, Hodges D, Zboralske FF. Movement of the feline esophagus associated with respiration and peristalsis. J Clin Invest. 1973;52:1–13.

34. Edmundowicz SA, Clouse RE. Shortening of the esophagus in response to swallowing. Am J Physiol. 1991;260:G512–5166.

35. Ghosh SK, Pandolfino JE, Rice J, Clarke JO, Kwiatek M, Kahrilas PJ. Impaired deglutitive OGJ relaxation in clinical esophageal manometry: a quantitative analysis of 400 patients and 75 controls. Am J Physiol. 2007;293:G878–85.

36. Clouse RE, Staiano A, Alrakawi A, et al. Application of topographical methods to clinical esophageal manometry. Am J Gastroenterol. 2000;95:2720–30.

37. Pandolfino JE, Leslie E, Luger D, Mitchell B, Kwiatek MA, Kahrilas PJ. The contractile deceleration point: an important physiologic landmark on oesophageal pressure topography. Neurogastroenterol Motil. 2010;22:395–400.

38. Massey BT, Dodds WJ, Hogan WJ, Brasseur JG, Helm JF. Abnormal esophageal motility. An analysis of concurrent radiographic and manometric findings. Gastroenterology. 1991;101:344–54.

39. Kahrilas PJ, Dodds WJ, Hogan WJ. Effect of peristaltic dysfunction on esophageal volume clearance. Gastroenterology. 1988;94:73–80.

40. Bulsiewicz WJ, Kahrilas PJ, Kwiatek MA, Ghosh SK, Meek A, Pandolfino JE. Esophageal pressure topography criteria indicative of incomplete bolus clearance: a

study using high-resolution impedance manometry. Am J Gastroenterol. 2011; 104(11):2721–8.

41. Ghosh SK, Pandolfino JE, Zhang Q, Jarosz A, Shah N, Kahrilas PJ. Quantifying esophageal peristalsis with high-resolution manometry: a study of 75 asymptomatic volunteers. Am J Physiol. 2006;290:G988–97.

42. Pandolfino JE, Kwiatek MA, Nealis T, Bulsiewicz W, Post J, Kahrilas PJ. Achalasia: a new clinically relevant classification by high-resolution manometry. Gastroenterology. 2008;135:1526–33.

43. Bredenoord AJ. Fox M. Kahrilas PJ. Pandolfino JE. Schwizer W. Smout AJ. International High Resolution Manometry Working Group. Chicago classification of esophageal motility disorders defined in high-resolution esophageal pressure topography. Neurogastroenterol Motil. 2012;24(Suppl 1):57–65.

10. Esophageal pH and Impedance Monitoring

Eytan Bardan

Abstract　Gastro Esophageal Reflux Disease (GERD) is most common and affects a significant part of the population. It is a multifactorial condition, with a wide clinical expression. Heartburn is the most common symptom, but other complaints such as acid regurgitation, dysphagia, and also atypical complaints: coughs, asthma and laryngitis can be caused by this pathology. Several diagnostic tests, including clinical trials, imaging techniques, endoscopies, esophageal manometry and reflux evaluation, are available. All of them have advantages and disadvantages. Several treatments are available for this disease, a lifestyle modification, medical, as well as surgical therapies. Wise use, proper question, knowing the limitations of various methods will help accurate diagnosis and optimal treatment matching.

Gastroesophageal reflux disease (GERD) is one of the most common diseases in the general population; it affects the patients' health and could significantly impair the quality of life.

Allison introduced the term "reflux esophagitis" in 1946 [1], directing the reflux of gastric content into the esophagus. With greater understanding of the GERD, clinicians noticed that the spectrum of the disease is wide, and many patients did not have anatomic or pathologic evidence of esophagitis. Other diagnostic modalities as well as different clinical approaches were needed.

In this chapter we will review the different aspects of GERD, including pathogenesis, clinical, diagnostic tools, and treatments options.

R. Shaker et al. (eds.), *Manual of Diagnostic and Therapeutic Techniques for Disorders of Deglutition*, DOI 10.1007/978-1-4614-3779-6_10, © Springer Science+Business Media New York 2013

Definition of GERD

Gastroesophageal Reflux (GER) is a common physiological phenomenon in which gastric content goes back up into the esophagus. It occurs multiple times, mainly after meals without producing any symptoms. When GER either causes esophageal macroscopic damage or affects quality of life, it becomes a disease—GERD.

The Montreal consensus, emanated from a panel of world experts, defined GERD as "a condition which develops when the reflux of stomach contents causes troublesome symptoms and/or complications" [2]. Symptoms are considered troublesome if heartburn episodes occur at least twice a week, but many times we cannot use arbitrary cutoffs for frequency or duration of the symptoms. If they adversely affect an individual's well-being, and regularly interferes with the patient's normal daily activities, it is troublesome.

Epidemiology

GERD is a common condition, which has been increasing in Western countries over the past 30 years [3]. In Gallup population based study, 44% of the responders reported of heartburn at least once a month [4]. In Olmsted County, Minnesota, the prevalence of heartburn was 42% within the past year, 20% reported of weekly GERD symptoms, although only 5.4% looked for medical assistance [5]. Combined data of 31 articles with a total number of 77,671 subjects, reports of 25% of people having heartburn at least once a month, 12% at least once per week, and 5% had daily symptoms [6]. GERD has different geographical distribution with lower prevalence in East Asian population, with 11% describing monthly episodes of heartburn, 4% weekly, and 2% daily [7].

Pathogenesis

Equilibrium between defensive factors, protecting the esophagus (lower esophageal sphincter, diaphragmatic crura, intra-abdominal segment of the esophagus, the phrenoesophageal ligaments, the angle of His, gravity, esophageal clearance, and tissue resistance), as opposed to the pro-reflux factors (intra-abdominal and intra-gastric pressure, negative esophageal pressure during inspiration) prevent GER. Failure of the anti-barrier factors could result in movements of gastric contents into the esophagus.

Some gastroesophageal refluxes are asymptomatic and considered physiological. However, several factors may predispose patients to pathologic reflux, including Transient LES Relaxation (TLESRs) which is consider to be the predominant mechanism by which gastric contents can back up into the esophagus [8, 9] hiatus hernia [10, 11], lower esophageal sphincter hypotension, loss of esophageal peristaltic function, obesity [11, 12], and delayed gastric emptying. Often multiple risk factors are present.

The lower esophageal sphincter is a segment of smooth muscle in the distal esophagus that tonically contracts so that the pressure in this area is at least 15 mmHg above intragastric pressure [13]. The sphincter relaxes in response to esophageal peristalsis to allow the passage of the swallowed bolus into the stomach. There are brief periods when the sphincter relaxes without preceding swallow or peristalsis. These events are termed transient lower esophageal sphincter relaxations (TLESRs). Physiological TLESRs appears mainly after eating, and are thought to be mediated via the vagovagal reflex pathway in response to the activation of stretch receptors in the stomach [14–16]. Most of these events are not associated with a significant acid reflux [17]. If reflux occurs, esophageal peristalsis and saliva will return the pH to normal. Increased number LESRs, excessive gastric refluxate volume, together with ineffective esophageal clearance, may result with pathological reflux events, causing symptoms and esophageal mucosa damage, erosions, and ulcers.

Other factors that increase the risk for pathological reflux include large hiatal hernia which decreases the pressure zone between the esophagus and the stomach [18–20], obesity [21], and smoking [22]. Alcohol [23], coffee [24], and fatty foods [25] have pharmacological effects that reduce the tone of the LES, predisposing the esophagus for reflux.

Clinical Manifestations

Reflux clinical manifestations could be divided into two groups; typical or classic esophageal symptoms, and atypical or extraesophageal symptoms (Fig. 10.1).

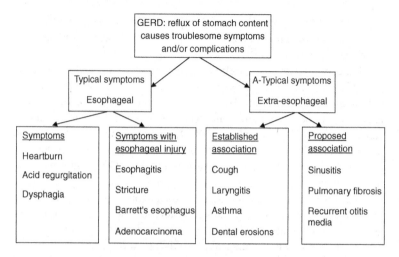

Fig. 10.1. Clinical manifestation pof GERD.

Heartburn is the classic symptom of GERD. A burning sensation rising up from the stomach into the chest, sometimes radiate toward the throat and the back [26]. Heartburn could be stimulated by large meal, certain foods (citrus, spicy and fatty foods, chocolates, alcohol). Reflux may impair sleep [27]. Sleep deprivation, no matter what causes it, may lower the threshold for symptom perception [28–30], and aggravates the patient's complaining. The frequency and severity of heartburn do not predict the severity of esophageal damage [31]. Acid regurgitation, which occurs mainly after meals, and dysphagia are also classic reflux symptoms. Dysphagia is reported by 30% of patients with GERD [32]. Other less common typical symptoms includes water brush, odynophagia, burping, hiccups, nausea, and vomiting [33]. Some patients, particularly elderly, are asymptomatic. They could present with esophagitis, stricture, or Barrett's esophagus.

Atypical, extraesophageal manifestation of GERD could be presented separately, or in combination with typical symptoms. The association between reflux and some of them is well established, and in others, the association is only proposed (Fig. 10.1). Noncardiac chest pain, asthma, posterior laryngitis, hoarseness, chronic cough and frequent throat cleaning, recurrent pneumonitis, sinusitis, recurrent otitis media, globus sensation, and dental erosions, could be attributed to GERD [34].

Diagnosis of GERD

Typical symptoms of GERD, heartburn or acid regurgitation are usually sufficient and specific for the diagnosis of reflux disease, and many times additional diagnostic tests are not practical and unnecessary [35–37]. However, in some cases the clinician has to establish the diagnosis of GERD. There are large numbers of diagnostic tests, and the clinician must tailor the appropriate test for each case. Empiric therapy is usually the first line of management, if the clinical presentation is compatible with uncomplicated GERD. Further testing is required when empiric trail with acid suppressing medications fails, when complication or other etiologies for the patient's symptoms are suspected. The important differential diagnosis includes coronary artery disease, gallbladder disease, gastric or esophageal malignancies, peptic ulcer disease, eosinophilic esophagitis, esophageal motility disorders, infectious and caustic esophagitis.

Several diagnostic tests are available:

> Empiric acid suppression test
> Endoscopy (including biopsies)
> Capsule endoscopy
> Barium esophagogram
> Esophageal manometry
> Esophageal pH monitoring
> Impedance (and pH) monitoring

Empiric Trial: Proton Pump Inhibitor Test

Empiric acid suppression is a simple, practical method for diagnosing GERD. Gastric refluxate is mainly acidic, so if symptoms respond to anti reflux therapy, the patient is likely to have GERD. The response to acid suppression favors a cause and effect relationship between the symptoms and acid related disease. Proton pump inhibitor (PPI) test has become the first test to use in patients without alarm signs. The initial PPI dose is usually high (omeprazole 40–80 mg/day) given usually for 1–4 weeks. Positive response is defined as at least 50% symptomatic improvement. If symptoms return when the treatment is discontinued, GERD diagnosis is established. The test is easily done, inexpensive, available as an office based, avoiding other unnecessary procedures. A review of 15 studies assessing the accuracy of PPI test (24 pH monitoring was used as a gold standard reference) reports of pooled sensitivity of 78% but poor specificity of 54% [38].

Upper Gastrointestinal Endoscopy

Acidic gastric juice that refluxes into the esophagus could cause mucosal damage. Endoscopy is the standard tool to evaluate the extent and the severity of the esophagitis, documenting the existing of esophageal complications (strictures, Barrett's esophagus, and carcinoma), and exclude other etiologies for the patient's symptoms. However, there is a poor correlation between the severity of the symptoms and the presence and severity of esophagitis [39]. Esophagitis is found in only 20–60% of patients with abnormal esophageal reflux, Thus, the sensitivity of endoscopy for GERD is poor, but it has excellent specificity at 90–95%" [40].

When endoscopic changes are accompanied by typical reflux symptoms, the specificity for GERD is even higher, 97% [41].

Endoscopy should be performed in patients who present with "alarm" symptoms: dysphagia, odynophagia, weight loss, gastrointestinal bleeding, anemia, and epigastric mass, in order to diagnose significant pathologies including esophageal malignancies [35].

Dysphagia can indicate of esophageal stricture, either benign or malignant. However, dysphagia was reported by 37% of 11,945 patients with esophagitis without stricture. In 83% of the patients the dysphagia resolved with PPI therapy [42]. For this reason, the Montreal consensus recommended that not all, but only "troublesome" (when patients need to change their eating patterns, episodes of food impaction and when the dysphagia does not resolve with PPI treatment), should be investigated [43].

Microscopic changes occur in the irritated esophageal mucosa, even when the mucosa endoscopically appears normal [44]. However, these changes are not specific for GERD. In patients with classic esophagitis, biopsies are usually not necessary.

Capsule Endoscopy

Esophageal capsule endoscopy (11 × 26 mm) obtains video images at 14 frames per second, using two cameras, on both tips of the capsule. The patient is instructed to swallow the capsule in supine position, and the images are transmitted to a receiver via digital radiofrequency. The capsule accuracy was compared with standard upper endoscopy. The reported sensitivity and specificity for the presence of Barrett's esophagus were 79 and 78%, for erosive esophagitis 50–79 and 90–94%, and for hiatal hernia 54 and 67%, respectively. As a screening tool, capsule endoscopy has good specificity; however, its sensitivity is not optimal [45, 46].

Barium Esophagogram

Barium esophagogram is most useful in demonstrating anatomic narrowing of the esophagus, strictures webs, rings as well as hiatal hernias. It also allows assessment of esophageal motor function and esophageal clearance. Barium esophagogram is a reasonable modality for the detection of moderate to severe esophagitis, with sensitivity of 79–100%, but mild esophagitis, as well as Barrett's esophagus, is usually missed [47, 48].

Esophageal Manometry

Manometry is not routinely indicated as part of the evaluation and assessment of GERD. It allows measurements of esophageal body motor activity and LES function. Manometry is used to define the exact location of the LES for accurate location of the pH probe, and before anti-reflux surgery, to document adequate esophageal peristalsis [49].

pH Monitoring

Indication

Current approach for patients with classical uncomplicated GERD favors empiric PPI trail over initial tests [50, 51]. Further investigations are needed in the following scenarios:

1. Refractory typical esophageal symptoms of GERD who have not responded to antisecretory therapy
2. Atypical symptoms of GERD (for initial evaluation or after a therapeutic trial)

3. Failure to response to medical therapy (not as part of short empiric high dose therapeutic test)
4. Medical therapy follow-up to assess the efficacy of the treatment, especially in asymptomatic esophagitis and Barrett's esophagus.
5. In case of surgical therapy — preassessment to confirm GERD, and postoperative effectiveness evaluation

Endoscopy is probably the most reasonable next step to evaluate such patients, but esophagitis which is almost always associated with increased esophageal exposure to acid occurs in only about half of the patients with reflux [52]. Assessing the diagnosis by symptomatology and endoscopic findings is problematic, and measurement of esophageal exposure to acidic gastric refluxate has become a key factor in the evaluation of patients with clinical suspicion of GERD.

Once a day PPI treatment is not effective in 25–42% of the patients. Of those, 20–25% will improve after doubling the dose [53, 54].

Assuming compliance is assuring, and endoscopy rules out other etiologies, reflux monitoring directs into three possible categories: (1) Partial, not sufficient acid suppression with ongoing reflux. (2) Adequate acid control with nonacid reflux. (3) No reflux at all, or no association between the patient's complaints and reflux events. In this case, other causes for the patient's symptomatology should be considered.

Instrumentation

Specter introduced the continuous intraesophageal pH monitoring technique in 1969 [55]. Accepted normal values that unify the interpretation of this study were established by Johnson and DeMeester in the mid-1970s [56]. Since then the technique has been widely spread, and ambulatory pH monitoring is the standard test for establishing pathologic reflux [57, 58].

Performance of pH monitoring requires one or more pH electrodes, recorder, and program software. Several types of reflux detectors electrodes are available; catheter based and wireless electrodes. Each one of them has its advantages as well as limitations. The pH probe has two electrodes that function as a galvanic cell. One electrode acts as a reference with constant potential, and the other one acts as an indicator electrode with potential changes according the hydrogen ion concentration. Translation of the potential differences between the two electrodes into a concentration gradient of hydrogen, gives the pH value.

Catheter-Based pH Monitoring

Esophageal pH catheters use either monocrystalline antimony or glass sensors.

Antimony electrodes have single or multichannel probes and are smaller than the glass electrodes, more flexible and less expensive. Their operation life is up to ten studies. Compared with glass electrodes, they have greater recording drift and less linear response [59–61]. Insertion of the antimony catheter is easier, and more tolerable by the patients.

Glass electrodes have long operational life (40–50 studies), rapid and linear response and are more accurate with less recording drift compared with the antimony probe. Glass electrodes have only one channel, they are stiffer and more expensive [59–62].

Both types of electrodes provide similar clinical results, and antimony electrodes are accepted as standard for use in clinical practice, with sensitivity around 60% in patients with normal endoscopy, and with a specificity of 85–90% [63].

Previous-generation electrodes required external reference electrode, while the newest type contains internal built-in electrode which make the procedure more reliable with less artifacts and easier for the patient.

Standard esophageal pH monitoring is an ambulatory procedure, and patients fast for 4–6h prior the procedure. The catheter is passed transnasally, and the pH sensor is placed in the distal esophagus. In the adult population the pH sensor is located 5cm above the manometrically determined proximal border of the LES [64]. The catheter is connected to a battery powered portable recorder, capable to collect pH values obtain from the pH probe, every 4–6 sec for 24h. The patient is instructed to mark, by push button located on the recorder, or in a diary, every relevant symptom, as well as meals, sleeping time, and body position changes.

Wireless pH Probe (Bravo)

Wireless pH probe consist of an antimony pH electrode, with an internal battery and transmitter located within a capsule ($6 \times 5.5 \times 25$ mm) [65]. After setup and calibration, very similar to the catheter based pH probe, a delivery system is inserted trans-orally (or less common transnasally) with conscious IV sedation, and places the attached capsule 6cm above the Z-line (the gastroesophageal junction). Previous endoscopy or manometry is needed for measuring the exact location of the gastroesophageal junction. A vacuum unit pulls the attached esophageal wall mucosa, into a small

Catheter free pH monitoring system (Bravo system).

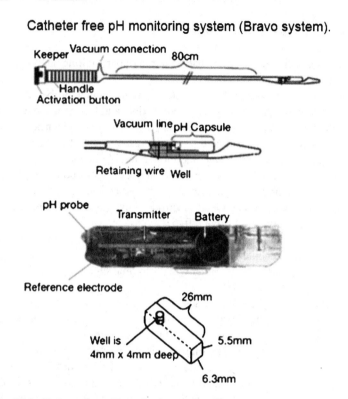

Fig. 10.2. Catheter free pH monitoring system (Bravo system).

well within the capsule, and secures it by a stainless pin. The capsule transmits pH data using radio telemetry to a portable receiver. The electrode samples pH data at 6s intervals. The patient is instructed to keep the recorder within 3–5 ft at all times. Routine recording time is 48h rather than 24h of the catheter base probes, should increase the sensitivity of the test [66, 67] (Fig. 10.2). The study may be performed off or on therapy for the entire 48h, but unlike the catheter base system, there is an option to study the patient off medical treatment for the first day, followed by on treatment for the second day, for more relevant complete data. After completion of the 48-h study, data are downloaded from the recorder. Patient diary information is entered into the computer-based record. Measurements of the total, upright, and supine percentage time when esophageal pH was below 4 are determined during day 1 and day 2 of the study. The capsule is detached spontaneously after 5–6 days. The performance of the wireless pH electrode was validated against catheter-based antimony pH electrode systems in simultaneous controlled trials

[68–70]. The wireless pH system detects less short reflux episodes, probably secondary to the lower sampling rate of the wireless pH compared with the catheter system. Such short events do not alter the overall acid exposure times, and its clinical significance is uncertain. The 95th percentile for distal esophageal acid exposure time for control subjects, recorded by the wireless devices was 5.3%, a value higher than values reported in some catheter-based system studies [63, 71, 72]. This higher acid exposure threshold may be the consequence of less limitation in daily activities. In fact, a major advantage of the wireless pH system is patient tolerability [66, 73, 74] providing more accurate and reliable information of the esophageal acid exposure profile. Nasally passed pH electrodes are uncomfortable, results in avoiding potentially reflux provoking stimuli such as certain foods and physical activity [73, 75].

The wireless sensing technique has some drawbacks: recording from a single probe only with all its consequences. Some patients do experience a mild foreign body sensation, and 5% complain of chest pain, odynophagia was reported in some cases as well. Early detachment can alter the results, and on the other hand failure of the capsule to detach, although rare, can necessitate endoscopic extraction [71, 76, 77].

pH Probes Limitations

pH recording, wireless or catheter based has some inherent limitations. The methods detect only reflux episodes during which the pH drops below 4.0, therefore providing limited information on nonacid reflux. This limitation has become even more important as PPI trials become many times, the first option in treating GERD patients, without any previous diagnostic tests. Many patients are referred for evaluation due to persistent GERD symptoms while treated. Conventional esophageal pH monitoring in patients taking acid-suppressive therapy is limited, unable to separate patients in whom persistent symptoms are associated with nonacid reflux, from those patients in whom symptoms are not associated with any type of reflux [78].

Multichannel Intraluminal Impedance (MII)

The impedance technique, first described in 1991 by Silny [79], measures the changes in resistance to electrical current across a pair of electrodes within the esophageal lumen. Since different type of boluses produce different current resistance, the system can recognize the presence of bolus inside the esophageal lumen, and the composition of the bolus: gas, liquid, or mixed bolus. Few pairs of electrodes are positioned in a serial manner along the catheter, usually spaced 2cm apart. The direction of the bolus movement can be determine, either antegrade to the stomach or retrograde. The impedance catheter, (2.1 mm in diameter) is inserted transnasally no different than catheter-based pH monitoring. Patients are usually monitored ambulatory for 24h (Fig. 10.3).

The conductivity of the esophageal lumen is relatively stable, with the electrical circuit values around $2,000–4,000\,\Omega$. Liquid bolus is recognized as a rapid drop in impedance (50%) as the increased ionic content of the bolus improves the electrical conductivity between the two electrodes. The impedance will remain low as long as the bolus is present between the pair of electrodes and will start rising once the bolus is cleared. The presence of gas is recognized by a simultaneously rise in impedance ($>5,000\,\Omega$), at least in two esophageal measuring segments, as there are no electrical charges to close the circuit when the two electrodes are encircled by air. Impedance will return to the baseline values once the air has passed and the electrodes are back in contact with the esophageal mucosa. Mixed gas liquid reflux is define when gas reflux occurring immediately before or during a liquid reflux.

The impedance technique is able to detect both acid as well as nonacid reflux. Impedance assembly is generally combined with pH probes. Different configurations are available. Ordinarily, the pH electrode is placed 5cm above the LES, similar to conventional pH testing probes. Additional pH electrodes in the stomach or the proximal esophagus are available. The combined monitoring technique has greater sensitivity than pH monitoring alone in the detection of reflux events.

By using the impedance–pH monitoring, all reflux events could be divided into three categories: acid, weakly acid, and weakly alkaline reflux [80, 81]. Acid refluxate has pH of less than 4, Weakly acidic reflux has been defined as a reflux event associated with a pH drop between 4 and 7, and weakly alkaline reflux as an impedance detected reflux event not associated with a pH drop below 7 (some studies use pH 6.5 instead of 7 as a limit) [13, 80, 81]. Reflux characteristics were studied in 60 healthy subjects, with ambulatory impedance, for 24h. The median number of reflux episodes was 30, most of them occurred in the upright position. Approximately two-thirds of the episodes were acid and another third weakly acidic reflux. Weakly alkaline refluxes were uncommon [82]. Similar findings were reported from a multicenter European study [83].

Impedance changes produced by liquid, mixed, or gas boluses.

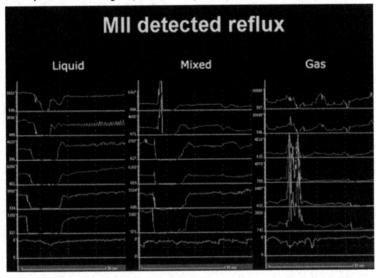

Fig. 10.3. Impedance changes produced by liquid, mixed, or gas boluses.

Overall, the frequency of reflux episodes is similar in GERD patients compared with healthy controls. However, the characteristics of the refluxate are different; patients with GERD had significantly more acid reflux episodes compared with the controls [84]. When symptomatic reflux evens were analyzed, 85% of them were associated with acid reflux, and the minority (15%) with weakly acidic reflux [85]. Omeprazole treatment diminished almost completely the number of acidic refluxes, but the total number of reflux events did not change, due to significant increase in the frequency of nonacid reflux episodes. Omeprazole did not change the overall frequency of symptomatic reflux events, although the number of heartburn episodes was decreased significantly, the number of regurgitation symptoms was increased [86]. Although impedance can detect those events, the clinical significance of nonacidic regurgitation is unclear.

The association between symptoms and reflux events of any type, acidic or nonacidic, was examined using combined pH and impedance monitoring, in a group of untreated typical GERD patients. The combined monitoring was more sensitive (77%) than pH testing alone (68%) for positive association between symptoms and reflux [85].

The yield of the combined pH-impedance test is more emphasize when GERD patients are studied on antisecretory treatment. A group of symptomatic patients underwent combined impedance -pH monitoring while taking PPIs at least twice daily. Positive association between symptoms and acidic reflux events was detected in 11% of the patients, compared with 37% who had positive association for nonacid refluxes. Regurgitation rather than heartburn was the predominant symptom. This information would have been interpreted as negative using pH monitoring only. When atypical symptoms were analyzed separately, the advantage of the combined pH impedance over pH only was even bigger (3% had a positive SI for acid reflux, and 19% had a positive SI for NAR) [87]. The diagnostic yield of combined pH–impedance monitoring over pH monitoring alone is higher when done on PPI therapy. An association between symptoms and nonacid reflux was found in 4.1 and 16.7% of subjects off and on PPI therapy, respectively [88].

Currently, Impedance–pH monitoring is considered by many experts as the most sensitive tool for measuring reflux, especially for PPI-refractory patients [89–93].

Impedance study limitations: Impedance study has the disadvantages of catheter based study and patients intolerability. Patients with Barrett's esophagus and esophagitis, present with low baseline impedance values generated by the mucosa, which make it difficult for interpretation. Esophageal motility disorders could result in intraluminal liquid retention, which may alter the impedance reading and causing recording artifacts. The technique is unable quantify refluxate volume, which is an important factor in the pathogenesis of GERD. Current automated analysis software is still not accurate enough, and requires manual data correction [94].

Multiple Sites pH Monitoring

Studies performed by catheter base pH monitoring, have the technical possibility of measuring the pH values at different esophageal sites simultaneously. The distal esophageal location, 5cm above the LES is always fixed, but other several additional locations for positioning the pH probes are used.

Esophago-Esophageal pH Monitoring

Dual-probe pH monitoring provides additional information concerning the occurrence of proximal esophageal reflux events. No consensus exists for the placement of the proximal probe. Various studies report probe placement at 15 or 20cm above the LES, or just below the upper esophageal sphincter (UES).

Establishment of normal values for proximal reflux depends on precise positioning of the pH probe within the esophagus. Because there is no consensus for probe placement for the proximal esophagus, each laboratory has developed its own standard procedure. Concurrent ambulatory esophageal pH recordings from 5 esophageal locations at 3, 5, 9, 12, and 15cm above the LES displayed a linear decrease in both the number of reflux events and the acid exposure time associated with progressively proximal positions [95]. The correlation between the proximal extent of reflux and symptoms in patients with GERD was investigated. Higher proportion of reflux events reached the proximal esophagus in patients with GERD than in healthy controls (20% vs. 11%) [96].

The normal range for total time with pH <4 is usually around 1% over 24h, when the probe is placed just distal to the lower margin of the UES, although there is no consensus regarding the normal values of proximal acid exposure. Proximal esophageal pH detection may serve as an indirect marker for the volume of gastroesophageal reflux [97], but such estimation is questionable. The reproducibility of the proximal reflux events recording was challenged by examining the same patients on two separate days. Abnormal proximal acid reflux pH values were reproducible in only 55% of studies in contrast to 82% for distal esophageal reflux [98].

Several studies have demonstrated abnormal proximal acid exposure in patients with pharyngeal, laryngeal, and pulmonary abnormalities such as asthma 197 and laryngitis [98, 99]. On the other hand, another study did not find a correlation between otolaryngeal pathologies and abnormal proximal esophageal acid exposure [100]. Intragroup variation and an extensive overlap between patient groups and normal controls make the measurement of proximal acid exposure unreliable for the diagnosis of supraesophageal complications of reflux in individual subjects. Proximal pH recording has very good specificity (91%) but poor sensitivity (55%) for identifying abnormal proximal acid reflux [100], and a negative test does not exclude proximal reflux.

Gastroesophageal pH Monitoring

Intragastric pH monitoring is performed by placing dual pH electrode in the gastric fundus 7–10cm below the LES, while the esophageal one is located 5cm above the sphincter [101]. Data that show a correlation between intragastric pH and gastroesophageal reflux is limited and inconsistent [102, 103]. Intragastric pH can help determine the efficacy of acid suppressive medications or suggest poor compliance, but its clinical significance and applicability is unclear [103].

Esophagopharyngeal pH Monitoring

In recent years there has been an increasing awareness of the role of gastroesophagopharyngeal reflux (GER) in the pathogenesis of numerous disorders of the aerodigestive tract [100, 104, 105].

Studies have shown that normal volunteers rarely have proximal reflux [100, 106]. Further, patients with laryngeal symptoms and proven laryngitis attributed to reflux have pH study results at the distal esophagus that are similar to those in controls [100]. Similar findings have been reported for patients with vocal cord nodules, unexplained persistent pulmonary symptoms [107], posterior laryngitis [100, 108], and patients with persistent laryngeal symptoms [99].

Some of the supraesophageal manifestations of GERD require direct contact of acid and/or gastric contents with the target organs (larynx, vocal cords, teeth, etc.). Although proximal acid exposure does not demonstrate pharyngeal exposure, direct measurement of acid reflux events at the level of the pharynx could provide this information. Pharyngeal acid exposure was measured by placing a pH probe 2cm proximal to the upper margin of the UES's high-pressure zone, in addition to placing both proximal and distal esophageal probes in patients with proven laryngitis and in controls. There was no difference in the reflux parameters at the distal esophagus between the groups. The number and duration of reflux episodes at the proximal esophagus and the pharynx were significantly higher in the laryngitis patient group compared with the control group [105]. Using a similar 3-site technique in patients with vocal cord nodules and healthy controls, distal and proximal acid reflux event parameters showed no difference between the 2 groups, while the number of pharyngeal acid reflux events and the percentage of pharyngeal acid exposure time were significantly greater in the patients with nodules [109]. A study conducted in patients with posterior laryngitis and healthy controls found that the laryngitis group demonstrated a significantly higher number of reflux events and pharyngeal acid exposure time compared with the control group [100]. Some pharyngeal reflux events occurred in most of the healthy subjects, mainly in the upright position. Based on these data, a value for the upper limit of normal for total pharyngeal acid exposure time was set at 0.9% (0.2% after exclusion of meal times) [110].

The location of the pH electrode in the pharynx may expose the probe to a false recording, mainly due to electrode drying, referred to as "pseudoreflux" [111–113]. In one study, 67% of proximal reflux events were artifacts, occurring independently of distal esophageal acidification [112]. In order to overcome these limitations, more stringent criteria be used to define pharyngeal reflux: (1) magnitude of change of pH >2 units, (2) nadir pH <4.0, (3) abrupt pH decrease (onset of pH decrease to nadir <30 s to exclude pseudo-reflux), and (4) pH decrease occurring during a period of distal esophageal acidification [112].

Pharyngeal acid reflux events may be significant in the pathogenesis of various supraesophageal manifestations of GERD; however, the clinical value of pharyngeal pH monitoring still remains uncertain.

Duodenoesophageal Monitoring (Bilitec)

Duodenogastroesophageal reflux exposes the esophagus to duodenal contents that may include biliary secretions, pancreatic enzymes, and bicarbonate. Earlier studies suggested esophageal pH values of >7 as a surrogate marker of this reflux. However, more recent studies have questioned the validity of this method, since saliva and esophageal bicarbonate secretion may be the origin of such events [114]. The development of a fiberoptic sensor that detect bilirubin (Bilitec system), allowed a more direct measure of duodenal reflux into the esophagus. Duodenal gastroesophageal reflux (DGER) occurred in 50% of patients with non-erosive reflux disease, 79% of patients with erosive esophagitis, and 95% of patients with Barrett's esophagus. Combined acid and bile reflux was the most common reflux pattern in patients with GERD [115, 116]. However, the significance of the duodenal content compared with the gastric content reflux is not clear. Today, with the development of the impedance technology, the role of bile measurement seems to be very limited in clinical practice.

Calibration and Setup

Calibration is performed on all pH systems prior to each study. The pH study setup starts with a two point calibration of the electrodes, using reference buffer solutions (usually pH 1 or 4 and pH 7). Post study calibration confirms or denies pH drift and provides information concerning the accuracy of the study.

The data logger samples esophageal pH every 4–5 s. An event marker can be activated by the patient for meals, recumbent periods as well as symptoms. The patient also records all the specific symptoms and all relevant events on a diary. The information can be correlated with the pH tracing for reflux-symptoms association. Since the event marking is crucial for the analysis and for establishing an accurate diagnosis, careful clear instructions for the patient is needed.

At the completion of the study, the catheter is removed, recalibration confirms that the reading is accurate, without any drift. (Not relevant for the wireless capsule). The data from the recorder is uploaded to the computer for analysis.

Electrodes Positioning

The pH catheter is passed through the nostril and positioned 5cm above the proximal margin of the lower esophageal sphincter.

The distance of 5cm was selected to avoid possible electrode displacement and movement into the stomach, especially during contraction of the longitudinal esophageal muscle and shortening of the esophagus induced by swallowing. Misplacing of the electrode changes the sensitivity of the test [117]. Placing the probe too proximal, may result in reading fewer reflux events, placing it more distal, closer to the stomach may expose the probe to more reflux events, compromising the sensitivity and accuracy of the study. Consistent placement of the pH electrode is crucial for reliable assessment and for the reproducibility of the esophageal pH data. Most of the standard normative diagnostic values were obtained from studies that used this position of 5cm above the LES.

Localization of the LES before the positioning of the pH probe is mandatory. Esophageal manometry considered to be the most reliable technique for measuring the exact location of the LES. Other methods, including endoscopy, fluoroscopy, pH catheter step up across the LES, and LES locater device within the pH catheter were offered. However, the accuracy of all these methods was questioned and esophageal manometry is considered to be the "gold standard" for the localization of the LES. Once the LES was located, the pH catheter is passed into the stomach, to document acidic pH below 4, than the probe is pulled back into the esophagus, to the desired location, and the study begin.

With the introduction of a wireless pH system, when the majority of capsule placements are done transorally, validation of the placing technique was needed. The position of the capsule with an endoscope was compared with the transnasal manometric based positioning of the catheter based pH probe. The average difference in position was negligible and did not have a significant influence on the total number of reflux events detected by both systems [68]. A correction factor of 3.74cm was reported and validated, which accounts for the difference in distance between trans nasal and trans oral insertion of the probes [118]. Practically, the wireless capsule should be placed 6cm above the endoscopic determination of the squamocolumnar junction (the Z-line), or 9cm above the proximal aspect of the LES via a transnasal manometric measurement.

Proximal Esophagus or Oropharyngeal Placement

Since the distal electrode location at the distal esophagus, 5cm above the LES is fixed, the proximal electrode location may vary, according the catheter configuration, usually 5, 10 or 15cm above the distal probe. In a prospective analysis of 661 proximal pH studies, in 9% of subjects, the proximal probe was in the hypopharynx, 55% in the cervical esophagus, and 36% at the UES [119]. For pharyngeal pH monitoring, the electrode is usually placed 2cm above the manometrically measured UES, but there is no consensus regarding the probe location. A different location of the electrode changes the reflux parameters and its interpretation.

Duration of the Study

The typical duration for clinical catheter-based reflux monitoring is 24h. Shortening the study, mainly because of patients intolerance, may reduce the sensitivity of the test [120–124]. Short study periods of 3h limited to the postprandial period were reported to have sensitivity ranged from 54 to 88% compared with 24-h pH studies [125]. The reproducibility of a 24-h pH test was estimated at 77–83% in various studies and has been shown to decrease significantly when studies are less than 10h [120, 123, 126–128]. The shorter studies may not provide adequate time to document a symptom-reflux correlation, and are lacking the supine and night time recording, which may affect the interpretation of the study.

The wireless pH monitoring system enables to extend the study beyond 24h. Extended studies are associated with greater sensitivity by distinguishing day-to-day variability and improving the symptom-reflux correlation. Prolongation of the study allow for comparison studies with the patient off and then on antisecretory medication, Defining GERD as the presence of erosive esophagitis and an abnormal pH study as greater than 5.3% exposure time, the sensitivity of day 1 testing was 74% and specificity 90%. By using the worst day of the two studied days, the sensitivity increased to 100%; however, the specificity was decreased to 85% and the false negative rate was high [71].

Diet and Activity While on Study

Early studies recommended on standard meals during the pH study, in order to avoid acidic products intake, which may mimic reflux events and produce false-positive results [129]. However, the effect of such food on esophageal pH is minimal. Combined MII-pH can differentiate reflux from swallow-induced pH changes and may not require any restrictions.

Patients should not be restricted to certain food, and are encouraged to maintain their usual activity and diet routine—normal diet and daily activities.

Excluding the eating period from the overall analysis eliminates the artifacts introduced by ingestion of foods or liquids with a pH <4.0 and improves the separation of normal from abnormal [130].

On/Off Therapy

Whether pH study should be performed with the patient on or off acid suppressive therapy is debated. Each option provides different information. The advantages and disadvantages of each setting must be considered.

Basically, pH studies are performed to answer two major questions: (1) Is the patient complains are caused by esophageal acid reflux? (2) In a patient who remains symptomatic despite medical therapy, has the reflux been controlled, and if not, are the symptoms due to esophageal acid reflux?

The three likely causes of treatment failure might be inadequate acid suppression [131], symptoms caused by weakly acidic reflux events [132–134], or erroneous diagnosis of GERD [135]. Thus, the main goal of the optimal diagnostic test is to determine which of these possibilities are most likely.

Off Therapy

Studying the patient off medication determine whether a patient has abnormal gastroesophageal reflux. Although GERD symptoms could be caused by nonacid reflux, with a pH >4, these reflux episodes are responsible for a very small portion of symptomatic events when patients are off medication [81]. Nonacid reflux is only relevant during acid suppression. Documenting abnormal reflux parameters while off medication could separate the majority of patients into normal or abnormal reflux.

MII-pH could detect all types of reflux events, regardless the pH value of the refluxate. However, evidence that the addition of impedance will improve documentation of abnormal reflux in patients while off medication is very little. For routine clinical purpose, pH study (catheter based or wireless) is sufficient to determine the presence or absence of abnormal reflux in refractory patients while off medication. If pH study while off medication is negative, GERD is very unlikely, and patients with heartburn as the main symptom may be labeled as "functional heartburn."

In studies performed off medical therapy, patients should stop acid suppressing as well as promotility drugs. PPI should be stopped for 5–7 days before the study and histamine 2 blockers for 2 day prior.

On Therapy

On-therapy testing is more commonly used to evaluate patients who remain symptomatic despite medical therapy. The rationale of the test is to investigate the possibility that the symptoms presenting by the patient are caused by esophageal acid exposure in spite of PPI therapy. The likelihood of continued abnormal acid reflux, while on optimal medical treatment, is very low. On twice-daily PPI therapy, only 4% of patients had abnormal pH study [78]. However, identifying the minority of patients who are truly refractory may support the use of more aggressive medical or surgical therapies for GERD [63, 136].

On therapy pH study should be interpreted very carefully. Thresholds for abnormal reflux events are not clear. One study reported of a threshold of 1.6% of acid exposure time at the distal esophagus, while on PPI treatment [137]. Other data that validate this cutoff is limited. The variability of esophageal acid exposure and the lack of outcome predictors of those patients, make the clinical interpretation ambiguous. Although the threshold for abnormality is unclear, in case of esophageal acid exposure high above normal ranges, more aggressive treatment or compliance evaluation should be considered. Negligible values while on PPI treatment, indicates that the patient will probably won't benefit from further acid suppression treatment. Negative test does not exclude GERD as a potential cause for the patients complains, because the reduction in

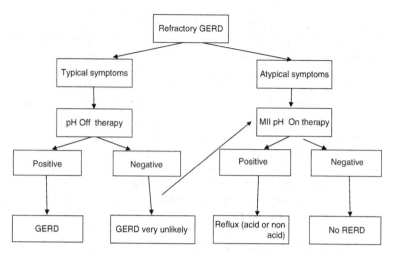

Fig. 10.4. On or off?—Summary.

gastric acidity converts acid to weakly acid or nonacid reflux episodes that are not detected by pH monitoring, and the patient may still have reflux related symptoms.

Impedance–pH monitoring is superior for testing patients with acid suppression because of its ability to detect acid as well as nonacid reflux. A normal impedance–pH test of the patient while on medication establishes that the patient's symptoms are not from GERD,

Wireless pH monitoring enable prolong pH study for 2 or even 4 days. Studying the patient while off and then while on PPI therapy on consecutive days, in a single test, may be helpful in documenting the presence of GERD, and whether the patient will require an escalation of therapy [138]. Still this technique is limited by the inability to detect nonacid refluxes (Fig. 10.4).

Normal Values

Normal esophageal pH is considered to be close to pH 7.0. Gastroesophageal reflux is defined as a sudden decrease in intraesophageal pH to below 4.0, with the nadir pH being reached within 30 s from the beginning of the drop. The cutoff limit of pH 4 has been chosen because pepsin, the main proteolytic enzyme of the gastric secretions, is inactive above this value [139], and GERD patients report of heartburn when the intraesophageal pH drops below 4 [140].

The measured parameters for pH study includes the following: (1) Percent of total time when pH is less than 4, (2) Percent of time, upright and supine when pH is less than 4, (3) The number of reflux events, (4) Duration of longest reflux episode, (5) The number of reflux episodes longer than 5 min [57]. The most reproducible parameter for GERD is the percent of the total time when pH is less than 4 (acid exposure time). The accepted upper limit of normal of this parameter ranges from 4 to 5.5% [57]. Johnson and DeMeester developed a scoring system which incorporates those parameters for easier interpretation. Values larger than 14.7 are considered abnormal [141]. Weakness of the score is that it does not include any information on association between symptom and reflux. Wireless pH studies reported similar values for acid exposure time, ranging from 4.4 to 5.3% for 48h [71, 142].

Normal values for impedance parameters includes the following: [82, 143]
Total number of reflux episodes: 73–75
Acid-reflux episodes: 50–59
Nonacid-reflux episodes: 27–48

The clinical utility of these cutoff values is unclear, especially when normal MII-pH validated values in acid-suppressed subjects, are not available. It is also not clear whether nonacid reflux can injure the esophageal mucosa, and the association between positive impedance test and patient's symptoms is still questionable.

Symptom-Reflux Correlation

Abnormal pH study does not necessarily indicate causality between the patient's complains and the results of the test. Cause and effect relationship are needed to prove this assumption. An attempt to improve the significance of the study incorporates the Symptom Index (SI) in order to express the relationship between symptoms and reflux episodes [144]. It defined as the percentage of symptom episodes that proceeded by acid reflux, within a 5-min time window (or 2 min window as reported in some studies [145]. Each symptom should be determined separately.

$$SI = \frac{\text{Number of symptoms with pH} < 4}{\text{Total number of symptoms}} \times 100$$

A value of >50% is considered positive (at least half of the symptoms are associated with pH drop below 4, within a 2 or 5-min time window). The disadvantage of the SI is that it does not take into account the number of reflux episodes. For example, a patient with many reflux events but only one symptomatic reflux event will have a SI of 100%. It is also possible that in patients with multiple reflux episodes and few symptoms, the association may occur by chance. For these reasons, another parameter, the Symptom Sensitivity Index, (SSI) was proposed [146]. It is defined as the percentage of reflux episodes associated with symptoms out of the total number of reflux episodes. A value of greater than 10% is considered to be positive.

$$SSI = \frac{Number\ of\ reflux - related\ symptoms\ episodes}{Total\ number\ of\ reflux\ episodes} \times 100$$

Another complex index for analyzing symptom–reflux correlation is the Symptom Probability Analysis (SAP) [147]. The SAP tries to estimate if association between reflux and symptoms during the study may have occurred by chance. The statistical program calculates four fields: (1) positive symptom, positive reflux; (2) negative symptom, positive reflux; (3) positive symptom, negative reflux; and (4) negative symptom, negative reflux. SAP indicates the statistical probability with which symptoms and reflux episodes are associated. Only a SAP greater than 95% (the probability of this association having occurred by chance is less than 5%) is considered positive.

The clinical use of all three indices is doubtful. SI, SSI, and SAP were compared with omeprazole test. The sensitivities were 35, 74, and 65% while the specificities were 80, 73, and 73%, respectively [148]. None of the symptom association schemes have been well validated; they should be used as complementary information, but do not guarantee response to antireflux therapy.

GERD Treatment

Lifestyle Modifications

Appropriate lifestyle adjustment in patients with reflux can be divided into three categories: (1) avoidance of foods that may stimulate reflux (coffee, alcohol, peppermint, chocolate, fatty foods), (2) avoidance of acidic foods that may promote heartburn (citrus, carbonated drinks, spicy foods), (3) adoption of lifestyle that may reduce esophageal acid exposure (weight loss, quitting smoking, raising the head of the bed, and avoiding from lying down for 2–3 h after meals). Most evidence supporting such recommendations is weak, and there are insufficient data to suggest a consistent benefit of lifestyle changes for all patients with GERD. However, it is also clear that there are subgroups of patients who may benefit from lifestyle changes, and it is good practice to make those recommendations to those patients.

Medication

Acid suppression is the mainstay of treatment in both the acute and long standing GERD. In a large meta-analysis of 136 randomized, controlled trials involving 35,978 patients with esophagitis, PPIs exhibit a better healing effect and faster symptom relief (83%) than histamine$_2$ receptor antagonists (H$_2$RAs) (52%), and both had higher healing rates than that with placebo (8%) [149]. That review also concluded that there is no significant difference in efficacy among the currently available PPIs (esomeprazole, lansoprazole, omeprazole, pantoprazole, rabeprazole) and that the gain achieved by doubling the standard dose of PPI therapy is modest.

Surgery

The principle of surgical treatment in GERD patients is strengthening the lower esophageal high pressure zone by wrapping the proximal stomach around the distal esophagus. The most common operation is Nissen funduplication. The effectiveness of the two methods of treatment, medication and surgery, seems to be similar.

Patients with esophagitis were randomized into two groups: surgery and PPI therapy. The rate of recurrent esophagitis was similar after 7 years follow-up (11.8 and 10.3% respectively) [150]. However, in another study, up to 60% of patients who underwent funduplication were using anti reflux medication after 10–12 years after surgery [151]. Refractory GERD patients have a lower probability of symptom resolution with antireflux surgery [152]. Probably because a large proportion of these patients are misdiagnosed and do not have abnormal GERD. Thus, surgery should only be recommended when there is strong evidence that the patient's symptoms are truly related to reflux despite PPI therapy.

GI societies recommendations of the treatment of GERD [153] (Table 10.1).

Table 10.1. Summary of management guidelines.

	First-line therapy[a]	When to use endoscopy	Step up/down therapy	Role of H. pylori	Other therapies
NICE (England and Wales)	PPI therapy	Endoscopy discouraged apart from alarm features and concern for malignancy in those older than 55 years	Low-dose PPI therapy and PPI on demand	H. pylori test and treatment recommended as part of management strategy of upper GI symptoms. No evidence H. pylori has a role in GERD	Surgery may be beneficial but not for routine use Prokinetics not recommended Endoscopic therapy not addressed
ACG (USA)	PPI therapy, H₂RA therapy in milder cases of GERD	Endoscopy for those with symptoms suggestive of complications and those at risk of Barrett's esophagus	The dose of PPI needed for symptom control This will be full dose PPI or even increased dose PPI in many cases	Not discussed	Surgery is an option for maintenance therapy by an experienced surgeon Prokinetics not recommended but monotherapy may be useful in select patients with acid suppression Endoscopic therapy controls symptoms in selected patients with well documented GERD
Genval (International)	PPI therapy or H₂RA therapy (PPI strongly preferred)	Endoscopy for all patients experiencing reflux symptoms at least twice a week for 6 months	The dose of PPI needed for symptom control Step down to H₂RA after low-dose PPI	H. pylori eradication not indicated in GERD	Indications for surgery not discussed but if performed should be by an experienced surgeon Prokinetics not usually indicated Endoscopic therapies not addressed

Asia-Pacific	PPI therapy	Symptoms persist despite PPI therapy, frequent relapses of symptoms with on-demand PPI therapy or alarm features present	On demand PPI therapy	H. pylori does not have a role in the pathogenesis in GERD. Advisable that H. pylori status checked and eradication given before long-term PPI therapy to reduce the risk of atrophic gastritis	Choice of surgery and medical therapy dependent on patient preference and available expertise. Prokinetics not recommended. Endoscopic therapy only in the context of a clinical trial
Candy (Canadian)	PPI or H₂RA therapy (PPI preferred)	Patients that have been on acid suppressive medication for 5–10 years. Alarm features	PPI or H₂RA therapy to control symptoms	H. pylori testing not required in GERD; however, it is reasonable on a case by case basis	Surgery is an option for patients on long-term acid suppression or have symptoms despite medical therapy. Prokinetics not recommended. Endoscopic therapies cannot be recommended for routine practice
Australian	PPI therapy	Alarm features, symptoms persist despite therapy, diagnosis unclear as symptoms are not characteristic	On-demand PPI therapy	Decision to test and treat for H. pylori needs to be individualized. No evidence H. pylori has a role in GERD. Long-term PPI therapy in presence of H. pylori may increase the risk of gastric atrophy	Surgery if fail to respond to medical therapy, side effects of therapy or patient desire not to take medication. Prokinetics not recommended. Endoscopic therapy only in the context of a clinical trial

PPI proton-pump inhibitor; *GI* gastrointestinal; *GERD* gastrointestinal–esophageal reflux disease; *NICE* National Institute of Clinical Excellence; *ACG* American College of Gastroenterology

[a] After lifestyle modification and antacid therapy have failed

[b] Dyspepsia guidelines that included the management of gastroesophageal reflux disease

Extraesophageal Manifestations of GERD (Cough, Chest Pain, Asthma)

Noncardiac Chest Pain

Ischemic heart disease, because of it curtail clinical importance, should be excluded before any other diagnosis, but once it has been ruled out, GERD may be the next most likely etiology [154–156]. Empirical therapy with twice-daily PPIs for 4 weeks is recommended [154, 157]. If a patient continues to have chest pain despite this course of therapy, diagnostic testing with esophageal manometry and pH or impedance–pH monitoring can exclude motility disorders or refractory reflux symptoms.

Extraesophageal Manifestations of GERD

Patients with suspected extraesophageal GERD syndromes may have GERD as a contributing etiology but rarely as the sole cause. Given the nonspecific nature of the extraesophageal symptoms and the poor sensitivity and specificity of diagnostic tests such as pH monitoring, laryngoscopy, or endoscopy for establishing an etiology of GERD [158] empirical therapy with twice-daily PPIs for 2–4 months become common practice [158, 159].

Chronic Laryngeal Symptoms

Patients with laryngeal symptoms, such as chronic cough, sore throat, hoarseness, globus sensation, and excessive throat clearing are often diagnosed with GERD. The majority will have typical esophageal GERD symptoms as well. Pharyngeal pH monitoring was offered for better identifying patients with laryngeal symptoms caused by gastro-esophagolaryngeal reflux. However, artifacts are common [113] normal values are poorly defined [160–162], and 10–30% of healthy subjects meet the criteria for abnormal pharyngeal reflux, suggesting some reflux into the hypopharynx may be a normal phenomenon [105]. The cutoff value of pH <4 may not be applied for pharyngeal reflux, but even less restrictive pH criteria not help discriminate healthy volunteers and patients with suspected reflux-related ENT symptoms [163]. The practical approach is an empiric trial with PPI for few months, reserving pH and impedance testing for patients with refractory symptoms [158].

Asthma

The prevalence of GERD in asthmatics ranges from 34 to 89% according to various reports. The reason for these differences is mainly due to different definitions of reflux, and differences diagnostic methods (symptoms or pH study). Reflux test was abnormal in 66% of asthmatic patients [164]. However, it is unclear whether reflux causes asthma, or if reflux is caused by decreased intrathoracic pressure during asthmatic attack. As with other extraesophageal manifestation of GERD, therapeutic trial should be the first step, followed by pH or impedance–pH study.

In Conclusion

Esophageal-reflux monitoring is the mainstay in the evaluation and management of GERD. And indeed, varieties of options are available. Understanding the strengths and limitations of each technique is essential. Asking the right questions, selecting the appropriate test, and tailoring the right setting for each patient will produce the most of every test. Each specific study can provide the medical staff important information regarding the presence of abnormal reflux and whether there is a consistent cause and effect relationship between reflux episodes and symptoms. All results should always be taken with a "grain of salt," and not infrequently, it is necessary to repeat the test in different circumstances, in order to adjust the medical policy and provide the best medical care.

References

1. Allison PR. Peptic ulcer of the esophagus. J Thorac Cardiovasc Surg. 1946;15:308–17.
2. Vakil N, van Zanten SV, Kahrilas P, Dent J, Jones R. The Montreal definition and classification of gastroesophageal reflux disease: a global evidence-based consensus. Am J Gastroenterol. 2006;101:1900–20.
3. Serag HB. Time trends for gastroesophageal reflux disease: a systematic review. Clin Gastroenterol Hepatol. 2007;5:17–26.

4. Gallup Organization. A Gallup Organization National Survey: heartburn across America. Princeton: The Gallup Organization; 1988.

5. Locke GR, Talley NJ, Fett SL, et al. Prevalence and clinical spectrum of gastroesophageal reflux: a population-based study in Olmsted County, Minnesota. Gastroenterology. 1997;112:1448.

6. Moayyedi P, Axon ATR. Gastro-oesophageal reflux disease: the extent of the problem. Aliment Pharmacol Ther. 2005;22 Suppl 1:11–9.

7. Hu WH, Hui WM, Lam CL, Lam SK. Anxiety and depression are co-factors determining health care utilisation in patients with dyspepsia: a Hong Kong population based study. Gastroenterology. 1997;112 Suppl 1:A153.

8. Dodds WJ, Dent J, Hogan WJ, et al. Mechanisms of gastroesophageal reflux in patients with reflux esophagitis. N Engl J Med. 1982;307:1547–52.

9. Dent J, Dodds WJ, Friedman RH, et al. Mechanism of gastroesophageal reflux in recumbent asymptomatic human subjects. J Clin Invest. 1980;65:256–67.

10. Kahrilas PJ, Shi G, Manka M, Joehl RJ. Increased frequency of transient lower esophageal sphincter relaxation induced by gastric distension in reflux patients with hiatal hernia. Gastroenterology. 2000;118:688–95.

11. de Vries DR, van Herwaarden MA, Smout AJ, Samsom M. Gastroesophageal pressure gradients in gastroesophageal reflux disease: relations with hiatal hernia, body mass index, and esophageal acid exposure. Am J Gastroenterol. 2008;103:1349–54.

12. Corley DA, Kubo A, Levin TR, et al. Abdominal obesity and body mass index as risk factors for Barrett's esophagus. Gastroenterology. 2007;133:34–41.

13. Kahrilas PJ. GERD pathogenesis, pathophysiology and clinical manifestations. Cleve Clin J Med. 2003;70 Suppl 5:S4–19.

14. Blackshaw LA. Receptors and transmission in the brain-gut axis: potential for novel therapies. IV. GABA(B) receptors in the brain-gastroesophageal axis. Am J Physiol Gastrointest Liver Physiol. 2001;281:G311–5.

15. Hirsch DP, Tytgat GN, Boeckxstaens GE. Transient lower oesophageal sphincter relaxations: a pharmacological target for gastro-oesophageal reflux disease? Aliment Pharmacol Ther. 2002;16:17–26.

16. Penagini R, Carmagnola S, Cantu P, et al. Mechanoreceptors of the proximal stomach: role in triggering transient lower esophageal sphincter relaxation. Gastroenterology. 2004;126:49–56.

17. Dent J. Patterns of lower esophageal sphincter function associated with gastroesphageal reflux. Am J Med. 1997;103(Suppl 5A):29S–32S.

18. Wajed SA, Streets CG, Bremner CG, DeMeester TR. Elevated body mass disrupts the barrier to gastroesophageal reflux. Arch Surg. 2001;136:1014–8.

19. Kahrilas PJ, Lin S, Chen J, et al. The effect of hiatus hernia on gastrooesophageal junction pressure. Gut. 1999;44:476–82.

20. van Herwaarden MA, Samsom M, Smout AJ. Excess gastroesophageal reflux in patients with hiatus hernia is caused by mechanisms other than transient LES relaxations. Gastroenterology. 2000;119:1439–46.

21. Barak N, Ehrenpreis ED, Harrison JR, Sitrin MD. Gastro-oesophageal reflux disease in obesity: pathophysiology and therapeutic considerations. Obes Rev. 2002;3:9–15.

22. Kahrilas PJ, Gupta RR. Mechanisms of acid reflux associated with cigarette smoking. Gut. 1990;31:4–10.

23. Vitale GC, Cheadle WG, Patel B, Sadek SA, Michel ME, Cuschieri A. The effect of alcohol on nocturnal gastroesophageal reflux. JAMA. 1987;258:2077–9.

24. Thomas FB, Steinbaugh JT, Fromkes JJ, Mekhjian HS, Caldwell JH. Inhibitory effect of coffee on lower esophageal sphincter pressure. Gastroenterology. 1980;79:1262–6.

25. Holloway RH, Lyrenas E, Ireland A, Dent J. Effect of intraduodenal fat on lower oesophageal sphincter function and gastro-oesophageal reflux. Gut. 1997;40:449–53.

26. Carlsson R, Dent J, Bolling-Sternevold E, et al. The usefulness of a structured questionnaire in the assessment of symptomatic gastroesophageal reflux disease. Scand J Gastroenterol. 1998;33:1023.

27. Shaker R, Castell DO, Schoenfeld PS, Spechler SJ. Nighttime heartburn is an under-appreciated clinical problem that impacts sleep and daytime function: the results of a Gallup survey conducted on behalf of the American Gastroenterological Association. Am J Gastroenterol. 2003;98:1487.

28. Fass R, Naliboff BD, Fass SS, et al. The effect of auditory stress on perception of intraesophageal acid in patients with gastroesophageal reflux disease. Gastroenterology. 2008;134:696–705.

29. Schey R, Dickman R, Parthasarathy S, et al. Sleep deprivation is hyperalgesic in patients with gastroesophageal reflux disease. Gastroenterology. 2007;133:1787–95.

30. Wright CE, Ebrecht M, Mitchell R, et al. The effect of psychological stress on symptom severity and perception in patients with gastro-oesophageal reflux. J Psychosom Res. 2005;59:415–24.

31. Johnson DA, Fennerty MB. Heartburn severity underestimates erosive esophagitis severity in elderly patients with gastroesophageal reflux disease. Gastroenterology. 2004;126:660–4.

32. Jacob P, Kahrilas PJ, Vanagunos A. Peristaltic dysfunction associated with non-obstructive dysphagia in reflux disease. Dig Dis Sci. 1990;35:939.

33. Brzana RJ, Koch KL. Gastroesophageal reflux disease presenting with intractable nausea. Ann Intern Med. 1997;126:704.

34. Richter JE. Extraesophageal presentations of gastroesophageal reflux disease. Am J Gastroenterol. 2000;25:S1.

35. DeVault KR, Castell DO. Updated guidelines for the diagnosis and treatment of gastroesophageal reflux disease. Am J Gastroenterol. 2005;100:190–200.

36. Armstrong D, Marshall JK, Chiba N, et al. Canadian Consensus Conference on the management of gastroesophageal reflux disease in adults—update 2004. Can J Gastroenterol. 2005;19:15–35.

37. Kahrilas PJ, Shaheen NJ, Vaezi M, et al. AGAI medical position statement: management of gastroesophageal reflux disease. Gastroenterology. 2008;135:1383–91.

38. Numans ME, Lau J, de Wit NJ, Bonis PA. Short-term treatment with proton-pump inhibitors as a test for gastroesophageal reflux disease: a meta-analysis of diagnostic test characteristics. Ann Intern Med. 2004;140:518–27.

39. Sonnenberg A, El-Serag HB. Clinical epidemiology and natural history of gastroesophagal reflux disease. Yale J Biol Med. 1999;72:81–92.

40. Richter JE. Severe reflux esophagitis. Gastrointest Endosc Clin N Am. 1994;4:677.

41. Terea L, Fein M, Ritter MP, et al. Can the combination of symptoms and endoscopy confirm the presence of gastroesophageal reflux disease? Am Surg. 1997;63:933–6.

42. Vakil NB, Traxler B, Levine D. Dysphagia in patients with erosive esophagitis: prevalence, severity, and response to proton pump inhibitor treatment. Clin Gastroenterol Hepatol. 2004;2:665–8.

43. Vakil N, van Zanten SV, Kahrilas P, et al. The Montreal definition and classification of gastroesophageal reflux disease: a global evidence-based consensus. Am J Gastroenterol. 2006;101:1900–20.

44. Dent J. Microscopic esophageal mucosal injury in nonerosive reflux disease. Clin Gastroenterol Hepatol. 2007;5:4–16.

45. Sharma P, Wani S, Rastogi A, et al. The diagnostic accuracy of esophageal capsule endoscopy in patients with gastroesophageal reflux disease and Barrett's esophagus: a blinded, prospective study. Am J Gastroenterol. 2008;103:525–32.

46. Galmish JP, Sacher-Huvelin S, Coron E, et al. Screening for esophagitis and Barrett's esophagus with wireless esophageal capsule endoscopy: a multicenter prospective trial with reflux symptoms. Am J Gastroenterol. 2008;103:528–45.

47. Thompson JK, Koehler RE, Richter JE. Detection of gastro-esophageal reflux: value of the barium studies compared with 24-hour pH monitoring. Am J Roentgenol. 1994;162:621.

48. Johnston BT, Troshinsky MB, Castell JA, Castell DO. Comparison of barium radiology with esophageal pH monitoring in the diagnosis of gastroesophageal reflux disease. Am J Gastroenterol. 1996;91:1181.

49. Waring JP, Hunter JG, Oddsdottir M. The preoperative evaluation of patients considered for laparoscopic antireflux surgery. Am J Gastroenterol. 1995;90:35.

50. Kahrilas PJ, Shaheen NJ, Vaezi MF. American Gastroenterological Association Institute technical review on the management of gastroesophageal reflux disease. Gastroenterology. 2008;135:1383–413.

51. Kenneth R, DeVault DOC. Updated guidelines for the diagnosis and treatment of gastroesophageal reflux disease. Am J Gastroenterol. 2005;100:190–200.

52. DeMeester TR, Peters JH, Bremner CG, et al. Biology of gastroesophageal reflux disease: pathophysiology relating to medical and surgical treatment. Annu Rev Med. 1999;50:469–506.

53. Carlsson R, Galmiche JP, Dent J, et al. Prognostic factors influencing relapse of oesophagitis during maintenance therapy with antisecretory drugs: a meta-analysis of long-term omeprazole trials. Aliment Pharmacol Ther. 1997;11:473–82.

54. Fass R, Murthy U, Hayden CW, et al. Omeprazole 40 mg once a day is equally effective as lansoprazole 30 mg twice a day in symptom control of patients with gastro-oesophageal reflux disease (GERD) who are resistant to conventional-dose lansoprazole therapy: a prospective, randomized, multi-centre study. Aliment Pharmacol Ther. 2000;14:1595–603.

55. Spencer J. Prolonged pH recording in the study of gastroesophageal reflux. Br J Surg. 1969;56:9–12.

56. Johnson LF, DeMeester TR. Twenty-four-hour pH monitoring of the distal esophagus. A quantitative measure of gastroesophageal reflux. Am J Gastroenterol. 1974;62:325–32.

57. Hirano I, Richter JE. ACG practice guidelines: esophageal reflux testing. Am J Gastroenterol. 2007;102:668–85.

58. Booth MI, Stratford J, Dehn TCB. Patient self-assessment of test-day symptoms in 24 hour pH metry for suspected gastroesophageal reflux disease. Scand J Gastroenterol. 2001;36:795.

59. McLauchlan G, Rawlings JM, Lucas ML, et al. Electrodes for 24 hour pH monitoring: a comparative study. Gut. 1987;28:935–9.

60. Smout AJPM. Ambulatory monitoring of esophageal pH and pressure. In: Castell DO, Richter JE, editors. The esophagus. 3rd ed. Philadelphia: Lippincott Williams & Wilkins; 1999. p. 119–33.

61. Kahrilas PJ, Quigley EMM. Clinical esophageal pH recording: a technical review for practice guideline development. Gastroenterology. 1996;100:1982–96.

62. McLauchlan G, Rawlings JM, Lucas ML, McCloy RF, Crean GP, McColl KE. Electrodes for 24 hours pH monitoring-a comparative study. Gut. 1987;28:935–9.

63. Kahrilas PJ, Quigley EMM. Clinical esophageal pH recording: a technical review for practice guidelines development. Gastroenterology. 1996;110:1982–96.

64. Chiocca JC, Olmos JA, Salis GB, Soifer LO, Higa R, Marcolongo M. Prevalence, clinical spectrum and atypical symptoms of gastro-oesophageal reflux in Argentina: a nationwide population-based study. Aliment Pharmacol Ther. 2005; 22:331–42.

65. Wenner J, Johnsson F, Johansson J, Oberg S. Wireless esophageal pH monitoring is better tolerated than the catheter-based technique: results from a randomized cross-over trial. Am J Gastroenterol. 2007;102:239–45.

66. Pandolfino JE, Kahrilas JP. Prolonged pH monitoring: Bravo capsule. Gastrointest Endosc Clin N Am. 2005;15:307–18.

67. Tseng D, Rizvi A, Fennerty MB, et al. Forty-eight-hour pH monitoring increases sensitivity in detecting abnormal esophageal acid exposure. J Gastroenterol Surg. 2005;9(8):1043–52.

68. Pandolfino JE, Schreiner MA, Lee TJ, et al. Comparison of the Bravo wireless and Digitrapper catheter-based pH monitoring systems for measuring esophageal acid exposure. Am J Gastroenterol. 2005;100:1466–76.

69. Pandolfino JE, Zhang Q, Schreiner MA, et al. Acid reflux event detection using the Bravo wireless versus the Slimline catheter pH systems: why are the numbers so different? Gut. 2005;54:1687–92.

70. des Varannes SB, Mion F, Ducrotte P, et al. Simultaneous recordings of oesophageal acid exposure with conventional pH monitoring and a wireless system (Bravo). Gut. 2005;54:1682–6.

71. Pandolfino JE, Richter JE, Ours T, et al. Ambulatory esophageal pH monitoring using a wireless system. Am J Gastroenterol. 2003;98:740–9.

72. Richter JE, Bradley LA, DeMeester TR, et al. Normal 24-hr ambulatory esophageal pH values. Influence of study center, pH electrode, age, and gender. Dig Dis Sci. 1992;37:849–56.

73. Wong WM, Bautista J, Dekel R, et al. Feasibility and tolerability of transnasal/peroral placement of the wireless pH capsule vs. traditional 24-h oesophageal pH monitoring: a randomized trial. Aliment Pharmacol Ther. 2005;21:155–63.

74. Sweis R, Fox M, Anggiansah R, et al. Patient acceptance and clinical impact of Bravo monitoring in patients with previously failed catheter-based studies. Aliment Pharmacol Ther. 2009;29:669–76.

75. Fass R. Effect of ambulatory 24-hour esophageal pH monitoring on reflux-provoking activities. Clin Cornerstone. 1999;1:1–17.

76. Prakash C, Jonnalagadda S, Azar R, et al. Endoscopic removal of the wireless pH monitoring capsule in patients with severe discomfort. Gastrointest Endosc. 2006; 64:828–32.

77. Bhat YM, McGrath KM, Bielefeldt K. Wireless esophageal pH monitoring: new technique means new questions. J Clin Gastroenterol. 2006;40:116–21.

78. Charbel S, Khandwala F, Vaezi MF. The role of esophageal pH monitoring in symptomatic patients on PPI therapy. Am J Gastroenterol. 2005;100:283–9.

79. Silny J. Intraluminal multiple electric impedance procedure for measurement of gastrointestinal motility. J Gastrointest Motil. 1991;3:151–62.

80. Sifrim D, Castell D, Dent J, et al. Gastro-oesophageal reflux monitoring: review and consensus report on detection and definitions of acid, non-acid, and gas reflux. Gut. 2004;53:1024–31.

81. Bredenoord AJ, Weusten BL, Curvers WL, et al. Determinants of perception of heartburn and regurgitation. Gut. 2006;55:313–8.

82. Shay S, Tutuian R, Sifrim D, et al. Twenty-four hour ambulatory simultaneous impedance and pH monitoring: a multicenter report of normal values from 60 healthy volunteers. Am J Gastroenterol. 2004;99:1037–43.

83. Zerbib F, Bruley des Barannes S, Roman S, et al. 24 hour ambulatory esophageal multichannel intraluminal impedance-pH in healthy European subjects. Gastroenterology. 2005;128:A396.

84. Sifrim D, Holloway R, Silny J, et al. Acid, nonacid, and gas reflux in patients with gastroesophageal reflux disease during ambulatory 24-hour pH-impedance recordings. Gastroenterology. 2001;120:1588–98.

85. Bredenoord AJ, Weusten BL, Timmer R, et al. Addition of esophageal impedance monitoring to pH monitoring increases the yield of symptom association analysis in patients off PPI therapy. Am J Gastroenterol. 2006;101:453–9.

86. Vela MF, Camacho-Lobato L, Srinivasan R, et al. Simultaneous intraesophageal impedance and pH measurement of acid and nonacid gastroesophageal reflux: effect of omeprazole. Gastroenterology. 2001;120:1599–606.

87. Mainie I, Tutuian R, Shay S, et al. Acid and non-acid reflux in patients with persistent symptoms despite acid suppressive therapy. A multicentre study using combined ambulatory impedance-pH monitoring. Gut. 2006;55:1398–402.

88. Zerbib F, Roman S, Ropert A, et al. Esophageal pH-impedance monitoring and symptom analysis in GERD. A study in patients off and on therapy. Am J Gastroenterol. 2006;101:1956–63.

89. Park W, Vaezi M. Esophageal impedance recording: clinical utility and limitations. Curr Gastroenterol Rep. 2005;7:182–9.

90. Sifrim D, Blondeau K. Technology insight: the role of impedance testing for esophageal disorders. Nat Clin Pract Gastroenterol Hepatol. 2006;3:210–9.

91. Tutuian R, Castell D. Review article complete gastro-oesophageal reflux monitoring — combined pH and impedance. Aliment Pharmacol Ther. 2006;24 Suppl 2:27–37.

92. Agrawal A, Castell D. Clinical importance of impedance measurements. J Clin Gastroenterol. 2008;42:579–83.

93. Bredenoord A, Tutuian R, Andre J, et al. Technology review: esophageal impedance monitoring. Am J Gastroenterol. 2007;102:187–94.

94. Shay S. Esophageal impedance monitoring: the ups and downs of a new test. Am J Gastroenterol. 2004;99:1020–2.

95. Weusten BL, Akkermans LM, vanBerge-Heneggouwen GP, Smout AJ. Spatiotemporal characteristics of physiological gastroesophageal reflux. Am J Physiol. 1994;266: G357–62.

96. Weusten BLAM, Akkermans LMA, Vanberge-Henegouwen GP, et al. Dynamic characteristics of gastro-oesophageal reflux in ambulatory patients with gastro-oesophageal reflux disease and normal control subjects. Scand J Gastroenterol. 1995;30:731–7.

97. Sifrim D. Relevance of volume and proximal extent of reflux in gastro-oesophageal reflux disease. Gut. 2005;54:175–8.

98. Vaezi MF, Schroeder PL, Richter JE. Reproducibility of proximal probe pH parameters in 24-hour ambulatory esophageal pH monitoring. Am J Gastroenterol. 1997;92:825–9.

99. Jacob P, Kahrilas PJ, Herzon G. Proximal esophageal pH-metry in patients with "reflux laryngitis". Gastroenterology. 1991;100:305–10.

100. Ulualp SO, Toohill RJ, Shaker R. Pharyngeal acid reflux in patients with single and multiple otolaryngologic disorders. Otolaryngol Head Neck Surg. 1999;121:725–30.

101. Katz PO. Ambulatory intragastric pH monitoring: clinical laboratory to clinical practice. Rev Gastroenterol Disord. 2003;3 Suppl 4:S3–9.

102. Bell NJ, Burget D, Howden CW, et al. Appropriate acid suppression for the management of gastro-oesophageal reflux disease. Digestion. 1992;50 Suppl 1: 59–67.

103. Fackler WK, Ours TM, Vaezi MF, et al. Long-term effect of H2RA therapy on nocturnal gastric acid breakthrough. Gastroenterology. 2002;122:625–32.

104. Koufman JA. The otolaryngologic manifestations of gastroesophageal reflux disease (GERD) a clinical investigation of 225 patients using ambulatory 24-hour pH monitoring and an experimental investigation of the role of acid and pepsin in the development of laryngeal injury. Laryngoscope. 1991;101:1–78.

105. Shaker R, Milbrath M, Ren J, et al. Esophagopharyngeal distribution of refluxed gastric acid in patients with reflux laryngitis. Gastroenterology. 1995;109:1575–82.

106. Dobhan R, Castell DO. Normal and abnormal proximal esophageal acid exposure results of ambulatory dual-probe pH monitoring. Am J Gastroenterol. 1999;88:25–9.

107. Patti MG, Debas HT, Pellegrini CA. Esophageal manometry and 24-hour pH monitoring in the diagnosis of pulmonary aspiration secondary to gastroesophageal reflux. Am J Surg. 1992;163:401–6.

108. Wilson JA, White A, von Haacke NP, et al. Gastroesophageal reflux and posterior laryngitis. Ann Otol Rhinol Laryngol. 1989;98:405–10.

109. Kuhn J, Toohill RJ, Ulualp SO, et al. Pharyngeal acid reflux events in patients with vocal cord nodules. Laryngoscope. 1998;108:1146–9.
110. Bove M, Ruth M, Cange L, Mansson I. 24-h pharyngeal pH monitoring in healthy volunteersa normative study. Scand J Gastroenterol. 2000;3:234–41.
111. Wiener GJ, Koufman JA, Wu WC, et al. Chronic hoarseness secondary to gastroesophageal reflux disease: documentation with 24-h ambulatory pH monitoring. Am J Gastroenterol. 1989;84:1503–8.
112. Williams RB, Ali GN, Wallace KL, et al. Esophagopharyngeal acid regurgitation: dual pH monitoring criteria for its detection and insights into mechanisms. Gastroenterology. 1999;117:1051–61.
113. Wo JM, Jabbar A, Winstead W, et al. Hypopharyngeal pH monitoring artifact in detection of laryngopharyngeal reflux. Dig Dis Sci. 2002;47:2579–85.
114. Singh S, Bradley LA, Richter JE. Determinants of oesophageal 'alkaline' pH environment in controls and patients with gastro-oesophageal reflux disease. Gut. 1993;34:309–16.
115. Ours TM, Fackler WK, Richter JE, et al. Nocturnal acid breakthrough: clinical significance and correlation with esophageal acid exposure. Am J Gastroenterol. 2003;98:545–50.
116. Vaezi MF, Richter JE. Role of acid and duodenogastroesophageal reflux in gastroesophageal reflux disease. Gastroenterology. 1996;111:1192–9.
117. Singh P, Taylor RH, Colin-Jones DG. Simultaneous two level oesophageal pH monitoring in healthy controls and patients with oesophagitiscomparison between two positions. Gut. 1994;35:304–8.
118. Lacy BE, O'Shana T, Hynes M, et al. Safety and tolerability of transoral Bravo capsule placement after transnasal manometry using a validated conversion factor. Am J Gastroenterol. 2007;102:24–32.
119. McCollough M, Jabbar A, Cacchione R, et al. Proximal sensor data from routine dual-sensor esophageal pH monitoring is often inaccurate. Dig Dis Sci. 2004;49: 1607–11.
120. Walther B, DeMeester T. Placement of the esophageal pH electrode for 24 hour esophageal pH monitoring. In: DeMeester T, Skinner DB, editors. Esophageal disorders: pathophysiology and therapy. New York: Raven; 1985. p. 539–41.
121. Dhiman RK, Saraswat VA, Naik SR. Ambulatory esophageal pH monitoring: technique, interpretations, and clinical indications. Dig Dis Sci. 2002;47:241–50.
122. Dobhan R, Castell DO. Prolonged intraesophageal pH monitoring with 16-hr overnight recording. Comparison with "24-hr" analysis. Dig Dis Sci. 1992;37:857–64.
123. Choiniere L, Miller L, Ilves R, et al. A simplified method of esophageal pH monitoring for assessment of gastroesophageal reflux. Ann Thorac Surg. 1983;36:596–603.
124. Fink SM, McCallum RW. The role of prolonged esophageal pH monitoring in the diagnosis of gastroesophageal reflux. JAMA. 1984;252:1160–4.
125. Galmiche JP, Guillard JF, Denis P, et al. A study of post-prandial oesophageal pH in healthy subjects and in patients with gastro-oesophageal reflux. Diagnostic value of a scoring index of acid reflux. Gastroenterol Clin Biol. 1980;4:531–9.
126. Johnsson F, Joelsson B. Reproducibility of ambulatory oesophageal pH monitoring. Gut. 1988;29:886–9.

127. Dalby K, Nielsen RG, Markoew S, et al. Reproducibility of 24-hour combined multiple intraluminal impedance (MII) and pH measurements in infants and children. Evaluation of a diagnostic procedure for gastroesophageal reflux disease. Dig Dis Sci. 2007;52:2159–65.

128. Dhiman RK, Saraswat VA, Mishra A, et al. Inclusion of supine period in short-duration pH monitoring is essential in diagnosis of gastroesophageal reflux disease. Dig Dis Sci. 1996;41:764–72.

129. Agrawal A, Tutuian R, Hila A, et al. Ingestion of acidic foods mimics gastroesophageal reflux during pH monitoring. Dig Dis Sci. 2005;50:1916–20.

130. Wo JM, Castell DO. Exclusion of meal periods from ambulatory 24-hour pH monitoring may improve diagnosis of esophageal acid reflux. Dig Dis Sci. 1994; 39:1601–7.

131. Furuta T, Shirai N, Watanabe F, et al. Effect of cytochrome P4502C19 genotypic differences on cure rates for gastroesophageal reflux disease by lansoprazole. Clin Pharmacol Ther. 2002;72:453–60.

132. Tutuian R, Vela M, Hill E, et al. Characteristics of symptomatic reflux episodes on acid suppressive therapy. Am J Gastroenterol. 2008;103:1090–6.

133. Zerbib F, Duriez A, Roman S, et al. Determinants of gastro-oesophageal reflux perception in patients with persistent symptoms despite proton pump inhibitors. Gut. 2008;57:156–60.

134. Tamhankar AP, Peters JH, Portale G, et al. Omeprazole does not reduce gastroesophageal reflux: new insights using multichannel intraluminal impedance technology. J Gastrointest Surg. 2004;8:888–96.

135. Smout AJPM. The patient with GORD and chronically recurrent problems. Best Pract Res Clin Gastroenterol. 2007;21:365–78.

136. DeVault KR, Castell DO. Updated guidelines for the diagnosis and treatment of gastroesophageal reflux disease. The Practice Parameters Committee of the American College of Gastroenterology. Am J Gastroenterol. 1999;94:1434–42.

137. Katzka DA, Paoletti V, Leite L, et al. Prolonged ambulatory pH monitoring in patients with persistent gastroesophageal reflux disease symptoms: testing while on therapy identifies the need for more aggressive anti-reflux therapy. Am J Gastroenterol. 1996;91:2110–3.

138. Hirano I, Zhang Q, Pandolfino J, et al. Four-day Bravo pH capsule monitoring with and without proton pump inhibitor therapy. Clin Gastroenterol Hepatol. 2005;3:1083–8.

139. Piper DW, Fenton BH. pH stability and activity curves of pepsin with special reference to their clinical importance. Gut. 1965;6:506–8.

140. Tuttle SG, Rufin F, Bettarello A. The physiology of heartburn. Ann Intern Med. 1961;55:292–300.

141. Johnson LF, DeMeester TR. Twenty four hour pH monitoring of distal esophagus. Am J Gastroenterol. 1974;62:323–32.

142. Wenner J, Johnsson F, Johansson J, et al. Wireless oesophageal pH monitoring: feasibility, safety and normal values in healthy subjects. Scand J Gastroenterol. 2005;40:768–74.

143. Zerbib F, des Varannes SB, Roman S, et al. Normal values and day-to-day variability of 24-h ambulatory oesophageal impedance-pH monitoring in a Belgian-French cohort of healthy subjects. Aliment Pharmacol Ther. 2005;22:1011–21.

144. Weiner GJ, Richter JE, Cooper JB, et al. The Symptom Index: a clinically important parameter of ambulatory 24-hour esophageal pH monitoring. Am J Gastroenterol. 1988;83:358–61.

145. Lam HG, Breumelhof R, Roelofs JM, Van Berge Henegouwen GP, Smout AJ. What is the optimal time window in symptom analysis of 24-hour esophageal pressure and pH data? Dig Dis Sci. 1994;39:402–9.

146. Breumelhof R, Smout AJPM. The Symptom Sensitivity Index: a valuable additional parameter in 24-hour esophageal pH recording. Am J Gastroenterol. 1991;86:160–4.

147. Weusten BL, Roelofs JM, Akkermans LM, et al. The symptom-association probability: an improved method for symptom analysis of 24-hour esophageal pH data. Gastroenterology. 1994;107:1741–5.

148. Taghavi SA, Ghasedi M, Saberi-Firoozi M, et al. Symptom association probability and symptom sensitivity index: preferable but still suboptimal predictors of response to high dose omeprazole. Gut. 2005;54:1067–71.

149. Khan M, Santana J, Donnellan C, Preston C, Moayyedi P. Medical treatments in the short term management of reflux esophagitis. Cochrane Database Syst Rev. 2007;(2):CD003244.

150. Lundell L, Miettinen P, Myrvold HE, et al. Seven-year follow-up of a randomized clinical trial comparing proton-pump inhibition with surgical therapy for reflux oesophagitis. Br J Surg. 2007;94:198–203.

151. Spechler SJ, Lee E, Ahnen D, et al. Long-term outcome of medical and surgical therapies for gastroesophageal reflux disease: follow-up of a randomized controlled trial. JAMA. 2001;285:2331–8.

152. Jackson PG, Gleiber MA, Askari R, et al. Predictors of outcome in 100 consecutive laparoscopic antireflux procedures. Am J Surg. 2001;181:231–5.

153. Moayyedi P, Tally NJ. Gastro-oesophageal reflux disease. Lancet. 2006;367(9528): 2086–100.

154. Cremonini F, Wise J, Moayyedi P, et al. Diagnostic and therapeutic use of proton pump inhibitors in non-cardiac chest pain: a metaanalysis. Am J Gastroenterol. 2005; 100:1226–32.

155. RC Ciriza de los, Garcia ML, Diez HA, et al. Role of stationary esophageal manometry in clinical practice. Manometric results in patients with gastroesophageal reflux, dysphagia or non-cardiac chest pain. Rev Esp Enferm Dig. 2004;96:606–8.

156. Dekel R, Pearson T, Wendel C, et al. Assessment of oesophageal motor function in patients with dysphagia or chest pain—the Clinical Outcomes Research Initiative experience. Aliment Pharmacol Ther. 2003;18:1083–9.

157. Wang WH, Huang JQ, Zheng GF, et al. Is proton pump inhibitor testing an effective approach to diagnose gastroesophageal reflux disease in patients with noncardiac chest pain?: a meta-analysis. Arch Intern Med. 2005;165:1222–8.

158. Vaezi MF, Hicks DM, Abelson TI, et al. Laryngeal signs and symptoms and gastroesophageal reflux disease (GERD): a critical assessment of cause and effect association. Clin Gastroenterol Hepatol. 2003;1:333–44.

159. Field SK, Sutherland LR. Does medical antireflux therapy improve asthma in asthmatics with gastroesophageal reflux?: a critical review of the literature. Chest. 1998;114:275–83.

160. Noordzij JP, Khidr A, Desper E, et al. Correlation of pH probe-measured laryngopharyngeal reflux with symptoms and signs of reflux laryngitis. Laryngoscope. 2002;112:2192–5.

161. Eubanks TR, Omelanczuk PE, Maronian N, et al. Pharyngeal pH monitoring in 222 patients with suspected laryngeal reflux. J Gastrointest Surg. 2001;5:183–90; discussion 190–1.

162. Maldonado A, Diederich L, Castell DO, et al. Laryngopharyngeal reflux identified using a new catheter design: defining normal values and excluding artifacts. Laryngoscope. 2003;113:349–55.

163. Shaker R, Bardan E, Gu C, et al. Intrapharyngeal distribution of gastric acid refluxate. Laryngoscope. 2003;113:1182–91.

164. Ahmed T, Vaezi MF. The role of pH monitoring in extraesophageal gastroesophageal reflux disease. Gastrointest Endosc Clin N Am. 2005;15:319–31.

11. Pharyngeal pH and Impedance Monitoring

Robert T. Kavitt and Michael F. Vaezi

Abstract Gastroesophageal reflux disease is increasingly associated with ear, nose, and throat symptoms, including laryngitis. Recent studies have assessed the increasing role of pharyngeal pH and impedance in the diagnosis of patients with laryngopharyngeal reflux and other disorders thought to be due to supraesophageal reflux of gastric and duodenal contents. Gastroenterology and otolaryngology specialty societies have released various guidelines in recent years addressing diagnostic and therapeutic approaches to these prevalent and often difficult to treat conditions. Further outcome studies are needed to assess the role of pharyngeal impedance and pH monitoring in this group of patients and to determine who might symptomatically benefit from medical or surgical intervention.

Introduction

Most patients with symptoms of gastroesophageal reflux disease (GERD), especially those with extraesophageal symptoms, are treated initially with acid-suppressive therapy; however, many ultimately require diagnostic testing to objectively assess the presence and degree of reflux of gastric contents into the esophagus and potentially the pharynx. Over the last three decades, esophageal function testing for GERD has significantly evolved, with enhanced patient comfort and improvements in the ambulatory nature of testing. Catheters were previously used to assess pH, whereas wireless devices with high sensitivity are now widely utilized. Combined esophageal and hypopharyngeal impedance/ph monitoring now allows detection of various constituents of refluxate and is considered the most sensitive test in the ambulatory arena to assess both acid and non-acid refluxate.

R. Shaker et al. (eds.), *Manual of Diagnostic and Therapeutic Techniques for Disorders of Deglutition*, DOI 10.1007/978-1-4614-3779-6_11, © Springer Science+Business Media New York 2013

Esophageal and hypopharyngeal reflux monitoring is typically conducted in patients with extraesophageal reflux syndrome in whom studies suggest an association between GERD and extraesophageal symptoms. In a population survey study, Locke et al. [1] showed that heartburn and acid regurgitation are significantly associated with chest pain, dysphagia, dyspepsia, and globus sensation. A subsequent VA-based case–control study [2] suggested that erosive esophagitis and esophageal stricture were associated with various extraesophageal symptoms such as sinusitis (OR 1.60; 95 % CI 1.51–1.70), pharyngitis (1.48; 1.15–1.89), aphonia (1.81; 1.18–2.80), and chronic laryngitis (2.01; 1.53–2.63), among others. The authors concluded that patients with reflux esophagitis are at an increased risk of harboring a large variety of extraesophageal signs and symptoms such as sinus, pharyngeal, laryngeal, and pulmonary diseases. As well, reflux of gastroduodenal contents into the laryngopharyngeal region is purported to be a significant cause of reflux-induced laryngitis often referred to as laryngopharyngeal reflux (LPR) [3]. This group of patients often present with symptoms of hoarseness, sore or burning throat, chronic cough, globus, dysphagia, postnasal drip, apnea, laryngospasm, and even laryngeal neoplasm, among other complaints [4–10].

In this chapter, we highlight the role of pharyngeal pH and impedance monitoring in the evaluation of patients with symptoms of extraesophageal reflux. The role of distal esophageal pH and impedance monitoring is not discussed here but is detailed in an accompanying chapter.

Pharyngeal pH Assessment

Esophageal exposure to gastric acidity may be measured by two main types of available devices: the traditional catheter-based pH monitor (Fig. 11.1a) and the wireless pH monitor (Fig. 11.1b). The catheter-based pH monitoring is the prototypical pH device which can be used for quantifying esophageal or hypopharyngeal acid exposure. Hypopharyngeal monitoring using this monitoring system often requires two separate catheters; one catheter positioned with two sensors in the esophagus (distal and proximal) and the second catheter with its sensor positioned at various intervals above the upper esophageal sphincter in the hypopharynx (Fig. 11.1c). Unlike the catheter pH monitoring which provides ambulatory 24-h data, the wireless device provides a continuous 48 h ambulatory monitoring of distal esophageal acid exposure and is better tolerated by most patients [11]. However, the limitation of the wireless device is that the collected data are only for distal esophageal acid exposure. Positioning of a second wireless device in the proximal esophagus is feasible, although controlled studies regarding their safety await confirmation. For obvious feasibility and safety issues, they cannot be used in the hypopharynx. The Restech Dx-pH Measurement System™ (Respiratory Technology Corp., San Diego, CA) is a relatively new device developed to detect acid reflux in the posterior oropharynx [12] (Fig. 11.1d). A nasopharyngeal catheter is utilized to assess pH in liquid or aerosolized droplets. The catheter employs

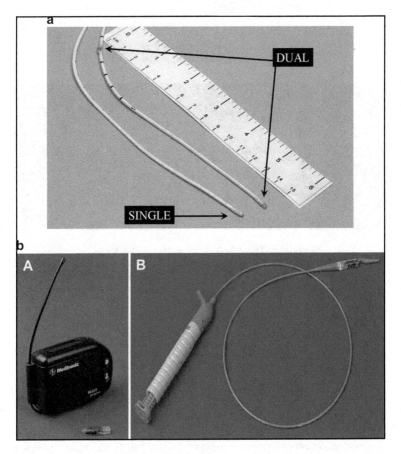

Fig. 11.1. (a) Catheter-based pH monitoring system showing both single sensor (distal esophageal) and dual sensor (distal and proximal esophageal) catheters. (b) Wireless pH capsule and recording device (*left*) and the introducing device (*right*). (c) Catheter-based hypopharyngeal pH catheter showing the position of distal and proximal esophageal as well as the

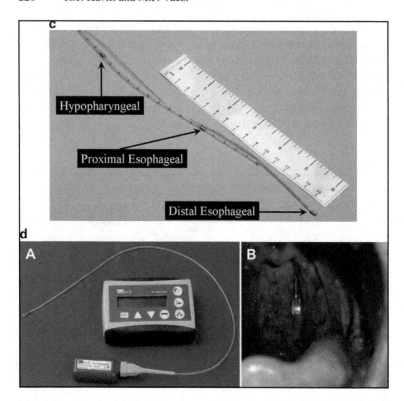

Fig. 11.1. (continued) hypopharyngeal sensors. (**d**) Restech catheter and recording device (*left*) and the oropharyngeal pH probe with transmitter and LED tip in the posterior aspect of the mouth. Figure (**d**) (adapted by permission from Wiley: The Laryngoscope [12], copyright 2009).

a 3.2-mm teardrop tip to aid in insertion and to ensure that the sensor is positioned in the airway. The tip has a colored light emitting diode (LED) for oral visualization. The special circuitry of this device prevents the inclusion of dry-out related "pseudo-reflux" events in the data obtained [13]. A comparison of this device to traditional pH catheters has shown a faster detection rate and a faster time to equilibrium pH. A recent prospective observational study [12] in healthy volunteers developed normative data for this device at a pH cutoff of 4, 5, and 6 for the distal esophagus and oropharynx. Although the initial studies with this device in patients with LPR are encouraging [14], controlled studies are needed to assess the future role of this new device in patients with extraesophageal reflux syndrome including those with LPR.

Clinical studies employing hypopharyngeal pH catheters are usually conducted in patients with suspected extraesophageal manifestations of reflux, such as asthma, laryngitis, chest pain, or cough [15]. Dual (esophageal and hypopharyngeal) pH probe monitoring is reported by some to have discriminatory ability in identifying those with LPR from healthy controls [7]. A meta-analysis of 16 studies involving a total of 793 subjects who underwent 24-h pH monitoring (529 patients with LPR, 264 controls) showed that the number of pharyngeal reflux events for the control group and for LPR patients differed significantly ($p < 0.0001$). The authors concluded that the "upper probe gives accurate and consistent information in normal subjects and patients with LPR" and that the acid exposure time and number of reflux events are most important in distinguishing normal subjects from patients with LPR [16]. However, there is a great degree of variability in the reported prevalence of pH abnormalities in the literature for patients with LPR (Table 11.1). This heterogeneity may be due to different patient populations and nonstandard pH probe placement [15], as some investigators utilized direct laryngoscopy for probe placement, while others utilized esophageal manometry to identify the upper and lower esophageal sphincters.

Current recommendations suggest that the hypopharyngeal probe be placed 1–2 cm above the upper esophageal sphincter as determined by manometry, while the distal and proximal pH probes be placed 5 and 15 cm above the manometric lower esophageal sphincter, respectively [3]. Hypopharyngeal pH catheter placement is more commonly used in research than clinical practice. pH probes in this area are prone to drying and causing an artificial drop in the detected pH (Fig. 11.2).

Measurement of hypopharyngeal pH exposure was initially used to objectively measure laryngeal extension of reflux. Koufman et al. [8] found that 7 of 16 (44 %) patients with laryngeal symptoms had abnormal hypopharyngeal reflux predominately in the upright position. Similarly, later studies by Shaker et al. [17] and Ylitalo et al. [18] using hypopharyngeal pH probes showed increased prevalence of pharyngeal reflux in patients with posterior laryngitis compared with control subjects and GERD patients. In addition another study suggested that hypopharyngeal pH assessment may be useful in conjunction with laryngoscopic findings to identify patients whose symptoms may be due to GERD [19]. In this study, 76 patients with respiratory complaints thought to be related to GERD were divided into three groups based on reflux finding score (RFS) and pharyngeal reflux events. The patients were classified as RFS+, if the score was greater than 7, and pharyngeal reflux positive, if they had greater than one episode of reflux noted during

Table 11.1. Prevalence of abnormal pH monitoring in distal and proximal esophagus and the hypopharynx.

Study, year, (reference)	Proportion of patients with LPR	Number of patients with reflux identified during proximal pH monitoring	Number of patients with reflux identified during distal pH monitoring	Number of patients with reflux identified during hypopharyngeal pH monitoring	Prevalence (%)
Ossakow et al. [40]	43/63	NR	43	NR	68
Koufman et al. [8]	24/32	NR	24	7	75
Wiener et al. [41]	12/15	NR	12	3	80
Wilson et al. [42]	17/97	17	NR	NR	18
Katz [43]	7/10	NR	7	7	70
Woo et al. [44]	20/31	20	20	NR	65
Metz et al. [45]	6/10	?	6	NR	60
Vaezi et al. [46]	21/21	11	21	NR	100
Chen et al. [47]	365/735	NR	229	255	50
Havas et al. [48]	10/15	NR	6	4	67
Ulualp et al. [31]	15/20	15	15	15	75
Smit et al. [49]	7/15	7	3	NR	47
Ulualp et al. [23]	28/39	28	28	28	72
Noordzij et al. [22]	29/42	NR	29	29	69
Park et al. [50]	33/78	20	28	NR	42
Cumulative	637/1,223	46 %	42 %	38 %	52

NR not reported; LPR laryngopharyngeal reflux; ? unclear how many patients tested.

Adapted by permission from Wiley-Blackwell (Kavitt RT, Vaezi MF. Gastroesophageal Reflux Laryngitis. In: Castell DO, Richter JE, eds. The Esophagus. 5th ed. Oxford: Wiley-Blackwell, copyright 2011.

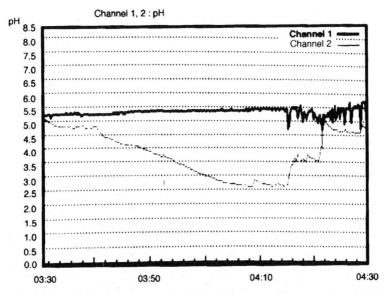

Fig. 11.2. pH tracing with a dual pH sensor (channel 1-esophageal and channel 2-hypopharyngeal) showing "pseudoreflux" due to drying out affect of the hypopharyngeal sensor which mimics a reflux event.

pH assessment. Controls were found to have a significantly lower RFS and fewer episodes of pharyngeal reflux. None of the controls had more than one episode of pharyngeal reflux during a 24-h period. Twenty-one patients had both an abnormal RFS and pharyngeal reflux, and these patients also had significantly higher heartburn scores and acid exposure in the distal esophagus. The authors conclude that agreement between detection of pharyngeal reflux by pH monitoring and an increased RFS greater than 7 help establish or refute the diagnosis of GERD as an etiology of laryngeal symptoms. When both are normal, GERD is most likely not playing a role in a patient's extraesophageal symptoms.

However, the initial enthusiasm about the diagnostic ability of hypopharyngeal reflux monitoring has now been replaced by skepticism. The positioning of the hypopharyngeal pH probe is operator-dependent and varies with regard to placement via direct visualization with laryngoscopy as compared to measurement by manometry [20]. Artifacts (Fig. 11.2) commonly occur and computer-driven interpretations must be manually reviewed [21]. Several studies have found that positive results of pharyngeal testing do not predict a favorable response to anti-reflux therapy [22, 23]. One study showed that the degree of improvement in symptoms among 19 of 27 patients with pharyngeal reflux was similar to the 8 patients not exhibiting pharyngeal reflux [23]. Furthermore, the largest placebo-controlled study to date in patients with LPR did not identify hypopharyngeal pH results as predictor of response to PPI therapy [24]. Additional difficulty in employing hypopharyngeal pH monitoring is that there are no universally accepted diagnostic criteria for abnormal pH in the hypopharynx. The range of normal pH values is not uniformly defined, and can vary from 0 to 4 pH drops less than 4 [22, 25, 26]. Less restrictive pH values, including a drop in pH of 1.0 or 1.5 units instead of 2.0 units, does not differentiate healthy volunteers from patients with suspected ENT complaints [27].

Recent studies evaluating the role of hypopharyngeal pH testing before surgical fundoplication have been conflicting. An earlier study evaluated patients with respiratory symptoms felt secondary to GERD before and after surgery. Patients underwent 24-h pharyngeal pH monitoring, in addition to esophageal manometry, both before and after undergoing laparoscopic Nissen fundoplication [28]. Pharyngeal exposure to acid was deemed abnormal when the pH was less than 4 outside of meal times and occurred at the same time as esophageal acidification. Of 15 patients who underwent pharyngeal pH testing preoperatively, 9 exhibited preoperative evidence of pharyngeal reflux. Fundoplication led to a decrease in pharyngeal reflux (from 7.9 to 1.6 episodes per 24-h period, $p<0.05$) and esophageal exposure to acid (7.5 to 2.1 %, $p<0.05$). Three patients (60 %) with pharyngeal reflux noted improvement of respiratory symptoms and resolved pharyngeal reflux. The authors concluded that an operative approach to GERD is effective at controlling extraesophageal reflux, and observation of pharyngeal reflux based on pH testing assists in identifying which patients with respiratory symptoms would benefit from fundoplication. However, a later prospective concurrent controlled study assessing 72 patients with laryngeal symptoms came to a different conclusion [29]. Patients with LPR refractory after 4 months of aggressive acid suppression (omeprazole 40 mg twice daily or lansoprazole 60 mg twice daily) were asked to undergo fundoplication and those who agreed were symptomatically and objectively followed for 1 year post surgery. Of the 25 patients in the study, 10 underwent fundoplication and 15 continued medical therapy with PPI. All patients had unremarkable pH studies at 3 and 12 months. Only 1/10 (10 %) patients who underwent fundoplication noted improvement in laryngeal symptoms 1 year postoperatively, similar to 1/15 (7 %) patients in the medical therapy group. The authors concluded that fundoplication did not reliably improve laryngeal symptoms among patients unresponsive to PPI therapy.

Thus, at the current time, there is inconclusive evidence that hypopharyngeal pH testing is helpful in the management of patients with extraesophageal reflux symptoms. This is due to complexity of patient presentations, multiple etiologies which may be responsible for patients' presenting symptoms as well as lack of sensitivity for hypopharyngeal pH monitoring.

Pharyngeal Impedance Monitoring

Given the increasing prevalence of partial or non-responders to aggressive acid suppression, "non-acid" or "weakly acid" reflux is implicated in patients' persistent symptoms. Impedance-pH monitoring is now the most sensitive ambulatory esophageal monitoring device which can measure gastric refluxate including gas, liquid, and mixed contents of acidic or non-acidic material into the esophagus or pharynx [27, 30–33]. Impedance refers to the resistance of a medium to the passage of alternating current [34]. Impedance is measured in ohms and is dependent on the characteristics of the medium (whether it is a liquid, solid, gas, or mixed gas/liquid) and on the contact surfaces between substances and electrodes. Air is resistant to current and exhibits a high impedance, while fluid has low resistance and exhibits a low impedance. Esophageal mucosa exhibits an intermediate impedance and serves as a baseline. Using electrodes within the impedance catheter and assessing changes in impedance of adjacent electrode pairs allow a determination of the direction of bolus transit. Abnormal migration of liquid or gas can be detected by the drop or increase in baseline impedance measurements, respectively, and the acidic nature of these events is measured by an integrated pH sensor (Fig. 11.3). The correlation between the acidic and less acidic refluxate and patients' symptoms are then established by either symptom index or symptom association probability [35].

One study found that impedance sensors are able to detect hypopharyngeal volume as small as 0.1 mL and are able to detect acidic liquid, nonacidic liquid, and mist reflux events when combined with a pH sensor [30]. The authors found that in the upright position, placement of the impedance sensor at the proximal margin of the upper esophageal sphincter yielded the greatest detection rate when compared to placement 2 cm proximally. Sensor position did not impact detection rate in the recumbent position. Nonacidic gaseous reflux was simulated by injecting 50 mL of air into the esophagus to induce belching, leading to gas ventilation into the pharynx. Acidic mist was simulated by infusing 0.1 N

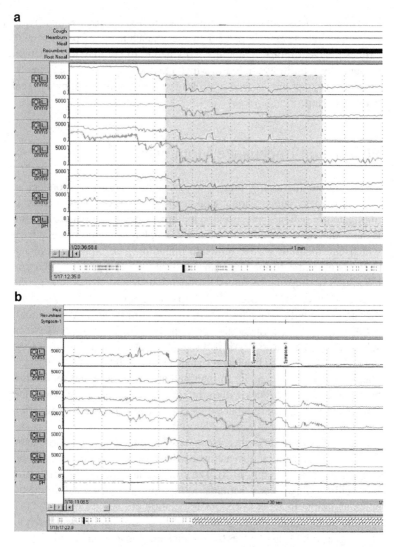

Fig. 11.3. (**a**) Impedance/pH monitoring showing an acidic liquid reflux event migrating to the proximal esophagus in the recumbent position with slow clearance of the acidic refluxate. (**b**) Non-acid liquid and gas reflux to the proximal esophagus associated with patient's report of symptoms.

hydrochloric acid into the esophagus before induction of belching, leading to ventilation of acidic mist. Combined pH impedance and sensors were able to record both acidic and nonacidic liquid and gaseous refluxate into the hypopharynx, highlighting test feasibility.

Another study assessed 24-h pharyngoesophageal impedance and pH monitoring of 31 patients, including 11 patients with GERD, 10 patients with reflux-attributed laryngitis, and 10 controls [33]. It was found that recording both impedance and pH values allows for the detection of significantly more reflux events in the pharynx than pH monitoring alone. The majority of these reflux events involve gaseous reflux, and those with weak acidity were more common among those with laryngeal lesions attributed to reflux compared to those with GERD and controls. This study implied that the pathophysiology of laryngeal signs and symptoms in LPR may be due to weakly acidic gaseous material which would not be detected by pH testing alone.

In order to further understand the impedance measurement findings in GERD and LPR, a study characterized pharyngeal impedance changes during patient-perceived belching events [36]. The authors evaluated 453 belch events in 11 patients with GERD, 10 patients with laryngitis attributed to GERD, and 16 controls. They found that in 15 % of belch events, impedance changes in the pharynx preceded the beginning of the impedance change in the proximal esophagus. In 12 % of events, these impedance changes occurred simultaneously, while in 73 % the pharyngeal impedance changes occurred after the proximal esophageal impedance change. A unique impedance signature was found for pharyngeal ventilation of gaseous contents from the stomach. This study helped better understand the physiologic impedance response of different group of patients to belching events. However, the clinical significance of abnormal impedance findings is as of yet uncertain given limited outcome data.

National Society Guidelines

The 2008 American Gastroenterological Association (AGA) Technical Review on the management of GERD suggested that the role of pH or impedance-pH monitoring in diagnosing extraesophageal reflux is controversial and unproven (Table 11.2) [37]. This evidence-based technical review concludes that the value of a negative pH or impedance-pH study is of greater clinical utility and states "In the absence of troublesome esophageal symptoms or endoscopic findings, with a failed 8-week therapeutic trial of twice-daily PPI therapy, and with normal esophageal acid exposure (PPI therapy withheld) on 24-h monitoring, one has gone as far as currently possible to rule out GERD as a significant contributor to these nonspecific syndromes. Such patients should have etiologies other than GERD explored" [37].

Table 11.2. Summary of AGA, AAOHNS, and ACG guidelines regarding pH testing and treatment modalities for patients with suspected LPR.

	AGA	AAOHNS	ACG
	American Gastroenterological Association Institute Technical Review on the Management of Gastroesophageal Reflux Disease, 2008 [37]	**Laryngopharyngeal Reflux: Position statement of the Committee on Speech, Voice, and Swallowing Disorders of the American Academy of Otolaryngology-Head and Neck Surgery, 2002 [38]**	**American College of Gastroenterology Practice Guidelines: Esophageal Reflux Testing, 2007 [20]**
pH testing	Role of pH or impedance-pH monitoring in diagnosing extraesophageal reflux is controversial and unproven	Diagnosis of LPR can be made based on symptoms and laryngeal findings, but ambulatory 24-h double-probe pH assessment is considered the gold standard diagnostic tool	"The accumulating data seriously question the clinical usefulness of esophageal or hypopharyngeal pH monitoring in the initial evaluation of patients with suspected acid-related ENT complaints"
	"In the absence of trouble some esophageal symptoms or endoscopic findings, with a failed 8-week therapeutic trial of twice-daily PPI therapy, and with normal esophageal acid exposure (PPI therapy withheld) on 24-h monitoring, one has gone as far as currently possible to rule out GERD as a significant contributor to these nonspecific syndromes. Such patients should have etiologies other than GERD explored"	Barium esophagraphy or esophagoscopy provide far less sensitive assessments of LPR, but may be advisable for screening of the esophagus for related pathology	"Studies using impedance pH monitoring in patients with extraesophageal symptoms unresponsive to PPI therapy show little evidence of nonacid reflux, except in the chronic cough patient"

| Treatment | Empiric therapy with twice-daily PPI for 2 months for patients with concomitant esophageal GERD syndrome and laryngitis remains a pragmatic clinical strategy. (USPSTF grade B, quality fair)

Do not support use of once- or twice-daily PPIs (or H$_2$RAs) for acute treatment of potential extra-esophageal GERD syndromes, including laryngitis and asthma, in absence of esophageal GERD. (USPSTF grade D, quality fair)

"Step-down therapy should be attempted in all patients with extraesophageal reflux syndromes after empirical twice-daily PPI therapy. Continuing maintenance PPI therapy should be predicated on either the requirements of therapy for concomitant esophageal GERD syndromes or extraesophageal syndrome symptom response. In both cases, maintenance therapy should be with the lowest PPI dose necessary for adequate symptom relief" | Treatment for LPR needs to be more aggressive and prolonged than that for GERD and depends on symptoms and severity of LPR and on response to therapy

Mild or intermittent LPR symptoms can be treated with dietary and lifestyle changes and H2-antagonists, while the majority of patients require at least twice-daily PPI (minimum of 6 months)

Fundoplication has been shown to be effective | "The practical and popular approach is an empiric trial with a BID PPI regimen for several months, reserving pH testing for patients with persistent symptoms. However, here again, the results of acid pH testing have limited clinical utility" |
|---|---|---|---|

Adapted by permission from Wiley-Blackwell (Kavitt RT, Vaezi MF. Gastroesophageal Reflux Laryngitis. In: Castell DO, Richter JE, eds. *The Esophagus.* 5th ed. Oxford: Wiley-Blackwell), copyright 2011.

This conclusion is in direct contrast to guidelines published by The American Academy of Otolaryngology-Head and Neck Surgery (AAOHNS) Committee on Speech, Voice, and Swallowing Disorders. The authors of the AAOHNS guidelines state that LPR can be diagnosed based on symptoms or laryngeal findings, but ambulatory 24-h double-probe (simultaneous esophageal and pharyngeal) pH assessment is considered the gold standard diagnostic tool (Table 11.2) [38]. They also suggested that barium esophagography or esophagoscopy provide far less sensitive assessments of LPR, but may be advisable for screening of the esophagus for related pathology [7, 38, 39]. However, in line with the AGA guidelines, the American College of Gastroenterology (ACG) Practice Guidelines [20] suggested that pH testing may not be the gold standard diagnostic test in this group of patients (Table 11.2). The authors refer to data indicating that the overall pre-therapy prevalence of an abnormal pH test in a population with chronic laryngeal symptoms is 53 % with the prevalence of excessive distal, proximal, and hypopharyngeal acid exposure being 42, 44, and 38 %, respectively [15], suggesting that this population may have abnormal reflux symptoms, but does not prove causality. In support of the ACG and AGA guidelines, a placebo-controlled study of 145 patients with suspected GERD-related ENT symptoms treated with high-dose esomeprazole or placebo for 16 weeks found that degree of symptomatic or laryngeal involvement was independent of pre-therapy pH findings and that neither esophageal nor hypopharyngeal acid reflux predicted a response to PPI use [24].

Summary

pH or impedance-pH studies can serve as diagnostic tools in patients whose symptoms are refractory to an empiric trial of PPIs. Hypopharyngeal pH or impedance monitoring are valuable tools in assessing continued acid or non-acid reflux in this group of patients. However, at the current time the data are limited by the observational nature of the studies and outcome data await multicenter trial. In this setting, the role of pH or impedance testing in patients refractory to PPI therapy is often to *rule out* reflux of any type (acid, non-acid, liquid, or gas). If these tests are normal on PPI therapy despite persistence of symptoms, other etiologies for abnormal laryngeal signs and symptoms should be investigated [3]. The value of a positive pH or impedance testing is as of yet unknown. In the infrequent cases of abnormal test results on therapy, clinical judgment should be exercised regarding the role of surgical fundoplication given the lack of controlled studies in this area. However, it is prudent to remember that patients with suspected extraesophageal GERD syndromes including those with LPR may have GERD as a contributing etiology, but rarely as the sole cause of their complaints [37]. Until we have better outcome data, initial empiric therapy with twice-daily PPI for 2 months is a reasonable starting point for patients with suspected extraesophageal reflux syndrome.

Key Points

- Pharyngeal pH and impedance monitoring are playing an increasing role in the diagnosis of patients with extraesophageal reflux syndrome.
- In patients who remain symptomatic despite aggressive acid-suppressive therapy, it is uncertain if non-acid reflux plays a significant role in their symptoms. However, the combination of impedance and pH monitoring allows for distinction between acid, weakly acidic, and weakly alkaline reflux in this group.
- Further outcome studies are needed to assess the role of impedance and pH monitoring in the pharynx in those remaining symptomatic despite PPI therapy.

References

1. Locke III GR, Talley NJ, Fett SL, Zinsmeister AR, Melton III LJ. Prevalence and clinical spectrum of gastroesophageal reflux: a population-based study in Olmsted County, Minnesota. Gastroenterology. 1997;112(5):1448–56.
2. el-Serag HB, Sonnenberg A. Comorbid occurrence of laryngeal or pulmonary disease with esophagitis in United States military veterans. Gastroenterology. 1997;113(3): 755–60.
3. Vaezi MF, Hicks DM, Abelson TI, Richter JE. Laryngeal signs and symptoms and gastroesophageal reflux disease (GERD): a critical assessment of cause and effect association. Clin Gastroenterol Hepatol. 2003;1(5):333–44.
4. Gaynor EB. Otolaryngologic manifestations of gastroesophageal reflux. Am J Gastroenterol. 1991;86(7):801–8.
5. Graser A. Gastroesophageal reflux and laryngeal symptoms. Aliment Pharmacol Ther. 1994;8:265–72.

6. Koufman J, Sataloff RT, Toohill R. Laryngopharyngeal reflux: consensus conference report. J Voice. 1996;10(3):215–6.

7. Koufman JA. The otolaryngologic manifestations of gastroesophageal reflux disease (GERD): a clinical investigation of 225 patients using ambulatory 24-hour pH monitoring and an experimental investigation of the role of acid and pepsin in the development of laryngeal injury. Laryngoscope. 1991;101(4 Pt 2 Suppl 53):1–78.

8. Koufman JA, Wallace CW, et al. Reflux laryngitis and its sequela. J Voice. 1988;2:78–9.

9. Richter JE. Typical and atypical presentations of gastroesophageal reflux disease. The role of esophageal testing in diagnosis and management. Gastroenterol Clin North Am. 1996;25(1):75–102.

10. Toohill RJ, Kuhn JC. Role of refluxed acid in pathogenesis of laryngeal disorders. Am J Med. 1997;103(5A):100S–6S.

11. Pandolfino JE, Richter JE, Ours T, Guardino JM, Chapman J, Kahrilas PJ. Ambulatory esophageal pH monitoring using a wireless system. Am J Gastroenterol. 2003;98(4): 740–9.

12. Sun G, Muddana S, Slaughter JC, et al. A new pH catheter for laryngopharyngeal reflux: normal values. Laryngoscope. 2009;119(8):1639–43.

13. Hong SK, Vaezi MF. Gastroesophageal reflux monitoring: pH (catheter and capsule) and impedance. Gastrointest Endosc Clin N Am. 2009;19(1):1–22; v.

14. Wiener GJ, Tsukashima R, Kelly C, et al. Oropharyngeal pH monitoring for the detection of liquid and aerosolized supraesophageal gastric reflux. J Voice. 2009;23(4): 498–504.

15. Ahmed T, Vaezi MF. The role of pH monitoring in extraesophageal gastroesophageal reflux disease. Gastrointest Endosc Clin N Am. 2005;15(2):319–31.

16. Merati AL, Lim HJ, Ulualp SO, Toohill RJ. Meta-analysis of upper probe measurements in normal subjects and patients with laryngopharyngeal reflux. Ann Otol Rhinol Laryngol. 2005;114(3):177–82.

17. Shaker R, Milbrath M, Ren J, et al. Esophagopharyngeal distribution of refluxed gastric acid in patients with reflux laryngitis. Gastroenterology. 1995;109(5): 1575–82.

18. Ylitalo R, Lindestad PA, Ramel S. Symptoms, laryngeal findings, and 24-hour pH monitoring in patients with suspected gastroesophago-pharyngeal reflux. Laryngoscope. 2001;111(10):1735–41.

19. Oelschlager BK, Eubanks TR, Maronian N, et al. Laryngoscopy and pharyngeal pH are complementary in the diagnosis of gastroesophageal-laryngeal reflux. J Gastrointest Surg. 2002;6(2):189–94.

20. Hirano I, Richter JE. ACG practice guidelines: esophageal reflux testing. Am J Gastroenterol. 2007;102(3):668–85.

21. Wo JM, Jabbar A, Winstead W, Goudy S, Cacchione R, Allen JW. Hypopharyngeal pH monitoring artifact in detection of laryngopharyngeal reflux. Dig Dis Sci. 2002; 47(11):2579–85.

22. Noordzij JP, Khidr A, Desper E, Meek RB, Reibel JF, Levine PA. Correlation of pH probe-measured laryngopharyngeal reflux with symptoms and signs of reflux laryngitis. Laryngoscope. 2002;112(12):2192–5.

23. Ulualp SO, Toohill RJ, Shaker R. Outcomes of acid suppressive therapy in patients with posterior laryngitis. Otolaryngol Head Neck Surg. 2001;124(1):16–22.

24. Vaezi MF, Richter JE, Stasney CR, et al. Treatment of chronic posterior laryngitis with esomeprazole. Laryngoscope. 2006;116(2):254–60.

25. Eubanks TR, Omelanczuk PE, Maronian N, Hillel A, Pope CE 2nd, Pellegrini CA. Pharyngeal pH monitoring in 222 patients with suspected laryngeal reflux. J Gastrointest Surg. 2001;5(2):183–90; discussion 190–1.

26. Maldonado A, Diederich L, Castell DO, Gideon RM, Katz PO. Laryngopharyngeal reflux identified using a new catheter design: defining normal values and excluding artifacts. Laryngoscope. 2003;113(2):349–55.

27. Shaker R, Bardan E, Gu C, Kern M, Torrico L, Toohill R. Intrapharyngeal distribution of gastric acid refluxate. Laryngoscope. 2003;113(7):1182–91.

28. Oelschlager BK, Eubanks TR, Oleynikov D, Pope C, Pellegrini CA. Symptomatic and physiologic outcomes after operative treatment for extraesophageal reflux. Surg Endosc. 2002;16(7):1032–6.

29. Swoger J, Ponsky J, Hicks D, et al. Surgical fundoplication in laryngopharyngeal reflux unresponsive to aggressive acid suppression: a controlled study. Clin Gastroenterol Hepatol. 2006;4(4):433.e431–41.

30. Aslam M, Bajaj S, Easterling C, et al. Performance and optimal technique for pharyngeal impedance recording: a simulated pharyngeal reflux study. Am J Gastroenterol. 2007; 102(1):33–9.

31. Ulualp SO, Toohill RJ, Hoffmann R, Shaker R. Pharyngeal pH monitoring in patients with posterior laryngitis. Otolaryngol Head Neck Surg. 1999;120(5):672–7.

32. Sifrim D, Dupont L, Blondeau K, Zhang X, Tack J, Janssens J. Weakly acidic reflux in patients with chronic unexplained cough during 24 hour pressure, pH, and impedance monitoring. Gut. 2005;54(4):449–54.

33. Kawamura O, Aslam M, Rittmann T, Hofmann C, Shaker R. Physical and pH properties of gastroesophagopharyngeal refluxate: a 24-hour simultaneous ambulatory impedance and pH monitoring study. Am J Gastroenterol. 2004;99(6):1000–10.

34. Ciriza-de-Los-Rios C, Canga-Rodriguez-Valcarcel F. High-resolution manometry and impedance-pH/manometry: novel techniques for the advancement of knowledge on esophageal function and their clinical role. Rev Esp Enferm Dig. 2009; 101(12): 861–9.

35. Bredenoord AJ, Weusten BL, Smout AJ. Symptom association analysis in ambulatory gastro-oesophageal reflux monitoring. Gut. 2005;54(12):1810–7.

36. Kawamura O, Bajaj S, Aslam M, Hofmann C, Rittmann T, Shaker R. Impedance signature of pharyngeal gaseous reflux. Eur J Gastroenterol Hepatol. 2007;19(1):65–71.

37. Kahrilas PJ, Shaheen NJ, Vaezi MF. American Gastroenterological Association Institute technical review on the management of gastroesophageal reflux disease. Gastroenterology. 2008;135(4):1392–413; 1413 e1391–5.

38. Koufman JA, Aviv JE, Casiano RR, Shaw GY. Laryngopharyngeal reflux: position statement of the committee on speech, voice, and swallowing disorders of the American Academy of Otolaryngology-Head and Neck Surgery. Otolaryngol Head Neck Surg. 2002;127(1):32–5.

39. Belafsky PC, Postma GN, Daniel E, Koufman JA. Transnasal esophagoscopy. Otolaryngol Head Neck Surg. 2001;125(6):588–9.

40. Ossakow SJ, Elta G, Colturi T, Bogdasarian R, Nostrant TT. Esophageal reflux and dysmotility as the basis for persistent cervical symptoms. Ann Otol Rhinol Laryngol. 1987;96(4):387–92.

41. Wiener GJ, Koufman JA, Wu WC, Cooper JB, Richter JE, Castell DO. Chronic hoarseness secondary to gastroesophageal reflux disease: documentation with 24-h ambulatory pH monitoring. Am J Gastroenterol. 1989;84(12):1503–8.

42. Wilson JA, White A, von Haacke NP, et al. Gastroesophageal reflux and posterior laryngitis. Ann Otol Rhinol Laryngol. 1989;98(6):405–10.

43. Katz PO. Ambulatory esophageal and hypopharyngeal pH monitoring in patients with hoarseness. Am J Gastroenterol. 1990;85(1):38–40.

44. Woo P, Noordzij P, Ross JA. Association of esophageal reflux and globus symptom: comparison of laryngoscopy and 24-hour pH manometry. Otolaryngol Head Neck Surg. 1996;115(6):502–7.

45. Metz DC, Childs ML, Ruiz C, Weinstein GS. Pilot study of the oral omeprazole test for reflux laryngitis. Otolaryngol Head Neck Surg. 1997;116(1):41–6.

46. Vaezi MF, Schroeder PL, Richter JE. Reproducibility of proximal probe pH parameters in 24-hour ambulatory esophageal pH monitoring. Am J Gastroenterol. 1997; 92(5):825–9.

47. Chen MY, Ott DJ, Casolo BJ, Moghazy KM, Koufman JA. Correlation of laryngeal and pharyngeal carcinomas and 24-hour pH monitoring of the esophagus and pharynx. Otolaryngol Head Neck Surg. 1998;119(5):460–2.

48. Havas T, Huang S, Levy M, et al. Posterior pharyngolaryngitis: double-blind randomised placebo-controlled trial of proton pump inhibitor therapy. J Otolaryngol. 1999;3:243.

49. Smit CF, Copper MP, van Leeuwen JA, Schoots IG, Stanojcic LD. Effect of cigarette smoking on gastropharyngeal and gastroesophageal reflux. Ann Otol Rhinol Laryngol. 2001;110(2):190–3.

50. Park W, Hicks DM, Khandwala F, et al. Laryngopharyngeal reflux: prospective cohort study evaluating optimal dose of proton-pump inhibitor therapy and pretherapy predictors of response. Laryngoscope. 2005;115(7):1230–8.

Part III
Management of Oral Pharyngeal Dysphagia in Adults

12. Oropharyngeal Strengthening and Rehabilitation of Deglutitive Disorders

Jacqueline A. Hind and JoAnne Robbins

Abstract This chapter provides an overview of the theory and evidence supporting oropharyngeal strengthening therapy for dysphagia rehabilitation based in principles of exercise, sensorimotor learning and neuromuscular functional interrelationships in the oropharynx. Comprehensive information is provided on anatomy and physiology of the tongue and related musculature/structures as well as therapeutic outcomes with healthy elders and specific patient populations including patients post-stroke and those with head and neck cancer. Strengthening protocol parameters such as frequency, repetition and duration are reviewed relative to published evidence as well as a side-by-side comparison of available devices for facilitation of oropharyngeal strengthening. Dysphagia therapy historically has focused on compensatory and dietary modification. While still useful options, evidence provided in this chapter supports the concept that patients with dysphagia caused, at least in part, by oropharyngeal weakness that complete progressive oropharyngeal strengthening exercises are capable of making significant gains in swallowing kinematics with associated improvements in bolus flow, safety and quality of life.

Introduction

Oromotor exercises have been widely used as a treatment modality in the practice of speech pathology for many decades [1]. However only in recent years have oropharyngeal *strengthening* exercises been applied to swallowing rehabilitation as several studies support their effectiveness [2–5]. As these therapeutic interventions are relatively new, they continue to be researched in order to elucidate the benefit to the patient's

R. Shaker et al. (eds.), *Manual of Diagnostic and Therapeutic Techniques for Disorders of Deglutition*, DOI 10.1007/978-1-4614-3779-6_12,
© Springer Science+Business Media New York 2013

swallowing function, as well as to better understand the neural and anatomic underpinnings which contribute to positive patient outcomes.

Anatomy and Physiology of the Tongue

The tongue often is the primary focus of oropharyngeal exercise because of the important role it plays in swallowing function and accessibility. The tongue is in a class of structures with unique biomechanical properties; that is, the tongue is composed entirely of muscle and lacks a stabilizing skeletal system to confine movement. As a muscular hydrostat, the tongue is incompressible as it is able to decrease in size in one dimension while creating a compensatory increase in size in at least one other dimension [6].

The tongue comprises four intrinsic muscles which include: the superior and inferior longitudinal, verticalis, and transversalis. The intrinsic muscles can alter the shape of the tongue by lengthening and shortening, curling and uncurling the apex and edges, as well as flattening and rounding the surface. In addition to the intrinsic muscles, there are four paired extrinsic muscles; the palatoglossus, hyoglossus, styloglossus, and genioglossus. The extrinsic muscles work together to protrude, retract, depress, and elevate the tongue [7].

Research studies to date have focused primarily on strengthening of the anterior and posterior tongue muscles in isolation or simultaneously. Systematic study evaluating isolated and simultaneous tongue muscle strengthening provides an understanding of the functional role of the anterior tongue vs. the posterior tongue and their distinct roles in swallowing. The anterior tongue acts as a critical anchor for positioning of lingual musculature during bolus formation and oral transit. In contrast, the posterior tongue or the tongue base has an important role in bolus propulsion into the pharynx. This complex organization and function of oropharyngeal swallowing and more specifically, the tongue muscles, is mediated by a widely distributed sensorimotor neural circuitry involving both cerebral hemispheres and the corticobulbar tracts in communication with the pons and medulla [8].

Cranial nerves play an important role in successful anterior and posterior tongue deglutitive function. The trigeminal nerve provides the sensory input to the anterior two-thirds of the tongue while the glossopharyngeal nerve provides the sensory input to the posterior third of the tongue. Tongue movement is integral in bolus manipulation and propulsion. Tongue base retraction, an essential component of bolus propulsion, is controlled by the medullary swallowing centers [7]. In contrast, the anterior two-thirds of the tongue is predominantly under volitional control, while the posterior one-third of the tongue coordinates with the pharyngeal response and is programmed by the brain stem central pattern generator. The differential understanding and diagnostic determination of whether a disorder involves responses that are volitional vs. reflexive is critical as the clinician designs therapeutic interventions that are appropriate and will result in improved functional outcomes.

Neuromuscular Functional Interrelationships in the Oropharynx

Lingual strengthening exercise has been found to result in positive physiologic change to other functions within the oropharynx thus improving deglutition. Palmer et al. evaluated the relationship between tongue-to-palate pressure and electromyographic (EMG) activity elicited during the tongue-to-palate pressure from the mylohyoid, anterior belly of the digastric, geniohyoid, medial pterygoid, velum, genioglossus, and intrinsic tongue muscles [9]. Increased EMG activation of the floor-of-mouth, tongue, and jaw closing muscles was reported with greater tongue-to-palate pressure. The floor-of-mouth muscles have an insertion point on the hyoid bone. The findings of this study found that suprahyoid muscle activation increased with greater tongue-to-palate pressure generation. Generalizing from the Palmer et al. study, tasks that generate greater tongue-to-palate pressure may strengthen weakened suprahyoid muscles. Strengthened suprahyoid muscles results in improved anterior hyolaryngeal excursion and greater anteroposterior deglutitive upper esophageal sphincter opening. The findings of this study support the use of a tongue-to-palate press exercise to strengthen the intrinsic tongue muscles and the muscles of the floor-of-mouth and jaw [9].

Principles of Exercise

Neuroplasticity refers to the ability of the brain and nervous system to change structurally and functionally. The change may occur because of input from many sources including the environment or as in the case of rehabilitation protocols, systematically designed exercise, that may facilitate neuroplastic alteration [10].

Table 12.1. Principles of neural plasticity, adapted from Kleim and Jones [11].

Principle	Description
Use it or lose it	Failure to drive specific brain functions can lead to degradation
Use it and improve it	Training that drives a brain function can lead to an enhancement of the function
Specificity[a]	The nature of the training experience dictates the nature of the plasticity
Repetition[a]	Induction of plasticity requires sufficient repetition
Intensity[a]	Induction of plasticity requires sufficient training intensity
Time	Different forms of plasticity occur at different times during training
Salience	The training experience must be sufficiently salient to induce plasticity
Age	Training-induced plasticity occurs more readily in younger brains
Transference	Plasticity in response to one training experience can enhance acquisition of similar behaviors
Interference	Plasticity in response to one experience can interfere with acquisition of other behaviors

[a]Three principles studied recently relative to rehabilitation of swallowing.

Ten principles of neuroplasticity have been identified by Kleim and Jones [11] (Table 12.1). These principles are reflected in research design and rehabilitation regimens applied to treatment of the limbs and in retraining locomotion. These principles have not been systematically studied in relation to human deglutition and its disorders. Three of the principles, repetition, intensity, and specificity, have been applied only recently to research studying the most efficient and effective treatments for rehabilitation of swallowing disorders.

Nudo et al. [12] and Kilgard and Merzenich [13] and others have illustrated the importance of repetition in inducing change. Regimens requiring systematic repetition, that is, defined as progressive repetitive isometric lingual exercise will result in positive change of swallow function. Determination of the number of repetitions performed in exercise protocols for swallow rehabilitation is based on exercise progression and regimens used in sports medicine research usually focused on striated corticospinal innervated musculature (e.g., lower extremity) [2, 3, 14]. Further research is needed to identify the optimal number of repetitions for exercise specific to rehabilitation of swallowing disorders.

The second principle, intensity of swallowing exercise, is important as it may impact swallowing rehabilitation outcomes [15, 16]. There appears to be a threshold of intensity consistent with the overload principle which when reached will result in muscle strengthening, tissue adaptation, and neural changes [13, 17]. Ironically, there is also the possibility of excitotoxicity which occurs when there is too great a level of stimulation. Excitotoxicity is the pathological process by which nerve cells are damaged by excessive stimulation by neurotransmitters [18]. Therefore, identifying the optimal exercise intensity level is critical in development of an exercise as well as in performance monitoring so as to insure improvement of the disorder.

And finally, specificity refers to directed exercise that results in changes to the targeted area or function. Specificity refers to change to the neural substrates involved only in the targeted behavior and implies little to no transference (another principle) to other behaviors (Table 12.1) [11].

Principles of Motor Learning and Rehabilitation of Deglutition

Schmidt and Wrisberg define motor learning as "the changes associated with practice or experience, in internal processes that determine a person's capability for producing a motor skill [19]." It is important to make a distinction between performance during acquisition (i.e., while exercising) and performance during retention/transfer (i.e., carryover to swallowing) [20].

Generalization refers to practice of one movement that carries over to related but untrained movement. An example of generalization would be isometric tongue strengthening exercise training affecting the tongue pressure generated during swallowing.

One aspect of motor learning that has received much attention is feedback [21]. Two types of feedback to consider in treatment are knowledge of performance and knowledge of results.

Knowledge of performance refers to feedback provided by the clinician that delivers specific information regarding accuracy of the movement performed by the patient or participant. This includes providing a correction to the specific movement such as "your tongue needs to press harder in front." Knowledge of results refers to the feedback from the clinician regarding overall performance such as "That wasn't correct, try it again." Some experts suggest that knowledge of performance is more appropriate in early treatment phases and knowledge of results more appropriate as the patient or participant gains some control [21]. The therapeutic goal is to develop intrinsic patient feedback and self-monitoring.

There is a risk to providing too much or too little external feedback. If too little is provided, the patient may fail to make progress because the system is not currently providing them with sufficient external feedback. If too much feedback is provided, the patient will not be taxed sufficiently to develop internal feedback loops and will possibly fail to take over the responsibility for independent processing. Several studies have compared outcomes from generalized motor program (GMP) learning between groups receiving various feedback frequency regimens (50 % vs.100 %). Reduced frequency of presentation regarding knowledge of results repeatedly has been associated with increased motor learning [22]. More research is needed to determine the optimal feedback type and frequency specific to oropharyngeal strengthening [20, 23, 24].

Oropharyngeal Strengthening in Healthy Adults: Effect of Isometric Lingual Exercise

Isometric lingual strengthening exercise is defined as active exercise performed against stable resistance, without change in the length of the muscle [25]. Strength is based on the ability to exert a force. Strength training requires high loads and low repetition, whereas progressive resistance entails periodically increasing the load. The outcome is manipulated with progressive loads and static repetitions.

Lazarus and colleagues examined the effects of two types of tongue strengthening exercises in a group of 31 healthy young subjects. Subjects were randomized to one of three groups: (1) no exercise; (2) 4 weeks of tongue strengthening exercises using a tongue depressor, or (3) 4 weeks of tongue strengthening exercises compressing an air-filled bulb between the tongue and hard palate using the Iowa Oral Performance Instrument (IOPI). Results revealed significantly greater maximum tongue strength in the groups that received lingual strengthening treatment compared with the group receiving no treatment and similar results between both exercise groups [4]. The results of this study pose the question of whether employing an exercise device is necessary for improved lingual strengthening. That is, is a device as effective or more effective in producing improved functional outcome when compared to a "low-tech" instrument such as a tongue blade? While certainly more cost-effective, the tongue blade provides no feedback or knowledge of performance to the patient allowing patient performance to be below the target goal.

Further discussion regarding the advantages and limitations of various exercise device options can be found in the "Devices" section.

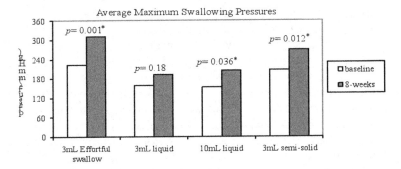

Fig. 12.1. Swallowing pressure changes after 8 weeks of progressive isometric lingual exercises. Adapted from Robbins et al. [2], with permission from John Wiley & Sons.

Robbins and colleagues enrolled ten older, non-dysphagic healthy men and women between the ages of 70 and 89 to complete 8-weeks of progressive lingual resistance exercises using the IOPI [2]. In addition to measuring isometric pressures at baseline and weeks 2, 4, and 6, pressure measurements during swallowing were collected and measurements of pre- and post-exercise lingual volume from magnetic resonance imaging (MRI) were completed. All subjects showed significant increase in isometric pressures and an increase in pressures generated during swallowing (Fig. 12.1). Pressures increased steadily from Week 1 to Week 6, indicating that no less than 6 weeks of exercise would have produced the extent of pressure gain achieved by this group. Additionally, the subset of patients who were able to complete the MRI demonstrated increased lingual volume of an average of 5.1 % suggesting muscle hypertrophy. Mean inter-rater measurement error was determined to be 1.2 % by repeating measures on 5 scans. Repeatability of measures taken from multiple scans for lingual volume was 0.22 %.

Clark and colleagues studied 39 healthy adults (mean age: 38 years) who completed three types of isometric lingual exercises: lingual elevation, protrusion, and lateralization [5]. Subjects completed 30 repetitions of a 1 sec push every day for 9 weeks. A portion of the subjects ($n=29$) were assigned to complete the three exercises sequentially (3 weeks of lingual elevation followed by 3 weeks of lingual protrusion and 3 weeks of lingual lateralization exercises), while the remaining subjects ($n=10$) were assigned to complete the exercises concurrently (one set of ten repetitions of each exercise daily). Significant increases in strength were observed for all three lingual exercise routines, although the increase was greater with lingual elevation exercise compared to protrusion or lateralization regimens. Post-training strength was the same for sequential vs. concurrent training protocols.

A study conducted by Steele sought to define tongue resistance training tasks that produced tongue pressure waveform characteristics most closely resembling bolus swallows in healthy young adults [26]. Participants performed water and nectar-thick juice swallows, effortful and non-effortful saliva swallows, and "half-maximum" tongue-palate partial-pressure tasks emphasizing either anterior or posterior tongue-palate contact at different speeds. Tasks that elicited pressures most similar to pressure waves observed in bolus swallows were (1) 50 %-maximum press with the anterior and posterior tongue (individually), (2) 100 % maximum posterior press, and (3) effortful swallow. These results provoke interesting discussion relative to principles of exercise in that two "non-specific" tasks (isometric press) and an "under load" task (50 % maximum press) elicited waveforms similar to those generated during swallowing.

Oropharyngeal Strengthening in Dysphagic Populations

Stroke

The contribution of improved muscle strength in stroke recovery has been shown in studies involving stroke and rehabilitation of limb musculature. Post-stroke patients who (Fig. 12.2) perform strengthening exercises for lower extremities have shown improvements in functional activities such as timed stair climbing, walking, and chair rising [27–30].

One analogous study focusing on the striated bulbar-innervated head and neck musculature included ten dysphagic stroke patients (six acute and four chronic) who completed an 8-week lingual strengthening regimen which entailed compressing an air-filled bulb between the tongue and the hard palate receiving knowledge of performance [3]. Subjects sequentially exercised portions of the tongue by performing ten repetitions of anterior tongue followed by posterior tongue, three times a day, three times per week consistent with recommendations for strength training by the American College of Sports Medicine [14]. As the patients became stronger, exercise targets were adjusted every 2 weeks to reflect 80 % of their maximum lingual press value. The clinically relevant result, reflected

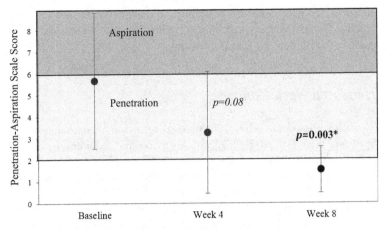

Fig. 12.2. Changes in penetration/aspiration scale scores after 8 weeks of isometric lingual exercises. *Filled circle* mean score, 10 mL liquid bolus condition. Adapted from Robbins et al. [3], with permission from Elsevier.

in the patient's Penetration-Aspiration Scale (PAS) scores [31, 32], were significantly reduced indicating increased swallowing safety for 3-mL thin liquid boluses after only 4 weeks of exercise. After 8 weeks of treatment, the PAS scores were significantly reduced for 10-mL thin liquid boluses (Fig. 12.2). Results were the same for acute and chronic stroke subjects. Following completion of the exercise protocol, there was a significant increase in maximum isometric pressures at the anterior and the posterior tongue locations with generalization to increased pressure during swallowing thin liquids. Reduced post-swallow residue with liquids was observed which lessens the probability for aspiration of material remaining in the oropharynx after the swallow. Two bolus timing measures were noted to change post-exercise regimen, that is, oral transit duration and duration of pharyngeal response. Oral transit duration, operationally defined as the time from beginning of posterior bolus movement until arrival of the bolus head at the ramus of mandible, decreased significantly indicating more efficient movement of the bolus through the oral cavity. Increased duration of the pharyngeal response (operationally defined as the time from beginning of hyoid excursion until the hyoid returns to rest) with thin liquid bolus conditions indicated a longer period of airway protection. Two of the three subjects who underwent MRI of the tongue showed increased total lingual volume after 8 weeks of lingual exercise, with an average increase of 4.35 %. Performance on a dysphagia-specific quality of life questionnaire (SWAL-QOL) [33–35] revealed increases for all subscales with statistically significant changes in the subscales of Fatigue, Communication, and Mental health. Substantial gains also were made in the Burden and Social subscales.

Head and Neck Cancer

Dysphagia occurs in 50 % of patients receiving chemoradiation for head and neck cancer (HNC) [36]. An associated reduction in lingual muscle strength has been observed in patients treated with primary chemoradiation for oral and oropharyngeal cancer [37]. Radiation fibrosis can lead to a decrease in range of motion and strength of the muscles involved in the field of treatment. Secondarily, resulting pathobiomechanics and incoordination can lead to disability and reduced quality of life for HNC patients. As fibrosis can begin to form within 3 months of treatment [38], clinicians generally begin a preventative series of range of motion and isometric lingual strengthening exercises as soon as the acute effects of radiation (i.e., mucositis) have resolved [39–41].

One study compared outcomes for patients with advanced squamous cell carcinoma of the oropharynx, hypopharynx, and larynx who exercised prior to chemoradiation ($n=9$) with those receiving standard treatment initiated after chemoradiation ($n=9$). Participants in the pretreatment group began swallowing exercises approximately 2 weeks prior to chemoradiation which included tongue-hold, tongue resistance using a tongue depressor, effortful swallow, Mendelsohn maneuver, and Shaker exercises. With the exception of the Shaker exercises, participants were instructed to perform ten repetitions, five times each day of each exercise. Results indicated that patients receiving pretreatment exercise maintained more normal epiglottal inversion than patients in the control group. Tongue base during swallowing was significantly closer to the posterior pharyngeal wall in patients receiving pretreatment swallowing therapy. Percutaneous endoscopic gastrostomy (PEG) tube removal rates did not significantly differ between groups [42].

Strengthening exercises with populations other than HNC are generally performed three to five times per week; however, with HNC patients having the additional challenge of decreased ROM due to radiation-induced fibrosis, exercises are often prescribed daily. Though exercises commonly are prescribed for patients after surgery or chemoradiation, little has been published about their effectiveness. Several clinical trials are ongoing with the aim of defining parameters such as the most effective type of exercise, frequency of performance, and duration of exercise to optimize rehabilitation for patients with HNC.

Detraining

Adherence to a maintenance program after the completion of progressive resistance exercise regimens can be of significant value to facilitate preservation of strength gains and performance. Despite the critical issue of maintaining motor and functional gains post-exercise, there is a paucity of literature regarding maintenance of muscle strength and functional outcomes even for healthy adults.

Detraining is defined in two ways: (a) withdrawal from training or (b) as the partial or complete loss of training-induced adaptations due to insufficient training stimuli. Detraining following resistance training programs in healthy older adults has been shown to result in significant decreases in muscle strength, muscle density, and flexibility [43].

Application of Detraining Principles to Tongue Exercises

Lingual elevation, protrusion, and lateralization strength measurements from 39 healthy participants were recorded before and after completion of 9 weeks of isometric lingual exercise. Results from this study by Clark et al. revealed that there were significantly greater immediate post-training effects compared to baseline ability. After 4 weeks of no training, strength measurements did not differ significantly from baseline ability indicating that the gains from exercise were lost in less than half the time it took to achieve the change [5]. Malandraki et al., published data from a longitudinal case study of a patient with Inclusion Body Myositis and Sjogren's Sydrome who completed eight weeks of lingual strengthening (three times per day, three days per week) with periods of detraining (no therapy) and maintenance (strengthening 3 times per day, one day per week). Conclusions from that study were that the lingual strengthening protocol slowed progression of the disease-related lingual strength loss during intense strengthening and during the maintenance period. One of the most common concerns of patients is how they will be able to maintain their gains after the completion of a progressive resistance exercise program, yet no definitive evidence-based guidance is available at this time.

Implementation of a Lingual Strengthening Protocol in Clinical Settings

Devices

There are various tools and devices available to use for oropharyngeal strengthening exercises. Deciding on the most appropriate method for a particular patient can depend on a variety of factors including (a) ease of use, (b) quantifiable information, and (c) cost. Figure 12.3 provides a comparative overview of devices including their advantages and limitations.

Developing a Patient-Specific Exercise Plan

Determining the Exercise Intensity Goal

When developing a progressive resistance isometric lingual exercise plan, the first step is to determine the patient's baseline lingual strength. Knowledge of the baseline performance allows the clinician to identify attainable yet challenging goals as well as provides a quantifiable reference for relevant and reportable outcome data. One method of identifying baseline pressures is to collect a one repetition maximum value [14].

One Repetition Maximum (1RM): is the highest amount of pressure a patient can generate in a single repetition for a given exercise [44]. 1RM can be used for determining an individual's maximum strength and also can be used as an upper limit, in order to determine the desired "load" for an exercise (as a percentage of the 1RM).

Variability of pressure data can be a challenge when collecting the 1RM because many patients with dysphagia are frail and not accustomed to maximum force exertion or may be less familiar or comfortable with electronic devices used to measure pressure. It is important that the 1RM be representative of what a patient can actually achieve and not a result of the device slipping or the patient misunderstanding the instructions given by the clinician. One method for obtaining accurate 1RM is to collect multiple samples of the maximum press. If, for example, a set of three repetitions result in values that vary by less than 5 %, then the data may be considered representative of the patient's ability. The highest value from the three

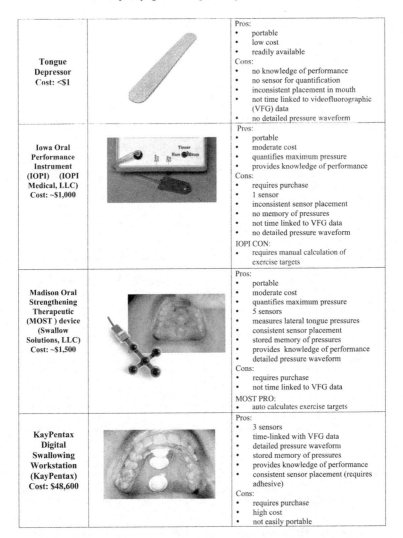

Tongue Depressor Cost: <$1		Pros: • portable • low cost • readily available Cons: • no knowledge of performance • no sensor for quantification • inconsistent placement in mouth • not time linked to videofluorographic (VFG) data • no detailed pressure waveform
Iowa Oral Performance Instrument (IOPI) (IOPI Medical, LLC) Cost: ~$1,000		Pros: • portable • moderate cost • quantifies maximum pressure • provides knowledge of performance Cons: • requires purchase • 1 sensor • inconsistent sensor placement • no memory of pressures • not time linked to VFG data • no detailed pressure waveform IOPI CON: • requires manual calculation of exercise targets
Madison Oral Strengthening Therapeutic (MOST) device (Swallow Solutions, LLC) Cost: ~$1,500		Pros: • portable • moderate cost • quantifies maximum pressure • 5 sensors • measures lateral tongue pressures • consistent sensor placement • stored memory of pressures • provides knowledge of performance • detailed pressure waveform Cons: • requires purchase • not time linked to VFG data MOST PRO: • auto calculates exercise targets
KayPentax Digital Swallowing Workstation (KayPentax) Cost: $48,600		Pros: • 3 sensors • time-linked with VFG data • detailed pressure waveform • stored memory of pressures • provides knowledge of performance • consistent sensor placement (requires adhesive) Cons: • requires purchase • high cost • not easily portable

Fig. 12.3. Comparison of devices available for oropharyngeal strengthening exercises.

would be used as the 1RM. If the values vary by more than 5 %, the data are considered too variable and additional sets of maximum values may be collected until values vary by less than 5 %. Allowing rest periods of several minutes between sets is imperative to reduce inconsistency in values.

Isometric Progressive Resistance Oropharyngeal (I-PRO) Therapy

1. Collect three repetitions of maximum lingual press at specific lingual location (i.e anterior or posterior tongue).
2. If pressures vary by <5%, collect pressures from next location.
3. If pressures vary by greater than 5%, collect an additional three maximum press repetitions.
4. Identify the maximum (MAX) value for each location from the values that vary by no more than 5%.
5. Have patient exercise with the goal of 60% of Max value for wk 1 and 80% of Max value at wks 2-8.
6. Begin exercises: 10 repetitions at each location (holding pressure at target value for 3 seconds). Exercises should be completed 3x/day, 3days/weeks for 8 weeks.
7. Repeat steps 1-5 at the beginning of week 3,5, and 7 to identify progressive exercise target values.

Example:

Step #1	Step #2	Step #3	Step #4
Set 1 25 24 24	25(max)-24(min) = 1 1/25 =.04=4% Values vary by 4%	No additional pressure collection required because values vary by < 5%	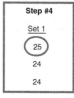

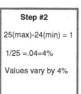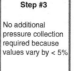

Step #5	Step #6	Step #7
25 x .6 =15 Week 1 target=15kPa 25 x.8 = 20 Week 2 target = 20kPa	- 10 repetitions of pressing to target and holding for 3sec - 3x day - 3 days/week - 8 weeks	Repeat steps 2-6 at week 3,5 and 7 to identify new exercise targets

Tips for successful exercising:

- Verbal encouragement when collecting maximum values has been shown to improve performance (i.e., higher pressures).
- Provide rest times between each trial as needed, If pressures vary by >5%, more rest time is probably necessary.
- Modify according to patient needs and performance.

Fig. 12.4. Isometric Progressive Resistance Oropharyngeal (I-PRO) Therapy courtesy. The UW/VA Swallowing Speech And Dining Enhancement Program (SSWAL-ADE) Program at the University of Wisconsin-Madison.

Once the 1RM has been identified, an exercise target may be calculated (Fig. 12.4).

If patients are asked to press to their maximum strength during each exercise repetition, they may fatigue quickly and may complain of muscle soreness. Uncomfortable and tired patients rarely appreciate the value of a prescribed intervention and may drop out of therapy all together. Compliance is a key to treatment success. Sports medicine literature reports that optimal exercises are 60–80 % of the 1RM [44]. In an 8-week protocol, patients may start exercising at 60 % of their 1RM and increase to 80 % at week two when they have become accustomed to the exercise regimen. In accordance with the overload principle of exercise [17], as patients become stronger, their exercise target values must be adjusted accordingly. This can be done every 2 weeks by re-measuring the 1RM and calculating the new exercise target (80 % of the new 1RM).

Determining Exercise Repetition and Frequency

Studies of oropharyngeal exercise, all of which report increases in pressure generation over the course of the protocol, have reported varying numbers of repetitions (trials in one sitting) and frequency (number of days/week). Repetitions ranged from 10 to 30 isometric presses lasting between 1 and 3 s. Frequency of exercise ranged from three times per week to daily [2–5, 42]. Intense exercise may cause acute trauma to the muscles and damage begins to proliferate within the fibers. Once muscles become damaged, the body immediately attempts to repair them. It is during this repair or rest period that muscles grow and become stronger; therefore daily exercise of the same muscles would be contraindicated [45]. Some protocols have included multiple exercise sites (i.e., anterior and posterior tongue) requiring more repetitions. Figure 12.4 provides an example of a protocol based on work by Robbins and colleagues in which patients completed ten repetitions, three times per day, three days per week.

Duration of Exercise Protocol

Improvement in swallowing outcomes has been reported in studies as limited in duration as 4 weeks [4]; however, studies of longer duration, that is, 8–9 weeks, report continual improvement in pressure gain until completion of the protocol [2, 3, 5]. The authors of a study on stroke patients who exercised for 8 weeks hypothesized that the pressure gains and reduction in aspiration observed after just 4 weeks of exercise reflected changes in underlying neural networks. Improvements in lingual strength and associated deglutitive outcomes observed after 8 weeks represented the positive effects of the exercise intervention on muscle hypertrophy [3, 45]. These results support that longer exercise regimen duration improves central as well as peripheral alterations in stroke patients. While at some point a pressure plateau no doubt exists for oropharyngeal strength gain completed for longer durations, a study has yet to be published that provides the important "dose response" piece of the exercise puzzle.

Conclusion

Dysphagia interventions historically have focused on compensatory strategies such as dietary modifications, and postural adjustments (i.e., head turn) and maneuvers (i.e., supraglottic swallow). Compensatory techniques continue to be useful options with positive functional swallow outcomes that often serve to permit safe oral intake; however, patients are required to continue to perform the compensatory techniques for months or years during every swallow for every meal. In skilled nursing facilities, 31 % of residents use compensatory dietary strategies to address their dysphagia [46, 47], despite the negative impact that dietary modifications may have on their quality of life. Subjects who perform oropharyngeal rehabilitative exercises, which include isometric lingual strengthening, effortful swallowing, and the Masako and Shaker exercises (described in subsequent chapters), report improved control of their health care and rehabilitation as they actively participate in their recovery. Evidence provided in this chapter supports the concept that patients with dysphagia caused at least in part by oropharyngeal weakness who complete progressive oropharyngeal strengthening exercises are capable of making significant gains in swallowing efficiency and safety with associated improvements in quality of life.

References

1. McCauley RJ, Strand E, Lof GL, Schooling T, Frymark T. Evidence-based systematic review: effects of nonspeech oral motor exercises on speech. Am J Speech Lang Pathol. 2009;18:343–60.
2. Robbins J, Gangnon R, Theis S, Kays SA, Hind J. The effects of lingual exercise on swallowing in older adults. J Am Geriatr Soc. 2005;53:1483–9.
3. Robbins J, Kays SA, Gangnon R, Hewitt A, Hind J. The effects of lingual exercise in stroke patients with dysphagia. Arch Phys Med Rehabil. 2007;88:150–8.
4. Lazarus C, Logemann J, Huang C, Rademaker A. Effects of two types of tongue strengthening exercises in young normals. Folia Phoniatr Logop. 2003;55:199–205.
5. Clark HM, O'Brien K, Calleja A, Corrie SN. Effects of directional exercise on lingual strength. J Speech Lang Hear Res. 2009;52:1034–47.
6. Kier WM, Smith KK. Tongues, tentacles and trunks: the biomechanics of movement in muscular-hydrostats. Zool J Linn Soc. 1985;83:307–24.
7. Gray H. Gray's anatomy. Philadelphia: Running Press; 1974.
8. Robbins J. The evolution of swallowing neuroanatomy and physiology in humans: a practical perspective. Ann Neurol. 1999;46:279–80.

9. Palmer PM, Jaffe DM, McCulloch TM, Finnegan EM, Van Daele DJ, Luschei ES. Quantitative contributions of the muscles of the tongue, floor-of-mouth, jaw, and velum to tongue-to-palate pressure generation. J Speech Lang Hear Res. 2008;51:828–35.

10. Shaw C, McEachern J. Toward a theory of neuroplasticity. Hove: Psychology Press; 2001.

11. Kleim JA, Jones TA. Principles of experience-dependent neural plasticity: implications for rehabilitation after brain damage. J Speech Lang Hear Res. 2008;51:S225–39.

12. Nudo RJ, Wise BM, SiFuentes F, Milliken GW. Neural substrates for the effects of rehabilitative training on motor recovery after ischemic infarct. Science. 1996; 272:1791–4.

13. Kilgard MP, Merzenich MM. Cortical map reorganization enabled by nucleus basalis activity. Science. 1998;279:1714–8.

14. American College of Sports Medicine. The recommended quantity and quality of exercise for developing and maintaining cardiorespiratory and muscular fitness in healthy adults. Med Sci Sports Exerc. 1990;22:265–74.

15. Martin RE. Neuroplasticity and swallowing. Dysphagia. 2009;24(2):218–29.

16. Carey JR, Kimberley TJ, Lewis SM, et al. Analysis of fMRI and finger tracking training in subjects with chronic stroke. Brain. 2002;125:773–88.

17. Powers S, Howley E. Exercise physiology: theory and application to fitness and performance. McGraw-Hill Humanities/Social Sciences/Languages; 2008.

18. Temple M, O'Leary D, Faden A. The role of glutamate receptors in the pathophysiology of traumatic CNS injury. In: Miller L, Hayes R, editors. Head trauma: basic, preclinical, and clinical directions. New York: Wiley; 2001. p. 87–113.

19. Schmidt RA, Wrisberg CA. Motor learning and performance: a situation-based learning approach. 4th ed. Human Kinetics: Champaign; 2008.

20. Maas E, Robin DA, Austermann Hula SN, et al. Principles of motor learning in treatment of motor speech disorders. Am J Speech Lang Pathol. 2008;17:277–98.

21. Wulf G, Shea C, Lewthwaite R. Motor skill learning and performance: a review of influential factors. Med Educ. 2010;44:75–84.

22. Lai Q, Shea CH, Wulf G, Wright DL. Optimizing generalized motor program and parameter learning. Res Q Exerc Sport. 2000;71:10–24.

23. Lai Q, Shea CH. Generalized motor program (GMP) learning: effects of reduced frequency of knowledge of results and practice variability. J Mot Behav. 1998;30:51–9.

24. Wulf G, Lee TD, Schmidt RA. Reducing knowledge of results about relative versus absolute timing: differential effects on learning. J Mot Behav. 1994;26:362–9.

25. Duchateau J, Hainaut K. Isometric or dynamic training: differential effects on mechanical properties of a human muscle. J Appl Physiol. 1984;56:296–301.

26. Steele CM. Pressure profile similarities between tongue resistance training tasks and liquid swallows. J Rehabil Res Dev. 2010;47:651–60.

27. Teixeira-Salmela LF, Olney SJ, Nadeau S, Brouwer B. Muscle strengthening and physical conditioning to reduce impairment and disability in chronic stroke survivors. Arch Phys Med Rehabil. 1999;80:1211–8.

28. Weiss A, Suzuki T, Bean J, Fielding RA. High intensity strength training improves strength and functional performance after stroke. Am J Phys Med Rehabil. 2000;79:369–76; quiz 391–4.

29. Engardt M, Knutsson E, Jonsson M, Sternhag M. Dynamic muscle strength training in stroke patients: effects on knee extension torque, electromyographic activity, and motor function. Arch Phys Med Rehabil. 1995;76:419–25.

30. Canning CG, Ada L, Adams R, O'Dwyer NJ. Loss of strength contributes more to physical disability after stroke than loss of dexterity. Clin Rehabil. 2004;18:300–8.

31. Rosenbek JC, Robbins JA, Roecker EB, Coyle JL, Wood JL. A penetration-aspiration scale. Dysphagia. 1996;11:93–8.

32. Robbins J, Coyle J, Roecker E, Rosenbek J, Wood J. Differentiation of normal and abnormal airway protection during swallowing using the penetration-aspiration scale. Dysphagia. 1999;14:228–32.

33. McHorney C, Bricker D, Kramer A, et al. The SWAL-QOL outcomes tool for oropharyngeal dysphagia in adults: I. Conceptual foundation and item development. Dysphagia. 2000;15:115–21.

34. McHorney CA, Bricker DE, Robbins JA, Kramer AE, Rosenbek JC, Chignell KA. The SWAL-QOL outcomes tool for oropharyngeal dysphagia in adults: II. Item reduction and preliminary scaling. Dysphagia. 2000;15:122–33.

35. McHorney CA, Robbins JA, Lomax K, et al. The SWAL-QOL outcomes tool for oropharyngeal dysphagia in adults: III. Extensive evidence of reliability and validity. Dysphagia. 2002;17:97–114.

36. Goguen LA, Posner MR, Norris CM, et al. Dysphagia after sequential chemoradiation therapy for advanced head and neck cancer. Otolaryngol Head Neck Surg. 2006;134:916–22.

37. Lazarus CL, Logemann JA, Pauloski BR, et al. Swallowing and tongue function following treatment for oral and oropharyngeal cancer. J Speech Lang Hear Res. 2000; 43:1011–23.

38. Murphy BA, Gilbert J. Dysphagia in head and neck cancer patients treated with radiation: assessment, sequelae, and rehabilitation. Semin Radiat Oncol. 2009; 19:35–42.

39. Lazarus C. Tongue strength and exercise in healthy individuals and in head and neck cancer patients. Semin Speech Lang. 2006;27:260–7.

40. Pauloski BR. Rehabilitation of dysphagia following head and neck cancer. Phys Med Rehabil Clin N Am. 2008;19:889–928; x.

41. Kammer R, Robbins J. Rehabiliation of heavily treated head and neck cancer patients. In: Bernier J, editor. Head and neck cancer: multimodality management. New York: Springer; 2011.

42. Carroll WR, Locher JL, Canon CL, Bohannon IA, McColloch NL, Magnuson JS. Pretreatment swallowing exercises improve swallow function after chemoradiation. Laryngoscope. 2008;118:39–43.

43. Fiatarone MA, O'Neill EF, Ryan ND, et al. Exercise training and nutritional supplementation for physical frailty in very elderly people. N Engl J Med. 1994; 330:1769–75.

44. Fiatarone MA, Marks EC, Ryan ND, Meredith CN, Lipsitz LA, Evans WJ. High-intensity strength training in nonagenarians. Effects on skeletal muscle. JAMA. 1990;263:3029–34.

45. Jones DA, Rutherford OM, Parker DF. Physiological changes in skeletal muscle as a result of strength training. Q J Exp Physiol. 1989;74:233–56.
46. Castellanos VH, Butler E, Gluch L, Burke B. Use of thickened liquids in skilled nursing facilities. J Am Diet Assoc. 2004;104:1222–6.
47. Groher ME, McKaig TN. Dysphagia and dietary levels in skilled nursing facilities. J Am Geriatr Soc. 1995;43:528–32.

13. Shaker Exercise

Caryn Easterling

Abstract The Shaker Exercise is a simple isometric and isotonic exercise that has been shown to strengthen the suprahyoid muscles resulting in changes in deglutition (Am J Physiol 272: G1518–G1522, 1997; Gastroenterology 122: 1314–1321, 2002). Those changes have been shown to include an increase in anterior laryngeal excursion and antero-posterior deglutitive opening of the upper esophageal sphincter in healthy older adults and in patients with dysphagia (Am J Physiol 272: G1518–G1522, 1997; Gastroenterology 122: 1314–1321, 2002). Dysphagic patients have also been shown to experience the elimination of post-deglutitive aspiration (Gastroenterology 122: 1314–1321, 2002). The exercise does result in mild muscular discomfort which dissipates over the first week of the 6-week treatment course. The progression of the Shaker Exercise regimen should be tailored to the individual abilities of each patient, that is, a gradual stepwise progression toward the isometric and isotonic exercise goals.

The evolution of the Shaker Exercise, a simple isometric and isotonic exercise that has been shown to increase maximum anterior laryngeal excursion and anteroposterior deglutitive opening of the upper esophageal sphincter (UES) resulting in elimination of post-deglutitive aspiration, is a model of interdisciplinary translational research [1, 2].

Researchers from the Medical College of Wisconsin (MCW) combined unique concepts from the scientific literature to design and validate the Shaker Exercise for use in rehabilitation of post-deglutitive disorders. A definitive chronology of the scientific findings leading to the development of the Shaker exercise is beyond the scope of this chapter; however, the unique pioneering quantification of relevant deglutitive physiologic swallow parameters by Dodds and colleagues over 30 years ago formed the foundation for the fundamental ideas and scientific principles on which the basis for the Shaker Exercise grew [3]. The fundamental principles of the Shaker Exercise began with the study and understanding of physiologic principles that contribute to the

R. Shaker et al. (eds.), *Manual of Diagnostic and Therapeutic Techniques for Disorders of Deglutition*, DOI 10.1007/978-1-4614-3779-6_13, © Springer Science+Business Media New York 2013

opening of the UES during deglutition. Understanding the deglutitive opening principles of the UES was foundational in the development of this unique exercise. The conditions required for successful UES opening and efficient bolus transport from the pharynx through the UES and into the esophagus are (a) distraction or the application of external traction force by supra-sphincteric structures, that is, the hyoid and larynx; (b) distensibility or compliance of the UES; (c) relaxation of the UES; (d) application of intrabolus pressure. Why are the traction forces important? Research findings support the notion that traction force on the UES is exerted by anterior movement of the hyoid and cricoid cartilages (laryngohyoid complex) and contributes to the opening of the sphincter [3]. Compliance or the intrinsic property of the muscle to stretch and accommodate the passage of the bolus from the pharynx to the proximal esophagus has been estimated as the measure of UES cross-sectional area and intrabolus pressure [4]. Relaxation of the UES takes place prior to the visual or radiographic documentation of the deglutitive opening of the sphincter. A precipitous drop in UES tone can be appreciated as a decrease in manometrically measured luminal pressure prior to the arrival of the bolus at the sphincteric segment [5]. Finally, intrabolus pressure or the pressure within the fluid bolus is distinct from the force exerted by the external pharyngeal musculature during pharyngeal closure. Intrabolus pressure can be measured by a solid state catheter as the bolus covers the pressure sensor. As the bolus traverses the UES, intrabolus pressure is also a measure of the force required to push the fluid bolus through the open sphincter (Fig. 13.1).

How Were These Principles Studied?

The principles of UES deglutitive opening began with the study of fluoroscopic images and the relationship of the superior and anterior movement of the hyoid and larynx with the anteroposterior UES opening diameter. Deglutitive excursion of the hyoid and larynx showed a significant correlation of anterior hyo-laryngeal movement and the AP diameter of the UES. The use of solid state or perfused manometry was used to evaluate the pressure along the pharyngo-esophageal lumen. Manofluorography allowed simultaneous measurement of both UES cross-sectional area and intrabolus pressure while deriving an estimate of deglutitive UES compliance to bolus passage. Measurable parameters

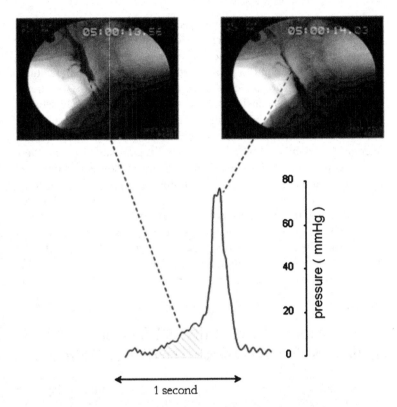

Fig. 13.1. Intrabolus pressure is indicated on the manometric pressure wave by the *hatched lines*. Intrabolus pressure is a measure of resistance to pharyngeal outflow.

such as hyoid and laryngeal excursion, UES anteroposterior deglutitive opening diameter, and intrabolus pressure can be used to evaluate and compare successful with failed swallows.

The Principle Inspiration

The principle inspiration for development of the Shaker Exercise came from studies of deglutitive UES opening in healthy elderly individuals. The primary focus of this research by the MCW group was to determine the effect of aging on the traction forces applied to the UES during deglutition. Hyoid and laryngeal excursion in the elderly was found to be significantly smaller than those of the young. This decrease in maximum anterior excursion was manifest in smaller anteroposterior opening of the UES [6]. Compliance of the UES segment was also found to be affected by aging. In a separate study, the intrabolus pressure associated with a particular UES cross-sectional area was found to be consistently greater in the tested elderly subjects compared to young subjects suggesting a stiffening of the sphincter muscles with age [4]. Further evidence of the effect of aging on UES opening was published by Shaker and colleagues showing that there was a significant increase in intrabolus pressure in the elderly compared to young subjects due to UES outflow compromise or smaller deglutitive UES opening dimensions in the elderly subjects [7]. Given the evidence of the interrelationship between hyo-laryngeal excursion, UES opening, and hydrodynamic resistance to flow, the notion of augmenting UES opening to effect flow through the sphincter by increasing the externally applied distractive or traction forces on the sphincter was conceived.

Augmentation of Deglutitive UES Opening in the Elderly by Exercise: The Shaker Exercise

The Shaker exercise was initially performed three times a day for 6 weeks by a cohort of 12 healthy elderly adults. View the steps of the Shaker Exercise: http://www.mcw.edu/ shakerexercise.html [8] (Fig. 13.2). Prior to and after completion of the 6-week exercise regimen, deglutitive UES anteroposterior opening diameter, maximum superior and anterior excursion of the larynx, and hyoid and hypopharyngeal intrabolus pressure were measured. A control group of age-matched healthy elderly subjects was also given a 6-week regimen of a sham exercise evaluated for the same deglutitive parameters as the real exercise group. The data revealed a significant increase in anteroposterior UES diameter, a significant increase in anterior laryngeal excursion, and a significant decrease in intrabolus pressure in the real exercise group. The study suggested that deglutitive UES anteroposterior opening is amenable to augmentation by exercise aimed at strengthening the UES opening muscles. This augmentation is associated with an increase in the swallow-induced anterior excursion of the larynx and results in a decrease in hypopharyngeal intrabolus pressure suggesting a decline in pharyngeal outflow resistance [1].

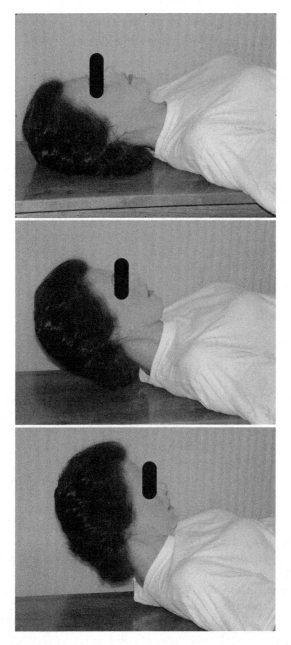

Fig. 13.2. The Shaker Exercise: the head is raised off of the floor or bed to allow the patient to look at their toes without raising their shoulders and continuing to breath while performing the exercise.

Suprahyoid Muscle Strengthening: Electromyographic Confirmation

Surface electromyographic studies have been used to evaluate specific muscle activation patterns and the relationship of the timing of hyolaryngeal excursion, UES opening, and activation of suprahyoid muscles (SHM) during swallowing [9–12]. Initial studies using sEMG allowed measurement of a shift in spectral analysis of sEMG activity indicating muscle fatigue and strengthening of the UES opening muscles or the SHM during performance of the isometric portion of the Shaker exercise [9–11]. Ferdjallah and colleagues identified post-isometric Shaker exercise fatigue of the suprahyoid, infrahyoid, and sternocleidomastoid muscles (SCM) through analysis of the sEMG spectral shift. All muscle groups fatigued with performance of the isometric portion of the Shaker exercise; however, the SCM fatigued before the SHM or infrahyoid muscles (IHM) indicating that the SCM may be limiting patient exercise and attainment of the goal of strengthening the SHM group [12].

Clinical Outcomes of the Shaker Exercise in Dysphagic Patients

The improvement in deglutitive function in the normal elderly provided the impetus for a study evaluating the effect of the Shaker exercise in dysphagic patients. Twenty-seven tube-fed dysphagic patients with post-deglutitive residue and aspiration confirmed by videofluoroscopic swallow study were enrolled. Prior to and following 6 weeks of the Shaker Exercise regimen anterior and superior hyoid and laryngeal maximum excursion, maximum AP UES opening diameter, height and width of pyriform sinus residue were measured. The Shaker Exercise was performed three times per day for 6 weeks. The patient was instructed to: (1) Perform 3 repetitive 1-min sustained head raises in supine position, interrupted by a 1-min rest period; (2) Perform 30 consecutive repetitions of head raising in the supine position; and (3) Breathe during the exercises and raise your head high and forward enough to see the toes without lifting the shoulders off the ground [1, 2]. The results of this study showed the effect of the Shaker Exercise significantly increased anterior laryngeal excursion and UES anteroposterior opening diameter following 6 weeks of exercise by the patients. In addition, the functional outcome assessment measure of swallowing (FOAMS) was used to measure functional outcome change from pre- to post-exercise. This was used to assign a pre- and post-exercise functional value. The FOAMS numerical scale: 1 = Profound dysphagia, 2 = Severe dysphagia, 3 = Moderate/severe, 4 = Moderate dysphagia, 5 = Mild/moderate dysphagia, 6 = mild dysphagia, 7 = Functional swallow dysphagia [13]. The median FOAMS score for all 27 patients before beginning the Shaker Exercise was 1 in contrast to the median score of 7 for all patients after completion of the exercise. All 27 patients discontinued tube feedings after completion of the exercise regardless of the etiology or duration of dysphagia. There was a significant decrease in both the height and width of pyriform sinus residue after completion of the Shaker Exercise. Prior to beginning the exercise, all patients experienced post-deglutitive aspiration while 2 of the 27 also experienced pre-deglutitive aspiration. Following 6 weeks of exercise, all 27 patients ceased experiencing post-deglutitive aspiration and two continued to have pre-deglutitive aspiration showing that the Shaker Exercise had an effect only on elimination of post-deglutitive aspiration. Deglutitive UES opening diameter showed significant increase after 6 weeks of exercise for all etiologies of dysphagia. Etiologies of dysphagia included nine patients with hemispheric CVA, seven patients with brainstem stroke, five patients post-pharyngeal radiation, and six patients with varied etiologies of dysphagia. Pyriform sinus residue showed a significant decrease in both height and width following the exercise for all patient etiology groups. Duration of dysphagia ranged from 2 to greater than 6 months duration. There was a significant increase in deglutitive UES anteroposterior opening diameter following 6 weeks of exercise for all patients regardless of duration of dysphagia. Width and height of pyriform sinus residue were significantly decreased in all patients regardless of duration of dysphagia after 6 weeks of exercise. Patient follow-up was conducted at 4–24 months after completion of the Shaker Exercise and revealed that all patients maintained their weight while some reported weight gain. Seventy percent continued the exercise protocol on a daily basis. Ninety-five percent maintained the diet consistency recommended when tube feedings were discontinued. No patients reported pneumonia or upper respiratory infections since resuming oral intake. The Shaker Exercise was effective in restoring oral feeding in patients with deglutitive failure due to abnormal UES opening irrespective of the underlying etiology and duration of dysphagia [2].

Shaker Exercise Compliance: Attaining and Maintaining the Exercise Goals

Exercise compliance is a major hurdle to achieving treatment success with any exercise program. A study was conducted to critically evaluate compliance with the Shaker exercise. The aim of this study was to determine (1) exerciser compliance with the Shaker Exercise among healthy elderly patients, (2) the number of days required to attain the isometric and isotonic exercise goals, (3) the rate and reason for dropout of subjects, and (4) exerciser complaints associated with performance of the exercise. The results of this study of healthy elderly participants confirmed the physiologic deglutitive changes measured in the previous Shaker Exercise findings. Duration to attain the performance goals of the Shaker Exercise, that is, the 60-s isometric hold repeated three times with equal rest periods between and the 30 consecutive head raises completed three times per day, was found to vary among participants. The isometric or 60-s hold portion took longest for all participants to attain. Seventy-four percent of enrollees were able to attain the goal by the end of 6 weeks. One hundred percent of participants were able to attain 30 consecutive repetitions by the end of the fifth week. Performance of the Shaker Exercise was associated with mild muscle discomfort that resolved spontaneously after the first week of exercise. The findings of this indicate the need for a more structured progressive plan for reaching the necessary exercise performance goals [14].

Shaker Exercise Effect on Vocal Function?

To critically evaluate the effect of the Shaker exercise on vocal function, a study was performed to determine if the Shaker Exercise which strengthens the SHM would have an effect on vocal function [15]. Eleven females and ten males from 65 to 78 years of age, mean age of 70 years ±4 years in good health, were enrolled in this study. Also enrolled were five age-matched controls that did not perform the Shaker Exercise during the 6-week period. Participants had a negative history for dysphagia and voice disorders and were non-smokers. Prior to and after 6 weeks of exercise, the group of 21 exercisers received an acoustic analysis of voice, biomechanical analysis of deglutition using videofluorographic frame-by-frame analysis measuring maximum anterior hyoid and laryngeal excursion, and anteroposterior UES deglutitive opening. As previously stated, the five controls performed the voice analysis only. Vocal function was determined using the Dysphonia Severity Index (DSI), a multivariate voice index yielding an objective measure of vocal quality which captures the multidimensional character of voice by means of multivariate statistics. DSI corrects for gender, therefore no additional analysis was needed to determine gender effects [16]. The voice analysis was used to compare vocal function prior to and after 6 weeks of exercise. The results showed that 10 of 21 participants had improved deglutitive biomechanical measures and DSI scores following 6 weeks of performing the Shaker Exercise. Eleven of twenty-one participants showed no significant change in deglutitive biomechanical measures or DSI. Five of the five control participants who did not perform the exercise and did the voice analysis at the beginning of the 6-week period and then after 6 weeks had no change in DSI scores. The study concluded that the lack of significant change in a large portion of the participant's DSI or deglutitive biomechanics may be due to inaccurate exercise performance, exercise regimen compliance, and/or undisclosed changes in physical health during the 6-week period. This study of healthy older adults concluded that it may be beneficial to include the Shaker Exercise regimen in exercise protocols for older adults in order to strengthen the extrinsic laryngeal resulting in improved vocal range and stability [15].

Confirmation of Suprahyoid Muscle Strengthening by the Shaker Exercise in Healthy Older Adults

In order to measure fatigue induced by the isometric Shaker exercise, White et al. utilized sEMG to calculate the rate of change in the median frequency of Power Spectral Density function at 20, 40, and 60 s. The rate of change in the median frequency of Power Spectral Density is interpreted as proportional to the rate of fatigue of suprahyoid, infrahyoid, and SCM. The results of the study confirmed previous findings that the first muscle to fatigue during the isometric portion of the Shaker exercise is the SCM. Muscle fatigue may occur as quickly as 20 s into the isometric portion of the exercise in elderly patients. After 6 weeks of exercise, the SCM had a decreased mean frequency rate. This indicated that the SCM had improved fatigue resistance, or muscle strengthening. The SHM and IHM showed increased mean frequency rates, indicating greater muscular exertion and increased fatiguing effort. The conclusion of this study indicated that the Shaker exercise initially leads to increased fatigue resistance in the SCM after which the isometric exercise loads the SHM and IHM that are less fatigue resistant muscle groups. It is at this point in the exercise regimen that the intended therapeutic effect on strengthening of the SHM occurs [17].

Shaker Exercise Compared to Traditional Therapy Regimen

In a recent study, Mepani and colleagues found that after completion of the Shaker Exercise protocol, dysphagic patients experienced suprahyoid strengthening and greater thyrohyoid shortening contributing to augmentation of deglutitive UES opening [18]. They enrolled 11 dysphagic patients with UES dysfunction. Six patients were randomized to a traditional therapy group while five were randomly assigned to the Shaker exercise group. Prior to beginning and after completion of their assigned therapy, measurements of anterior hyoid and laryngeal excursion, anteroposterior deglutitive UES opening, and thyrohyoid shortening were completed for each patient using frame-by-frame analysis of their videofluoroscopic swallow study images. Maximum thyrohyoid shortenting corresponded to maximum excursion. Prior to the therapy regimen, there was no significant difference in thyrohyoid shortening when comparing the two groups. After completion of 6 weeks of traditional and Shaker exercise therapy, there was a significant increase in thyrohyoid shortening for the Shaker exercise group compared to the traditional therapy participants. The results of this patient outcome study suggest that the Shaker exercise increases thyrohyoid shortening, strengthens the SHM, and contributes to augmentation of the UES.

Shaker Exercise Compared to Traditional Therapy Regimen: Diminished Incidence of Aspiration

In a randomized controlled study of a group of 19 patients with a 3-month or greater history of dysphagia with UES dysfunction, the effects of traditional therapy vs. Shaker Exercise were compared [19]. Three mL and 5 mL of liquid and 3 mL paste were administered to each of the patient participants prior to and after completion of their randomly assigned therapy regimen. Superior hyoid and laryngeal excursion, anterior hyoid and laryngeal excursion, pharyngeal residuals, presence or absence of aspiration, and anteroposterior deglutitive UES opening diameter were evaluated before and after treatment. After completion of 6 weeks of therapy or exercise, patients undergoing traditional therapy experienced significantly greater superior hyoid and laryngeal excursion for 3 mL pudding while the Shaker exercise group experienced significantly less aspiration. Both groups experienced increased deglutitive anteroposterior UES opening diameter with 3 mL paste and greater anterior laryngeal excursion with the 3 mL liquid bolus swallow.

Conclusion

The Shaker Exercise has been shown to significantly improve anterior laryngeal excursion and deglutitive anteroposterior UES opening diameter in healthy elderly and those with dysphagia. The Shaker Exercise treatment effect is to eliminate post-deglutitive aspiration. The effect of the Shaker Exercise on vocal function requires further investigation by randomized controlled studies. The Shaker Exercise should be administered with consideration of the appropriate dose to allow the patient progress in individualized exercise increments to avoid excessive muscle discomfort. A patient exercise journal will guide the individual patient to the prescribed exercise goal for each portion of Shaker Exercise over the 6-week exercise period. To view the Shaker Exercise for instruction purposes and patient review, please refer to the following Internetresource: http://www.mcw.edu/shakerexercise.htm [8].

References

1. Shaker R, Kern M, Bardan E, Taylor A, Stewart ET, Hoffmann RG, et al. Augmentation of deglutitive upper esophageal sphincter opening in the elderly by exercise. Am J Physiol. 1997;272:G1518–22.
2. Shaker R, Easterling C, Kern M, Nitschke T, Massey B, Daniels S, et al. Rehabilitation of swallowing by exercise in tube-fed patients with pharyngeal dysphagia secondary to abnormal UES opening. Gastroenterology. 2002;122:1314–21.
3. Dodds WJ, Man KM, Cook IJ, Kahrilas PJ, Stewart ET, Kern MK. Influence of bolus volume on swallow-induced hyoid movement in normal subjects. Am J Roentgenol. 1988;150:1307–9.

4. Shaw DW, Cook IJ, Gabb M, Holloway RH, Simula ME, Panagopoulos V, et al. Influence of normal aging on oral pharyngeal and upper esophageal sphincter function during swallowing. Am J Physiol. 1995;268:G389–96.

5. McConnell FM, Cerendo D, Jackson RT, Guffin Jr TN. Timing of major events of pharyngeal swallowing. Arch Otolaryngol Head Neck Surg. 1988;114:1413–6.

6. Kern M, Bardan E, Arndorfer R, Hofmann C, Ren J, Shaker R. Comparison of upper esophageal sphincter opening in healthy asymptomatic young and elderly volunteers. Ann Otol Rhinol Laryngol. 1999;108:982–9.

7. Shaker R, Ren J, Podvrsan B, Dodds WJ, Hogan WJ, Kern M, et al. Effect of aging and bolus variables on pharyngeal and upper esophageal sphincter motor function. Am J Physiol. 1993;264:G427–32.

8. The Shaker Exercise. http://www.mcw.edu/shakerexercise.html (2011). Accessed 1 Jan 2011.

9. Jurell KC, Shaker R, Mazur A, Haig AJ, Wertsch JJ. Spectral analysis to evaluate hyoid muscles involvement in neck exercise. Muscle Nerve. 1996;19:1224.

10. Jurell KC, Shaker R, Mazur A, Haig AJ, Wertsch JJ. Effect of exercise on upper esophageal sphincter muscles: a spectral analysis. Gastroenterology. 1997;112:A757.

11. Alfonso M, Ferdjallah M, Shaker R, Wertsch JJ. Electrophysiologic validation of deglutitive UES opening head lift exercise. Gastroenterology. 1998;114:G2942.

12. Ferdjallah M, Wertsch JJ, Shaker R. Spectral analysis of surface electromyography (EMG) of upper esophageal sphincter opening muscles during head lift exercise. J Rehabil Res Dev. 2000;37:335–40.

13. Easterling C, Grande B. Wisconsin Speech And Hearing Association (WSHA) Madison, WI. Dysphagia network pilot project: functional outcome assessment measure of swallowing. Language Pathology and Audiology Association Convention Brief 1. 1999. p. 2–3.

14. Easterling C, Grande B, Kern M, Sears K, Shaker R. Attaining and maintaining isometric and isokinetic goals of the Shaker exercise. Dysphagia. 2005;20:133–8.

15. Easterling C. Does and exercise designed to improve swallow function effect voice? Dysphagia. 2008;23:317–26.

16. Wuyts FL, De Bodt MS, Molenberghs G, Remacle M, Heylen L, Millet B, et al. The Dysphonia severity index: an objective measure of vocal quality based on a multiparameter approach. J Speech Lang Hear Res. 2000;43:796–809.

17. White KT, Easterling C, Roberts N, Wertsch J, Shaker R. Fatigue analysis before and after Shaker exercise: physiologic tool for exercise design. Dysphagia. 2008;23:385–91.

18. Mepani R, Antonik S, Massey B, Kern M, Logemann J, Pauloski B, et al. Augmentation of deglutitive thyrohyoid muscle shortening by the Shaker Exercise. Dysphagia. 2009;24:26–31.

19. Logemann JA, Rademaker A, Pauloski BR, Kelly A, Stangl-McBreen C, Antinoja J, et al. A randomized study comparing the shaker exercise with traditional therapy: a preliminary study. Dysphagia. 2009;24:403–11.

14. Mendelson Maneuver and Masako Maneuver

Cathy Lazarus

Abstract This chapter reviews the effects of the Masako (aka, tongue-hold) and Mendelsohn swallow maneuvers on swallow physiology for patients with dysphagia. The indications for use of these maneuvers are reviewed, as is treatment efficacy. Future research needs are also discussed.

Normal Pharyngeal Phase Swallow Physiology

Patients with oropharyngeal dysphagia often demonstrate difficulty during the pharyngeal phase of swallowing. Specifically, they can demonstrate motor impairment that can affect various components of the pharyngeal motor response during the swallow. These components or neuromuscular events include velopharyngeal closure, rapid posteriormotion of the tongue base, sequential contraction of the pharyngeal constrictor musculature and shortening of the pharynx, elevation and anterior motion of the hyo-laryngeal complex, and relaxation and opening of the upper esophageal sphincter (UES) r [1]. Tongue base posterior motion and an aborally propagated contraction of the pharyngeal constrictors in the horizontal plane occur as the bolus tail reaches the oropharynx. This sequential pharyngeal contraction results in an anterior bulging of the posterior pharyngeal wall [2–4]. The retraction of the tongue base to the sequentially contracting pharyngeal constrictors provides the driving force to propel a bolus of food or liquid through the pharynx [2–5]. There is simultaneous shortening of the pharynx in the vertical plane to assist in bolus clearance through the pharynx [4, 5]. During the pharyngeal motor response, the hyoid and larynx move in a vertical and anterior direction, providing anterior

R. Shaker et al. (eds.), *Manual of Diagnostic and Therapeutic Techniques for Disorders of Deglutition*, DOI 10.1007/978-1-4614-3779-6_14, © Springer Science+Business Media New York 2013

traction on the UES that assists with mechanical opening of the UES [6–8]. In addition, the anterior-superior motion of the larynx physically assists in tucking the larynx under the tongue base to assist in airway protection [1, 6]. Airway protection during the pharyngeal phase of swallowing involves closure of the supraglottic larynx, or laryngeal vestibule, as well as closure at the level of the true vocal folds [9–13]. Closure of the laryngeal vestibule during swallowing involves two mechanisms: (1) inversion or lowering of the epiglottis, with downward tilting past horizontal to maximally protect the larynx, and (2) contact of the epiglottic base to the arytenoids [9–11, 13]. The supraglottic closure involves apposition of the epiglottic base to the arytenoid cartilages as a result of active muscular movement involving anterior tilting of the arytenoid cartilages to meet a bulging epiglottic base [9, 12–14]. Closure of the larynx also occurs at the level of the glottis, with approximation of the true vocal cords [11, 15]. Vocal cord closure typically occurs as the larynx elevates approximately 50 % of maximum during the swallow [16].

Passage of a bolus into the esophagus during swallowing is accomplished by (1) cessation of resting neural input and muscular contraction in the cricopharyngeus muscle that comprises the UES [7]; (2) opening of the UES region, as a result of the forward traction on the relaxed, compliant muscular region by the anterior displacement of the larynx, as described above; and (3) further distention of the muscular region by intrabolus pressure [7, 17, 18].

Changes in Pharyngeal Phase Swallow Functioning with Age and Impairment: Tongue Base/Pharyngeal Wall and Hyo-Laryngeal Components: Indications for Use of Maneuvers

Tongue base to pharyngeal wall pressures during swallowing have been found to correlate with percent pharyngeal residue in the healthy elderly, with lower manometric pressures correlating with poorer bolus clearance and increased pharyngeal residue [19, 20]. Pharyngeal constriction impairment has also been found in the non-specific dysphagic elderly population, with an incidence of 18 % post-swallow aspiration due to pharyngeal residue [21]. Hyo-laryngeal motion has been found to be reduced in excursion and duration in the healthy elderly population as compared to the young healthy population [22–25]. Tightly coupled to hyo-laryngeal motion, UES opening anteroposterior diameter and duration has been found to be reduced in the healthy elderly as compared to younger counterparts [24–27].

Pharyngeal phase swallow impairment, specifically reduced tongue base posterior motion, reduced pharyngeal contraction, and reduced hyo-laryngeal motion and UES opening, can also occur after stroke, progressive neurologic disease, head and neck surgery, and radiotherapy [20, 26, 28–37]. In addition, medically debilitated patients who are weak can also demonstrate pharyngeal phase swallow impairment [38, 39].

Assessment of Tongue Base and Pharyngeal Wall Motion

Tongue base posterior motion and pharyngeal anterior motion can be assessed indirectly by using the pharyngeal constriction ratio (PCR), a measure of pharyngeal area during the swallow [40]. This measure can be made fluoroscopically in the lateral plane and has been found to be a useful surrogate for pharyngeal strength [40]. This measure has been validated using simultaneous manometry and fluoroscopy to examine pharyngeal clearance pressures during swallowing [40]. Pharyngeal manometry can be utilized with or without fluoroscopy to assess pharyngeal clearance pressures [20, 41–43]. Pharyngeal manometric variables have been found to correlate significantly with pharyngeal phase variables measured with videofluoroscopy [20]. Tongue base posterior motion and pharyngeal constrictor activity can also be viewed endoscopically with flexible endoscopic evaluation of swallowing (FEES) and pharyngeal residue can be viewed, with symmetry of pharyngeal constrictor weakness easily identifiable [44, 45].

The Masako (Tongue-Hold) Maneuver

The Masako maneuver was developed to improve swallow physiology in those patients who demonstrate impaired bolus clearance in the upper pharynx due to reduced tongue base posterior motion and reduced pharyngeal constrictor motion. Specifically, the Masako maneuver was developed to improve anteriorward motion of the pharyngeal constrictor musculature [46, 47]. Fujiu and colleagues [47] found that patients with oral tongue resections had a 30 % increase in

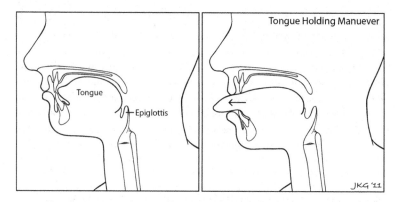

Fig. 14.1. Illustration of tongue at rest and using Masako (tongue-hold) maneuver.

anterior bulging of the posterior pharyngeal wall during swallows as compared to pre-operative swallows. This bulging correlated with extent of tongue resection, with greater bulging seen as more tongue tissue was resected. The anterior bulging was seen as a compensatory mechanism for when the tongue base is situated more anteriorly, as after partial tongue resection. Fujiu and colleagues [46] subsequently developed this maneuver to simulate having the tongue base in a more anterior position, thus potentially forcing the pharyngeal constrictor musculature to compensate and bulge further anteriorly to meet the tongue base. These authors found significantly increased posterior pharyngeal wall bulging in healthy individuals who utilized this maneuver during swallowing on videofluoroscopy [46]. The instruction for this maneuver is to place the tongue between the teeth (or between the lips for the edentulous patient) and swallow while keeping the tongue in an anterior position (Fig. 14.1).

The Masako maneuver has been found to be effective for patients with reduced pharyngeal clearance pressures. This may be due to reduced pharyngeal constrictor motion, reduced tongue base posterior motion or both. Lazarus and colleagues [35] examined use of this maneuver with simultaneous manofluoroscopy in a group of dysphagic head and neck cancer patients. These authors found increased pharyngeal pressures with use of the Masako maneuver as compared to baseline swallows [35]. They also found that the Masako maneuver generated higher pharyngeal pressures than the Super Supraglottic swallow and Mendelsohn maneuver [35]. However, Doeltgen and colleagues [48] found lower pharyngeal peak pressures with use of the Masako maneuver in healthy subjects. These authors hypothesized that the immediate effects with use of this maneuver may be less than with practice over time. No difference in pharyngeal pressures was found with or without the Masako maneuver in healthy adults by Umeki and colleagues [49]. The Masako maneuver is typically used as a swallow exercise to improve anterior range of motion of the posterior pharyngeal wall for swallowing, rather than during meals or with a bolus. This exercise should only be performed with dry swallows, as aspiration can occur with use of this maneuver during bolus swallows [46].

Assessment of Hyo-Laryngeal Motion and Upper Esophageal Sphincter Function

Hyoid and laryngeal motion during swallowing can be assessed fluoroscopically in the lateral plane, utilizing the Modified Barium Swallow procedure [50, 51]. Structural kinematics of vertical and anterior components of movement can be measured and quantified utilizing computerized methods [8, 27, 30, 52]. Laryngeal motion can also be assessed clinically using FEES; however, there are no current techniques to quantify the extent of motion. UES activity can be assessed electromyographically, to assess neural input and activity of the cricopharyngeus muscle [7, 53]. Esophageal sphincter pressures can be assessed via manometry [17, 43] to examine resting pressures, relaxation pressures during opening, and intrabolus pressures within the UES region [17, 18, 43]. High resolution manometry, which incorporates multiple sensors, is now being used to correlate coordination and timing of UES pressure events with the rapidly changing pharyngeal pressure events during the swallow [54, 55].

The Mendelsohn Maneuver

The Mendelsohn maneuver was developed to increase laryngeal motion and improve opening within the UES region during swallowing for those with impaired functioning. Specifically, the maneuver has been found to increase vertical and anterior duration and extent of hyoid and laryngeal motion as well as increase the anteroposterior opening diameter and opening duration of UES during swallowing [8, 56, 57]. The

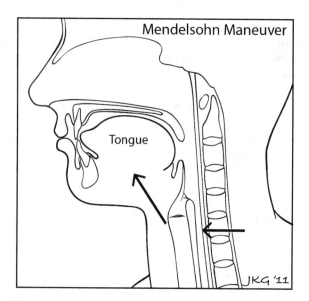

Fig. 14.2. Illustration of effects of Mendelsohn maneuver, with increased duration and extent of vertical and anterior laryngeal motion and increased width and duration of upper esophageal sphincter opening.

Mendelsohn maneuver has also been shown to improve coordination and timing of the pharyngeal events during the swallow [58]. Surface electrode electromyography (EMG) assessment of the submental and infrahyoid musculature during normal swallows and those with the Mendelsohn maneuver in healthy adults has revealed significantly longer duration of laryngeal elevation with the Mendelsohn maneuver [59]. In addition, these authors found significantly higher maximum amplitude and duration of EMG activity for the submental and the infrahyoid musculature during Mendelsohn swallows as compared to normal swallows [59]. Although not a specific target of the maneuver, duration of lateral pharyngeal wall motion medialward has been found to significantly increase with use of the maneuver in healthy subjects, likely due to shared muscle attachments and the muscular effort utilized with the maneuver [60].

The Mendelsohn maneuver has also been found to improve swallow functioning in patient populations. In a group of head and neck cancer patients treated with primary radiotherapy or chemoradiotherapy, results revealed increased duration and extent of laryngeal motion with the Mendelsohn maneuver as compared to baseline swallows [61] (Fig. 14.2). In addition, frequency and occurrence of pharyngeal phase motility disorders as well as aspiration were reduced with use of the Mendelsohn maneuver in this study [61]. Although not a targeted outcome, duration of tongue base-pharyngeal wall contact as well as pharyngeal pressures was increased with use of the Mendelsohn maneuver in a group of head and neck cancer patients treated surgically and with primary chemoradiotherapy [35]. Another unexpected but beneficial outcome with use of the Mendelsohn is improvement in coordination and timing of structural movement during the swallow. In a case study examining effects of maneuvers on swallowing in a dysphagia oral cancer patient [58], duration and extent of laryngeal motion as well as duration and width of UES opening improved as compared to baseline swallows [58]. Use of the Mendelsohn maneuver has been found to be effective in improving swallow functioning and in reestablishing oral nutrition in the chronic and severely dysphagic brainstem stroke population [26, 29, 36].

Biofeedback Usage for Training with the Mendelsohn Maneuver

The Mendelsohn maneuver can be difficult to accomplish, as the instruction includes several steps and is rather complex: "Swallow normally. When you feel your adam's apple lift, try to grab and hold it up with your throat muscles" [56]. Clinicians typically show patients how to perform this maneuver by having the patient feel the laryngeal motion on the clinician as they perform the maneuver. The clinician then typically palpates the patient's larynx and coaches the patient to "hold," in order to effect prolonged and increased laryngeal elevation during the swallow. Visual biofeedback utilizing surface electrode EMG has been used to help patients perform this maneuver, as the prolonged duration and increased excursion of the larynx can be easily visualized on the graphic output [36]. Use of surface electrode EMG has been beneficial for establishment of accurate performance of the Mendelsohn in the chronic dysphagic brainstem stroke population [36]. Use of the Mendelsohn maneuver combined with compensatory techniques, including postures and dietary modifications, was examined in a group of neurologically impaired dysphagic patients with cricopharyngeal dysfunction [62]. These authors found 95 % of the patients had improved swallow function resulting greater swallowing safety, type of feeding route (i.e., oral vs. non-oral), and diet type [62].

Cortical activation has been observed with use of the Mendelsohn maneuver [63], which is significant activation in the bilateral postcentral gyrus, bilateral precentral gyrus, bilateral cingulate gyrus, bilateral medial frontal gyrus, left inferior parietal lobe, left supramarginal gyrus, and right insula. The increased activation with the Mendelsohn maneuver as compared to dry swallows lends support to the notion of potential neural plasticity with use of this maneuver [64].

As opposed to the use of the Masako maneuver only with dry swallows, the Mendelsohn maneuver can be used with bolus swallows and during meals [65]. Some patients practice the Mendelsohn maneuver as a strengthening and range of motion exercise for the larynx. However, others must use the Mendelsohn maneuver during meals (i.e., with liquids and/or foods) in order to ensure swallow safety and efficiency. In some cases, patients are instructed to limit the volume per bolus when eating or drinking using this maneuver to avoid compromising swallow safety and/or efficiency. This is because UES opening may be improved but not normal with use of the maneuver, and boluses that are too large or too viscous may not clear completely through the UES region, potentially resulting in residue and potential post-deglutitive aspiration (see Chapter 3iib on bolus characteristics).

Summary

The Masako and Mendelsohn maneuvers are two swallow maneuvers that have been shown to improve pharyngeal phase swallow physiology and improve overall functioning in terms of swallow safety (i.e., elimination of aspiration) and improving diet outcomes. Future studies need to examine the impact of these maneuvers on swallow physiology, medical outcomes (i.e., aspiration pneumonia), oral intake type and diet, and quality of life outcomes in randomized controlled clinical trials to evaluate treatment efficacy for the medically debilitated, neurogenic, as well as treated head and neck cancer populations.

References

1. Dodds WJ, Stewart ET, Logemann JA. Physiology and radiology of the normal oral and pharyngeal phases of swallowing. AJR Am J Roentgenol. 1990;154(5):953–63.
2. Cerenko D, McConnel FM, Jackson RT. Quantitative assessment of pharyngeal bolus driving forces. Otolaryngol Head Neck Surg. 1989;100(1):57–63.

3. Kahrilas PJ, Lin S, Logemann JA, Ergun GA, Facchini F. Deglutitive tongue action: volume accommodation and bolus propulsion. Gastroenterology. 1993;104(1):152–62.

4. Kahrilas PJ, Logemann JA, Lin S, Ergun GA. Pharyngeal clearance during swallowing: a combined manometric and videofluoroscopic study. Gastroenterology. 1992;103(1): 128–36.

5. Palmer JB, Tanaka E, Siebens AA. Motions of the posterior pharyngeal wall in swallowing. Laryngoscope. 1988;98(4):414–7.

6. Ramsey GH, Watson JS, Gramiak R, Weinberg SA. Cinefluorographic analysis of the mechanism of swallowing. Radiology. 1955;64(4):498–518.

7. Asoh R, Goyal RK. Manometry and electromyography of the upper esophageal sphincter in the opossum. Gastroenterology. 1978;74(3):514–20.

8. Kahrilas PJ, Logemann JA, Krugler C, Flanagan E. Volitional augmentation of upper esophageal sphincter opening during swallowing. Am J Physiol. 1991;260(3 Pt 1): G450–6.

9. Martin BJ, Logemann JA, Shaker R, Dodds WJ. Normal laryngeal valving patterns during three breath-hold maneuvers: a pilot investigation. Dysphagia. 1993;8(1): 11–20.

10. Ardran GM, Kemp FH. The protection of the laryngeal airway during swallowing. Br J Radiol. 1952;25(296):406–16.

11. Ardran GM, Kemp FH. Closure and opening of the larynx during swallowing. Br J Radiol. 1956;29(340):205–8.

12. Ardran GM, Kemp FH. The mechanism of the larynx. II. The epiglottis and closure of the larynx. Br J Radiol. 1967;40(473):372–89.

13. Logemann JA, Kahrilas PJ, Cheng J, et al. Closure mechanisms of laryngeal vestibule during swallow. Am J Physiol. 1992;262(2 Pt 1):G338–44.

14. Ekberg O. Closure of the laryngeal vestibule during deglutition. Acta Otolaryngol. 1982;93(1–2):123–9.

15. Ohmae Y, Logemann JA, Kaiser P, Hanson DG, Kahrilas PJ. Timing of glottic closure during normal swallow. Head Neck. 1995;17(5):394–402.

16. Flaherty RF, Seltzer S, Campbell T, Weisskoff RM, Gilbert RJ. Dynamic magnetic resonance imaging of vocal cord closure during deglutition. Gastroenterology. 1995; 109(3):843–9.

17. Kahrilas PJ, Dodds WJ, Dent J, Logemann JA, Shaker R. Upper esophageal sphincter function during deglutition. Gastroenterology. 1988;95(1):52–62.

18. Cook IJ, Dodds WJ, Dantas RO, et al. Opening mechanisms of the human upper esophageal sphincter. Am J Physiol. 1989;257(5 Pt 1):G748–59.

19. Dejaeger E, Pelemans W, Ponette E, Joosten E. Mechanisms involved in postdeglutition retention in the elderly. Dysphagia. 1997;12(2):63–7.

20. Pauloski BR, Rademaker AW, Lazarus C, Boeckxstaens G, Kahrilas PJ, Logemann JA. Relationship between manometric and videofluoroscopic measures of swallow function in healthy adults and patients treated for head and neck cancer with various modalities. Dysphagia. 2009;24(2):196–203.

21. Kendall KA, Leonard RJ. Pharyngeal constriction in elderly dysphagic patients compared with young and elderly nondysphagic controls. Dysphagia. 2001; 16(4):272–8.

278   C. Lazarus

22. Logemann JA, Pauloski BR, Rademaker AW, Kahrilas PJ. Oropharyngeal swallow in younger and older women: videofluoroscopic analysis. J Speech Lang Hear Res. 2002;45(3):434–45.
23. Rademaker AW, Pauloski BR, Colangelo LA, Logemann JA. Age and volume effects on liquid swallowing function in normal women. J Speech Lang Hear Res. 1998;41(2):275–84.
24. Bardan E, Kern M, Arndorfer RC, Hofmann C, Shaker R. Effect of aging on bolus kinematics during the pharyngeal phase of swallowing. Am J Physiol Gastrointest Liver Physiol. 2006;290(3):G458–65.
25. Logemann JA, Pauloski BR, Rademaker AW, Colangelo LA, Kahrilas PJ, Smith CH. Temporal and biomechanical characteristics of oropharyngeal swallow in younger and older men. J Speech Lang Hear Res. 2000;43(5):1264–74.
26. Prosiegel M, Heintze M, Sonntag EW, Schenk T, Yassouridis A. Kinematic analysis of laryngeal movements in patients with neurogenic dysphagia before and after swallowing rehabilitation. Dysphagia. 2000;15(4):173–9.
27. Leonard RJ, Kendall KA, McKenzie S, Goncalves MI, Walker A. Structural displacements in normal swallowing: a videofluoroscopic study. Dysphagia. 2000; 15(3):146–52.
28. Robbins J, Levine RL, Maser A, Rosenbek JC, Kempster GB. Swallowing after unilateral stroke of the cerebral cortex. Arch Phys Med Rehabil. 1993;74(12):1295–300.
29. Robbins J, Levine R. Swallowing after lateral medullary syndrome plus. Clin Commun Disord. 1993;3(4):45–55.
30. Troche MS, Okun MS, Rosenbek JC, et al. Aspiration and swallowing in Parkinson disease and rehabilitation with EMST: a randomized trial. Neurology. 2010;75(21):1912–9.
31. Pauloski BR, Logemann JA, Fox JC, Colangelo LA. Biomechanical analysis of the pharyngeal swallow in postsurgical patients with anterior tongue and floor of mouth resection and distal flap reconstruction. J Speech Hear Res. 1995;38(1):110–23.
32. McConnel FM, Mendelsohn MS, Logemann JA. Manofluorography of deglutition after supraglottic laryngectomy. Head Neck Surg. 1987;9(3):142–50.
33. Logemann JA, Pauloski BR, Rademaker AW, et al. Swallowing disorders in the first year after radiation and chemoradiation. Head Neck. 2008;30(2):148–58.
34. Kotz T, Abraham S, Beitler JJ, Wadler S, Smith RV. Pharyngeal transport dysfunction consequent to an organ-sparing protocol. Arch Otolaryngol Head Neck Surg. 1999;125(4):410–3.
35. Lazarus C, Logemann JA, Song CW, Rademaker AW, Kahrilas PJ. Effects of voluntary maneuvers on tongue base function for swallowing. Folia Phoniatr Logop. 2002;54(4):171–6.
36. Huckabee ML, Cannito MP. Outcomes of swallowing rehabilitation in chronic brainstem dysphagia: a retrospective evaluation. Dysphagia. 1999;14(2):93–109.
37. Easterling CS, Bousamra II M, Lang IM, et al. Pharyngeal dysphagia in postesophagectomy patients: correlation with deglutitive biomechanics. Ann Thorac Surg. 2000;69(4):989–92.
38. Barquist E, Brown M, Cohn S, Lundy D, Jackowski J. Postextubation fiberoptic endoscopic evaluation of swallowing after prolonged endotracheal intubation: a randomized, prospective trial. Crit Care Med. 2001;29(9):1710–3.

39. Altman KW, Yu GP, Schaefer SD. Consequence of dysphagia in the hospitalized patient: impact on prognosis and hospital resources. Arch Otolaryngol Head Neck Surg. 2010;136(8):784–9.

40. Leonard R, Rees CJ, Belafsky P, Allen J. Fluoroscopic surrogate for pharyngeal strength: the pharyngeal constriction ratio (PCR). Dysphagia. 2011;26(1):13–7.

41. McConnel FM. Analysis of pressure generation and bolus transit during pharyngeal swallowing. Laryngoscope. 1988;98(1):71–8.

42. McConnel FM, Hester TR, Mendelsohn MS, Logemann JA. Manofluorography of deglutition after total laryngopharyngectomy. Plast Reconstr Surg. 1988;81(3):346–51.

43. Castell JA, Dalton CB, Castell DO. Pharyngeal and upper esophageal sphincter manometry in humans. Am J Physiol. 1990;258(2 Pt 1):G173–8.

44. Langmore SE, Schatz K, Olsen N. Fiberoptic endoscopic examination of swallowing safety: a new procedure. Dysphagia. 1988;2(4):216–9.

45. Leder SB, Acton LM, Lisitano HL, Murray JT. Fiberoptic endoscopic evaluation of swallowing (FEES) with and without blue-dyed food. Dysphagia. 2005;20(2):157–62.

46. Fujiu M, Logemann J. Effect of a tongue-holding maneuver on posterior pharyngeal wall movement during deglutition. Am J Speech Lang Pathol. 1996;5:23–30.

47. Fujiu M, Logemann J, Pauloski B. Increased postoperative posterior pharyngeal wall movement in patients with anterior oral cancer: preliminary findings and possible implications for treatment. Am J Speech Lang Pathol. 1995;4:24–30.

48. Doeltgen SH, Witte U, Gumbley F, Huckabee ML. Evaluation of manometric measures during tongue-hold swallows. Am J Speech Lang Pathol. 2009;18(1):65–73.

49. Umeki H, Takasaki K, Enatsu K, Tanaka F, Kumagami H, Takahashi H. Effects of a tongue-holding maneuver during swallowing evaluated by high-resolution manometry. Otolaryngol Head Neck Surg. 2009;141(1):119–22.

50. Logemann JA. Role of the modified barium swallow in management of patients with dysphagia. Otolaryngol Head Neck Surg. 1997;116(3):335–8.

51. Martin-Harris B, Brodsky MB, Michel Y, et al. MBS measurement tool for swallow impairment—MBSImp: establishing a standard. Dysphagia. 2008;23(4):392–405.

52. Wheeler-Hegland KM, Rosenbek JC, Sapienza CM. Submental sEMG and hyoid movement during Mendelsohn maneuver, effortful swallow, and expiratory muscle strength training. J Speech Lang Hear Res. 2008;51(5):1072–87.

53. Elidan J, Shochina M, Gonen B, Gay I. Electromyography of the inferior constrictor and cricopharyngeal muscles during swallowing. Ann Otol Rhinol Laryngol. 1990;99(6 Pt 1):466–9.

54. Mielens JD, Hoffman MR, Ciucci MR, Jiang JJ, McCulloch TM. Automated analysis of pharyngeal pressure data obtained with high-resolution manometry. Dysphagia. 2011;26:3–12.

55. Ghosh SK, Pandolfino JE, Zhang Q, Jarosz A, Kahrilas PJ. Deglutitive upper esophageal sphincter relaxation: a study of 75 volunteer subjects using solid-state high-resolution manometry. Am J Physiol Gastrointest Liver Physiol. 2006;291:G525–31.

56. Logemann JA. Swallowing physiology and pathophysiology. Otolaryngol Clin North Am. 1988;21(4):613–23.

57. Logemann JA, Kahrilas PJ. Relearning to swallow after stroke—application of maneuvers and indirect biofeedback: a case study. Neurology. 1990;40(7):1136–8.

58. Lazarus C, Logemann JA, Gibbons P. Effects of maneuvers on swallowing function in a dysphagic oral cancer patient. Head Neck. 1993;15(5):419–24.
59. Ding R, Larson CR, Logemann JA, Rademaker AW. Surface electromyographic and electroglottographic studies in normal subjects under two swallow conditions: normal and during the Mendelsohn manuever. Dysphagia. 2002;17(1):1–12.
60. Miller JL, Watkin KL. Lateral pharyngeal wall motion during swallowing using real time ultrasound. Dysphagia. 1997;12(3):125–32.
61. Lazarus CL. Effects of radiation therapy and voluntary maneuvers on swallow functioning in head and neck cancer patients. Clin Commun Disord. 1993;3(4):11–20.
62. Bartolome G, Neumann S. Swallowing therapy in patients with neurological disorders causing cricopharyngeal dysfunction. Dysphagia. 1993;8(2):146–9.
63. Peck KK, Branski RC, Lazarus C, et al. Cortical activation during swallowing rehabilitation maneuvers: a functional MRI study of healthy controls. Laryngoscope. 2010;120(11):2153–9.
64. Robbins J, Butler SG, Daniels SK, et al. Swallowing and dysphagia rehabilitation: translating principles of neural plasticity into clinically oriented evidence. J Speech Lang Hear Res. 2008;51(1):S276–300.
65. Lazarus CL. Management of swallowing disorders in head and neck cancer patients: optimal patterns of care. Semin Speech Lang. 2000;21(4):293–309.

15. Effortful Swallow

Maggie-Lee Huckabee and Phoebe Macrae

Maggie-Lee Huckabee and Phoebe Macrae

Abstract   As one of the first techniques to emerge in the management of the patient with swallowing impairment, the effortful swallow technique provides an excellent example of how our thinking has evolved in this area of clinical practice. This chapter will summarize the literature related to the application of effortful swallowing first as a compensatory mechanism, then as a task emphasizing strength training and finally representing the paradigm shift to skill training in dysphagia rehabilitation. Despite potential positive influences on swallowing physiology, no intervention is without potential for complication, thus clinicians are encouraged to understand potential adverse ramifications and judiciously apply this technique to patient populations.

Introduction

Current approaches to management of the patient with swallowing impairment are rapidly maturing as the knowledge base expands. This evolution in clinical thinking and the consequent paradigm shifts in management approaches can be no better illustrated than through a discussion of the effortful swallowing technique.

Early approaches to management of the patient with swallowing impairment focused very heavily on application of compensatory techniques to allow for ingestion of oral intake in the presence of oral pharyngeal swallowing impairment [1]. Although "exercise" was referred to in the literature, this focused heavily on oral motor exercises for oral phase impairment, rather than addressing pharyngeal pathophysiology. The technique of effortful swallowing was very simply described as a technique of swallowing "with effort." It was applied as a compensatory strategy with the ultimate goal of providing an immediate increase in

R. Shaker et al. (eds.), *Manual of Diagnostic and Therapeutic Techniques for Disorders of Deglutition*, DOI 10.1007/978-1-4614-3779-6_15,
© Springer Science+Business Media New York 2013

pharyngeal pressure, thereby facilitating bolus flow through the hypopharynx and upper esophageal sphincter (UES) and minimizing pharyngeal residual. Much of the research (to be summarized in the following sections) represents pharyngeal response to effortful swallowing during the execution of the maneuvre [2–7].

Over time, increased interest was directed toward the potential application of effortful swallowing as a rehabilitative approach for pharyngeal pathophysiology. This paradigm shift was founded on basic principles of muscle strengthening. It is well accepted that skeletal muscle, consisting of striated muscle fibers, is capable of generating greater force and increased bulk with repetitive execution of suprathreshold motor tasks [8, 9]. As the muscles involved in pharyngeal swallowing are classed as striated muscle [10], application of an exercise based on swallowing with maximal effort was hypothesized to yield increased muscle strength during pharyngeal swallowing. This assumption was predicated by yet a further assumption that the nature of the pathophysiology was due to muscle weakness. Regardless, the urgency to rehabilitate provided a strong motivating force for the recommendation of rehabilitation techniques. As such, these techniques have emerged into clinical practice ahead of supportive, empirical evidence for application [11–13]. Very few studies exist in support of this approach, and they are limited to case series reports and describe treatment outcomes from rehabilitation programs rather than a single technique.

Clinical practice is now perhaps on the cusp of another paradigm expansion. With an emerging' interest in cortical modulation of the swallowing response and the increasing recognition that not all dysphagia is associated with muscle weakness, effortful swallowing is gaining recognition as a skill training task, with the presumed effect of the technique extending from changes at the muscle, to changes in cortical motor planning. Research is currently underway to investigate how execution of this technique influences motor skill in swallowing. The end of this chapter summarizes a few of the basic principles surrounding this application.

Much of current practice in dysphagia rehabilitation is based on presumption and well-founded hypotheses. There is progress in substantiating clinical practice with well-designed empirical research, but the innate variability within and across individuals provides considerable challenges to this work. This chapter will outline the evidence that has been acquired to support application of the effortful swallow in rehabilitation programs and will provide foundation knowledge for further development.

Immediate Effects of Effortful Swallowing

Effects of Effortful Swallow on Submental Muscle Recruitment

Greater submental muscle activation has been documented with effortful swallowing [6, 14]. This increase in sEMG amplitude may consequently have implications for a number of biomechanical events including airway protection and UES pressures. The submental muscles, specifically the floor of mouth muscles (geniohyoid, anterior belly of digastrics, mylohyoid), are responsible during the pharyngeal swallow for anterior and/or superior excursion of the hyolaryngeal complex. As such, one would anticipate that increased sEMG amplitude would signal increased hyolaryngeal excursion and the biomechanical consequences of this action: namely epiglottic deflection for airway protection and UES opening via the traction force of anterior movement.

The observation that the duration of laryngeal closure increases with effortful swallowing fits with the assumption that airway protection is facilitated by effortful swallowing [4, 15]. Earlier onset of submental muscle activation is seen during effortful swallowing [14] and provides explanation for the earlier onset of laryngeal and hyoid elevation prior to execution of effortful swallowing compared with non-effortful swallowing [2, 14].

While pre-swallow activation of the submental muscles appears to increase the amount of time the airway is protected, it doesn't necessarily have the same influence on the magnitude of hyoid and laryngeal displacement. Documentation of the extent of hyoid and laryngeal displacement varies slightly from study to study, but a general trend of either unchanged [14] or decreased displacement [2, 4] is seen for effortful, when compared with non-effortful swallowing. It is difficult to assess whether this decrease has functional negative implications for swallowing. A reduction in laryngeal displacement may result in less effective closure of the airway, despite increased duration of closure. However, effortful swallowing has been shown to reduce the depth of penetration into the larynx and trachea [3], providing some support that this technique does not compromise laryngeal closure.

A decrease in hyolaryngeal displacement may also cause a biomechanical decrease in UES opening, but the width of UES at maximal opening is reportedly unchanged in the face of this decrease in displacement [4]. Furthermore, an increase in the magnitude of UES relaxation [6, 16], and an increase in UES relaxation duration [4, 15, 17], has been documented during effortful swallowing. Increased magnitude of UES relaxation represents less resistance for bolus transfer into the esophagus. Additionally, the increase in sEMG amplitude documented with effortful swallowing has been correlated with the increased UES relaxation magnitude [6]. These findings suggest that effortful swallowing assists with UES opening during swallowing [16], resulting in more favorable pressures for bolus transfer.

Effects on Pharyngeal Pressure Generation

Despite the positive modifications on swallowing biomechanics documented during effortful swallowing, there are discrepancies in the literature regarding how these changes affect pharyngeal pressures. The discrepancies raise questions about the application of effortful swallowing as both a compensatory and rehabilitation technique for heterogeneous populations.

There are many biomechanical events that contribute to pharyngeal pressures, including: pharyngeal and oral muscle contraction, closure of the larynx, lips and velopharyngeal port, and tongue movement [18]. These actions together are responsible for bolus propulsion and effective bolus clearance [18, 19]. When reporting the effects of effortful swallowing on healthy participants, various studies using manometry to quantify peak and nadir pressures in the pharynx have documented a significant increase in pharyngeal pressures [6, 15, 20] and pharyngeal pressure duration [2, 4, 15–17, 21]. These findings suggest that effortful swallowing may be effective for treating dysphagia resulting from decreased bolus propulsion and clearance. However, as decreased pharyngeal pressure can be the consequence of individual or combined contributions of pharyngeal and oral muscle contraction, closure of the larynx, lips and velopharyngeal port, and tongue movement, more information is needed about which of these mechanisms are influenced by effortful swallowing.

Tongue movement is presumably greater during effortful swallowing, based on findings of increased oral pressures with effortful swallowing [4, 22]. The finding that anterior bulging of the posterior pharyngeal wall decreases with effortful swallowing, but base of tongue to posterior pharyngeal wall contact pressure increases [15] implies that increases in pharyngeal pressure at the level of the base of tongue in healthy [15, 23] and dysphagic participants [7] are also likely to result from altered tongue movement during the effortful swallowing.

Early studies into the effects of effortful swallowing on pharyngeal pressures by Bulow and colleagues report findings that contradict later investigations [6, 20]. Bulow and colleagues found no significant pressure or duration of pressure differences in the pharynx and UES when effortful swallows were compared with non-effortful swallows [2, 3]. Although no findings reached significance, suggesting no differences between the two conditions, trends of decreased pressure at the level of the inferior constrictor during effortful swallowing were reported for both dysphagic [3] and healthy participants [2]. This finding raises questions regarding the use of this technique for the purpose of enhancing bolus propulsion and clearance.

The studies by Bulow and colleagues [2, 3] also show a trend for a decrease in the magnitude of UES relaxation during effortful swallows, suggesting the technique may result in greater resistance for the bolus in the transfer from pharynx to esophagus. For dysphagic patients, a trend towards decreased duration of UES relaxation was also documented for effortful swallows [3], with the opposite seen for healthy participants [2], suggesting some differences in the way healthy and disordered systems respond to the technique. Given that other studies of healthy participants have also found increases in UES relaxation duration [4, 17], this seems a plausible explanation. However, many trends reported in the Bulow study of healthy participants [2] are in contrast to other studies of healthy participants [6, 20], suggesting clarification of the discrepancies is essential before drawing conclusions about the application of effortful swallowing in dysphagia management. Furthermore, as the technique potentially influences measured swallowing biomechanics, clarification is essential to avoid exacerbation of physiologic deficits.

Catheter assembly is an important factor to take into account when determining the cause of discrepancies in manometric evaluations of pharyngeal pressures. The studies by Bulow et al. [2, 3] utilized solid-state transducers similar to those used in studies that have rendered conflicting findings [6, 20]. However, a point of difference in the catheter assembly of these studies is the diameter of the catheter, brought about by the incorporation of circumferential transducers in the Bulow studies. These differences must be considered when interpreting UES pressures specifically given the reduced lumen of this area compared with the pharynx. Further discrepancies exist between studies and warrant discussion.

Another consideration when comparing the Bulow studies to those with conflicting findings is the statistical power achieved. While studies to date haven't typically reported power statistics, the larger number of participants and trials utilized in the Huckabee studies may contribute to the different findings reported to those completed by Bulow and colleagues. As studies with similar participant numbers and trials have also rendered conflicting findings, alternative factors that differ between studies also warrant consideration.

Varied instructions on how an effortful swallow is to be executed may also contribute to these discrepancies [6]. An effortful swallow is typically completed following the instruction to "swallow hard," but the emphasis on whether tongue or pharyngeal muscles should be maximally contracted may change the observed effects on pharyngeal pressures [20, 21]. The observation that similar instructions have yielded dissimilar results suggests this variable alone is unlikely to explain the contrasting findings [2, 3, 6, 16, 20].

The use of a bolus during effortful swallowing in studies may also influence the differential effects on reported pharyngeal pressures [16]. Early investigations involved execution of the maneuvre with a bolus [2–4, 7, 23, 24], while more recent studies utilized saliva swallows and reported some contrasting results to those reported previously [6, 17, 20, 21]. To further investigate if the presence of a bolus could influence the findings, Witte et al. [16] investigated the effect of effort on both saliva and 10 mL water boluses. They concluded that the effects on pharyngeal pressures are the same for both bolus and non-bolus conditions, with the exception of one significant difference. This study suggested a role of the bolus in decreasing the magnitude of UES relaxation. The study also added to the pool of conflicting findings, reporting no increase in pharyngeal pressures associated with effortful swallowing, suggesting alternative confounds in studies to date.

Witte et al. [16] postulated that the use of biofeedback during training of the technique was a possible cause of their conflicting findings to those found previously in the same laboratory [6, 20]. However, there are contradictory findings from studies that have not used biofeedback in training the technique [2, 21].

The differences in anatomic location of pharyngeal pressure measurement may also explain uncertainty around the effects of effortful swallowing [16]. For the series of studies by Bulow and colleagues [2, 3, 24], measurement was at the level of the lower pharynx only. Other studies have reported increased pressure [7, 23] and increased duration of pressure generation [7] at the level of the base of tongue for the technique. Although it is possible that pressure changes at the level of the base of tongue went undetected in the Bulow studies, their findings at the level of the lower pharynx still differed to other studies [6, 20], suggesting other sources of conflict. Measurement of pharyngeal pressure in the lower pharynx may be heavily influenced by catheter selection, with Bulow and colleagues using a strain gauge catheter rather than the more frequently utilized solid-state catheter.

There is the possibility that effortful swallowing influences men and women differently. Witte et al. [16] found that greater duration of pressure generation at the oropharynx occurred with non-effortful swallowing for men, but with effortful swallowing for women. Another study found no differences in gender responses to effortful swallowing [6]. A study including a larger number of participants does not report gender effects; however, this study does not state whether gender was equally represented, and so these effects may not have been analyzed [4]. Other studies have included only one gender in the participant group [20, 21], or not stated the gender of participants [17], meaning gender differences cannot be ruled out as a possible cause for opposing results.

It is also possible that the effects of effortful swallowing vary with age. Studies investigating the effects of the technique have used participant groups of varying ages. One study controlled for this variable and found pyriform sinus residual was greater after effortful swallowing than in non-effortful for elderly participants, and the opposite in younger participants [4].

Although effortful swallowing is considered an intervention for pharyngeal swallowing, one investigation acknowledged the inherent links between pharyngeal and esophageal pressures and assessed the effect of effortful swallowing on esophageal peristalsis [22]. This study found an increase in peristaltic amplitudes associated with effortful swallowing, with the authors suggesting a place for the technique in the treatment of esophageal disorders. An additional consideration from these findings is the possibility that non-volitional aspects of swallowing can be influenced by execution of a volitional, oropharyngeal maneuvre. Interestingly, this study found increased peristaltic amplitudes of the distal (smooth) muscles but not the proximal (striated) muscles. These findings suggest promise for modulating reflexive aspects of swallowing and highlight the robust integration of all swallowing components.

Contraindications of Effortful Swallowing

Although effortful swallowing would appear to be, at first inspection, a fairly benign intervention, a recognition of the delicate balance of biomechanical movements underlying swallowing suggests that there is the potential for unanticipated adverse outcomes. As with any treatment, if it is powerful enough to engender a positive outcome, then it is likewise powerful enough to engender a negative one. Careful scrutiny of all biomechanical features of swallowing is thus required.

Substantial nasal redirection (redirection of food or fluid into the nasal cavity) has been reported during a rehabilitation program that resolved once effortful swallowing practice ceased [25]. After viewing videofluoroscopic images of the execution of the technique, the authors concluded that the timing of base of tongue contact with the posterior pharyngeal wall was altered, creating an obstruction to bolus flow in the upper pharynx. This obstruction prior to closure of the velopharyngeal port resulted in nasal redirection on 100 % of swallows. An alternative explanation is that compromised velopharyngeal closure may have been exacerbated with increased force of the pharyngeal musculature. With the various mechanisms available to patients to perceptively increase the "strength" of a swallow, there are possibilities for incorrect execution to combine with physiologic impairment, resulting in aggravation of an existing problem, or initiation of a new one.

A study by Bulow et al. [3] also reports a case in which severe pharyngeal dysfunction was exacerbated by effortful swallowing. All participants were reported to have either severe or moderate pharyngeal dysfunction; however, the variable of underlying physiologic deficits causing the dysphagia was not controlled, making it difficult to determine the specific physiologic impairment aggravated by the technique. The findings of these two studies stress the need for an understanding of the effects of treatment techniques on various physiologic deficits and for cautious application of this technique in the patient population in the interim.

Cumulative Effects of Effortful Swallowing

The studies discussed thus far highlight the biomechanical modifications that take place during effortful swallowing and provide valuable information about the compensatory possibilities of the technique; that is, what immediate changes in swallowing biomechanics occur during implementation. As introduced in this chapter, clinical application of effortful swallowing has evolved to the utilization of this technique in rehabilitation programs. This has been based on the assumption that repeated execution of the task will result in cumulative improvements in underlying swallowing physiology. A small number of studies have looked at the lasting effects of effortful swallowing and other techniques on swallowing biomechanics within the context of a clinical treatment paradigm. These studies have documented positive outcomes for dysphagic patients using the technique as part of a rehabilitation plan, including a decrease in aspiration-related pulmonary symptoms, removal of enteral feeding tubes and a return to full oral intake, increased activation of swallowing musculature, and continued functional improvements in swallowing following termination of therapy [26–28]. Although these findings suggest rehabilitative promise for the technique, the treatment protocols evaluated have all included additional exercises in conjunction with effortful swallowing and, therefore, positive outcomes cannot necessarily be attributed to effortful swallowing per se.

Applying Effortful Swallowing in the Rehabilitation Plan

The research summarized above provides an overview of known, although not undisputed, effects of effortful swallowing on deglutitive biomechanics. For ease of application, these findings are summarized in Table 15.1. Clinicians may use this information to guide decisions on development of treatment plans. However, the inconsistencies in the literature confuse this process. These discrepancies can be attributed to methodological differences in research design, execution, and interpretation of the subsequent data. Factors such as the age, gender, etiology, and presenting characteristics of the populations studied may heavily influence stated outcomes of research and thereby influence application to patient populations.

Not only is there inconsistency in the supporting literature, but there is inconsistency in the swallowing behavior of patient populations. As a result, the astute clinician will carefully question decisions to apply this technique to patients in their care. Caution is extended to avoid application of any technique based on a single presentation. Effortful swallowing may well be appropriate for a patient with pharyngeal residual as a primary feature of impairment. However, if that feature presents in conjunction with reduced hyolaryngeal excursion, effortful swallowing may be problematic. A prerequisite for development of a rehabilitative plan, whether including or excluding effortful swallowing, is a clear

Table 15.1. Summary of key research findings related to effortful swallowing from 2000 forward.

	A	B	C	D	E	F	G	H	I	J	K	L	M	N
Huckabee et al. [6]							✓		✓				✓	
Wheeler-Hegland et al. [14]		✓	✓				✓		✓					
Ohmae et al. [15]				✓				✓			✓			
Hind et al. [4]	✓			✓	✓			✓			✓			
Bulow et al. (1999)			✓		✓			✓			✓			
Bulow et al. (2001)						✓						✓		
Witte et al. [16]								✓						✓
Hiss and Huckabee [17]	✓							✓					✓	
Huckabee and Steele [20]		✓						✓	✓		✓			
Steele and Huckabee [21]	✓							✓						
Lever et al. [22]										✓				
Lazarus et al. [7]														✓

A = Increased oral pressures, B = Earlier onset of submental muscle sEMG, C = Earlier onset of hyolaryngeal elevation, D = Increased duration of laryngeal closure, E = Decreased displacement of hyolaryngeal complex, F = Reduced depth of laryngeal & tracheal penetration, G = Increased amplitude of submental muscle sEMG, H = Increased pressure duration in pharynx, I = Increased pressure in pharynx, J = Nasal Redirection, K = Increased duration of UES relaxation, L = Decreased duration of UES relaxation, M = Decreased pressure in UES, N = Increased opening of UES.

understanding of all pathophysiologic features underlying the clinical presentation of signs and symptoms and consideration of how modification in behavior may influence all features.

An Expansion on Rehabilitative Paradigms for Effortful Swallowing: Skill Training

Past presumptions have been that the effortful swallow technique influenced swallowing at the level of the periphery—that the muscles involved in swallowing were recruited to a greater degree. More current thinking proposes that effortful swallowing may also achieve improved swallowing skill through motor learning. Effortful swallowing is carried out in the context of functional swallowing and is therefore a task-oriented exercise in that the technique replicates the desired task. Thus, the technique can consequently be defined as a task-oriented form of skill training, with a strength component resulting from greater muscle activation than produced during regular swallowing [10]. This can be contrasted to another swallowing muscle strengthening exercise—the head-lift maneuvre—that targets isolated strengthening of one set of muscles (submental) involved in the swallowing process, i.e., hyolaryngeal excursion, but is not executed in the context of the targeted task. Head-lift maneuvre is consequently defined as a non-task-oriented form of strength training.

Background information follows in the subsequent section to support the emerging application of effortful swallowing as a skill training task. To date, no empirical research has carefully extracted the differential effects of skill vs. strength produced with this task in swallowing recovery.

The Effects of Skill Training on Neural Plasticity

Improvements in motor function have been associated with plasticity of cortical regions such as the primary motor cortex and supplementary motor area [29]. Changes in representation in the motor cortex have been shown to result from both spontaneous recovery of motor impairment [30] and functional movement training [31]. Animal studies evaluating arm and auditory exercises have documented similar altered representations in the motor [32] and somatosensory cortices [33] following training. These alterations can last for at least several days following termination of exercise practice [32, 34], suggesting that lasting effects of rehabilitation are reflected in the plasticity of these regions and mimic that seen in natural recovery.

Skill training programs that challenge routine motor execution have been shown to influence neural control of movement [35, 36]. There is increasing evidence that limb rehabilitation following stroke is most effective when exercise is incorporated into functional movements [37, 38]. These findings are based on both post-treatment functional movement outcomes, changes in neuroimaging measures such as positron emission tomography (PET) [38] and transcranial magnetic stimulation (TMS)-induced motor-evoked potentials (MEPs) [39]. Increased amplitude and/or decreased latency of MEPs has been shown following functional rehabilitation programs in patients with hemiplegia of the arm and/or leg secondary to stroke [40, 41], suggesting increased excitability in the corticospinal pathways as a result of such rehabilitation programs. Greater representation for a movement in the motor cortex [39] and reorganized activation of brain structures involved in motor programming and execution [38] has also been documented after rehabilitation involving functional movement practice.

Specific to muscles involved in swallowing, a series of studies have documented increased tongue representation in the motor cortex after a tongue protrusion exercise (see Sessle et al. [42] for review). Despite this increase in the tongue motor cortex, the authors report that no increase was seen in representation of the "cortical masticatory area/swallow cortex" (Sessle et al. [43], pg 111). This lends support to the "specificity of practice" hypothesis proposed by Barnett and colleagues [44], which states that specific motor skills are developed and stored through practice, and that these motor skills do not generalize across tasks. Task specificity would appear to apply as well to plasticity in the motor cortex. In relation to neural plasticity associated with recovery of swallowing impairment, plasticity of the undamaged hemisphere appears to be related to natural recovery of swallowing function following stroke [30, 45, 46].

One study aimed to evaluate the effects of effortful swallowing on excitability of cortical projections to the swallowing muscles [47] and found significant increases after 1 week of daily practice lasting 15 min. While this study indicates some promise for the effects of effortful swallowing on neural control mechanisms, baseline values were not reported and different stimulation methods were used for pre- and post-treatment time-points, making objective evaluation of their findings difficult.

The Role of Sensory Feedback in the Recovery of Motor Function

Proprioception consists of afferent feedback supplied to the brain from muscle mechanoreceptors [48] and is facilitated by visual and vestibular information [49]. Proprioceptive information during a movement may be disrupted by injury to the mechanoreceptors located in the muscle [48], the neural regions responsible for the processing of this information, or the pathways connecting the two [50]. Deficiencies of proprioceptive acuity result in delayed reflexive muscle contraction [51] and decreased functional motor performance [52, 53]. The interplay between motor output and sensory input is further highlighted by the finding that proprioceptive deficits seen following injury move towards restoration with functional rehabilitation [54].

Task-oriented training programs inherently incorporate proprioceptive facilitation [52]. They provide an opportunity for task-specific proprioceptive systems to be stimulated through repetition of meaningful activity. A specificity of learning phenomena has also been shown with afferent stimuli, with a lack of improvements generalizing from trained to untrained sensory skills [33, 34]. This suggests that task-specific proprioceptive experiences during training are important for generalization to functional outcomes. Rose and Christina [49] argue that if proprioceptive information encountered during practice contributes considerably to accuracy of the target movement, it will be integrated into the centrally stored motor pattern, regardless of whether it is explicit or implicit in nature. The development of centrally stored motor patterns is highly dependent on the proprioceptive feedback encountered during repetitive practice [49, 52], as are the neural plasticity mechanisms that aid functional recovery [55]. For these reasons, facilitation of proprioception is considered critical in functional rehabilitation programs [54, 56].

Some studies have investigated the function of proprioception in the swallowing process. Proprioceptive signals from the jaw muscles (through trigeminal afferent fibers) are necessary for coordination of the jaw with muscles of the larynx [57], tongue [58, 59], and visceral processes such as saliva production and respiratory changes [57]. Other swallowing literature has shown that the afferent information from the face, pharynx, and esophagus contributes significantly to motor output of the swallowing musculature [60, 61].

Because effortful swallowing is task-oriented, it provides task-specific neuromuscular control training and proprioceptive facilitation relevant to swallowing. Therefore, effortful swallowing may result in a greater degree of impact on swallowing neural control and functional motor outcomes than other rehabilitation techniques that are not completed within context, such as head-lift exercise. The finding that skill training techniques assist with strength and coordination of movement may suggest that effortful swallowing could be assumed to strengthen not only the swallowing musculature but possibly also coordination of swallowing.

Conclusions

Great progress has been made in the understanding of swallowing physiology, pathophysiology, and management. With this increased understanding, a clearer picture emerges of appropriate application of rehabilitation techniques. Research is sparse, but what is available would suggest that effortful swallowing has the potential to influence pharyngeal biomechanics positively, and perhaps negatively, as both a compensatory maneuvre and a rehabilitative exercise.

Summary Points

1. Effortful swallowing may have applications in both compensatory and rehabilitative realms.
2. Data generally support that execution of the maneuvre increases pharyngeal pressure and duration of oral pressure, hyolaryngeal excursion, airway protection, and UES opening.
3. There are potential, but not fully investigated, adverse effects of the technique; with the suggestion of inhibition of degree of anterior hyolaryngeal excursion and nasal redirection from improper timing of upper pharyngeal pressure generation.
4. Data are as yet limited regarding cumulative effects of effortful swallowing as exercise.
5. Emerging paradigm expansion into skill training may offer new applications for this well-used technique.

References

1. Logemann JL. Treatment for aspiration related to dysphagia: an overview. Dysphagia. 1986;1(1):31–8.

2. Bulow M, Olsson R, Ekberg O. Videomanometric analysis of supraglottic swallow, effortful swallow, and chin tuck in healthy volunteers. Dysphagia. 1999;14(2):67–72.

3. Bulow M, Olsson R, Ekberg O. Videomanometric analysis of supraglottic swallow, effortful swallow, and chin tuck in patients with pharyngeal dysfunction. Dysphagia. 2001;16(3):190–5.

4. Hind JA, Nicosia MA, Roecker EB, Carnes ML, Robbins J. Comparison of effortful and noneffortful swallows in healthy middle-aged and older adults. Arch Phys Med Rehabil. 2001;82(12):1661–5.

5. Doeltgen SH, Witte U, Gumbley F, Huckabee ML. Evaluation of manometric measures during tongue-hold swallows. Am J Speech Lang Pathol. 2009;18(1):65–73.

6. Huckabee ML, Butler SG, Barclay M, Jit S. Submental surface electromyographic measurement and pharyngeal pressures during normal and effortful swallowing. Arch Phys Med Rehabil. 2005;86(11):2144–9.

7. Lazarus C, Logemann JA, Song CW, Rademaker AW, Kahrilas PJ. Effects of voluntary maneuvers on tongue base function for swallowing. Folia Phoniatr Logop. 2002;54(4):171–6.

8. Folland JP, Williams AG. The adaptations to strength training: morphological and neurological contributions to increased strength. Sports Med. 2007;37(2):145–68.

9. Rasch PJ, Morehouse LE. Effect of static and dynamic exercises on muscular strength and hypertrophy. J Appl Phys. 1957;11(1):29–34.

10. Burkhead LM, Sapienza CM, Rosenbek JC. Strength-training exercise in dysphagia rehabilitation: principles, procedures, and directions for future research. Dysphagia. 2007;22(3):251–65.

11. Langmore SE. Efficacy of behavioral treatment for oropharyngeal dysphagia. Dysphagia. 1995;10(4):259–62.

12. Robbins J, Butler SG, Daniels SK, et al. Swallowing and dysphagia rehabilitation: translating principles of neural plasticity into clinically oriented evidence. J Speech Lang Hear Res. 2008;51(1):S276–300.

13. Rosenbek JC. Efficacy in dysphagia. Dysphagia. 1995;10(4):263–7.

14. Wheeler-Hegland KM, Rosenbek JC, Sapienza CM. Submental sEMG and hyoid movement during Mendelsohn maneuver, effortful swallow, and expiratory muscle strength training. J Speech Lang Hear Res. 2008;51(5):1072–87.

15. Ohmae Y, Sugiura M, Matumura Y. Role of anterior tongue as an anchor during swallow. In: Yoshimura H, Kida A, Arai T, Niimi S, Kaneko M, Kitahara S, editors. Bronchology and bronchoesophagology: State of the Art; Proceedings of the 11th World Congress for Bronchology (WCB) & the 11th World Congress for Bronchoesophagology (WCBE). Elsevier; 2001. p. 433–5.

16. Witte U, Huckabee ML, Doeltgen SH, Gumbley F, Robb M. The effect of effortful swallow on pharyngeal manometric measurements during saliva and water swallowing in healthy participants. Arch Phys Med Rehabil. 2008;89(5):822–8.

17. Hiss SG, Huckabee ML. Timing of pharyngeal and upper esophageal sphincter pressures as a function of normal and effortful swallowing in young healthy adults. Dysphagia. 2005;20(2):149–56.

18. Perlman AL, Christensen J. Topography and functional anatomy of the swallowing structures. In: Perlman AL, Schulze-Delrieu K, editors. Deglutition and its disorders: Anatomy, physiology, clinical diagnosis, and management. New York: Thompson Delmar Learning; 1997.

19. Miller AJ. The neuroscientific principles of swallowing and dysphagia. San Diego: Singular Publishing Group; 1999.

20. Huckabee ML, Steele CM. An analysis of lingual contribution to submental surface electromyographic measures and pharyngeal pressure during effortful swallow. Arch Phys Med Rehabil. 2006;87(8):1067–72.

21. Steele CM, Huckabee ML. The influence of orolingual pressure on the timing of pharyngeal pressure events. Dysphagia. 2007;22(1):30–6.

22. Lever TE, Cox KT, Holbert D, Shahrier M, Hough M, Kelley-Salamon K. The effect of an effortful swallow on the normal adult esophagus. Dysphagia. 2007;22(4):312–25.

23. Pouderoux P, Kahrilas PJ. Deglutitive tongue force modulation by volition, volume, and viscosity in humans. Gastroenterology. 1995;108(5):1418–26.

24. Bulow M, Olsson R, Ekberg O. Supraglottic swallow, effortful swallow, and chin tuck did not alter hypopharyngeal intrabolus pressure in patients with pharyngeal dysfunction. Dysphagia. 2002;17(3):197–201.

25. Garcia JM, Hakel M, Lazarus C. Unexpected consequence of effortful swallowing: case study report. J Med Speech Lang Pathol. 2004;12(2):59–66.

26. Bryant M. Biofeedback in the treatment of a selected dysphagic patient. Dysphagia. 1991;6(3):140–4.

27. Crary MA. A direct intervention program for chronic neurogenic dysphagia secondary to brain-stem stroke. Dysphagia. 1995;10(1):6–18.

28. Huckabee ML, Cannito MP. Outcomes of swallowing rehabilitation in chronic brainstem dysphagia: a retrospective evaluation. Dysphagia. 1999;14(2):93–109.

29. Aizawa H, Inase M, Mushiake H, Shima K, Tanji J. Reorganization of activity in the supplementary motor area associated with motor learning and functional recovery. Exp Brain Res. 1991;84(3):668–71.

30. Hamdy S, Aziz Q, Rothwell JC, et al. Recovery of swallowing after dysphagic stroke relates to functional reorganization in the intact motor cortex. Gastroenterology. 1998;115(5):1104–12.

31. Tyc F, Boyadjian A, Devanne H. Motor cortex plasticity induced by extensive training revealed by transcranial magnetic stimulation in human. Eur J Neurosci. 2005;21(1):259–66.

32. Nudo RJ, Milliken GW, Jenkins WM, Merzenich MM. Use-dependent alterations of movement representations in primary motor cortex of adult squirrel monkeys. J Neurosci. 1996;16(2):785–807.

33. Recanzone GH, Schreiner CE, Merzenich MM. Plasticity in the frequency representation of primary auditory-cortex following discrimination-training in adult owl monkeys. J Neurosci. 1993;13(1):87–103.

34. Karni A, Bertini G. Learning perceptual skills: behavioral probes into adult cortical plasticity. Curr Opin Neurobiol. 1997;7(4):530–5.

35. Jensen JL, Marstrand PCD, Nielsen JB. Motor skill training and strength training are associated with different plastic changes in the central nervous system. J Appl Phys. 2005;99(4):1558–68.

36. Remple MS, Bruneau RM, VandenBerg PM, Goertzen C, Kleim JA. Sensitivity of cortical movement representations to motor experience: evidence that skill learning but not strength training induces cortical reorganization. Behav Brain Res. 2001;123(2):133–41.

37. Hogan N, Krebs HI, Rohrer B, et al. Motions or muscles? Some behavioral factors underlying robotic assistance of motor recovery. J Rehabil Res Dev. 2006;43(5):605–18.

38. Nelles G, Jentzen W, Jueptner M, Muller S, Diener HC. Arm training induced brain plasticity in stroke studied with serial positron emission tomography. Neuroimage. 2001;13(6):1146–54.

39. Ziemann U, Muellbacher W, Hallett M, Cohen LG. Modulation of practice-dependent plasticity in human motor cortex. Brain. 2001;124:1171–81.

40. Koski L, Mernar TJ, Dobkin BH. Immediate and long-term changes in corticomotor output in response to rehabilitation: Correlation with functional improvements in chronic stroke. Neurorehabil Neural Repair. 2004;18(4):230–49.

41. Piron L, Piccione F, Tonin P, Dam M. Clinical correlation between motor evoked potentials and gait recovery in poststroke patients. Arch Phys Med Rehabil. 2005;86(9):1874–8.

42. Sessle BJ, Adachi K, Avivi-Arber L, et al. Neuroplasticity of face primary motor cortex control of orofacial movements. Arch Oral Biol. 2007;52(4):334–7.

43. Sessle BJ, Yao D, Nishiura H, et al. Properties and plasticity of the primate somatosensory and motor cortex related to orofacial sensorimotor function. Clin Exp Pharmacol Physiol. 2005;32(1–2):109–14.

44. Barnett ML, Ross D, Schmidt RA, Todd B. Motor skills learning and the specificity of training principle. Res Q. 1973;44(4):440–7.

45. Barritt AW, Smithard DG. Role of cerebral cortex plasticity in the recovery of swallowing function following dysphagic stroke. Dysphagia. 2009;24(1):83–90.

46. Hamdy S, Rothwell JC, Aziz Q, Thompson DG. Organization and reorganization of human swallowing motor cortex: implications for recovery after stroke. Clin Sci. 2000;99(2):151–7.

47. Gallas S, Marie JP, Leroi AM, Verin E. Impact of swallowing and ventilation on oropharyngeal cortical representation. Respir Physiol Neurobiol. 2009;167(2):208–13.

48. Moreau CE, Moreau SR. Chiropractic management of a professional hockey player with recurrent shoulder instability. J Manipulative Physiol Ther. 2001;24(6):425–30.

49. Rose DJ, Christina RW. A multilevel approach to the study of motor control and learning. 2nd ed. San Francisco: Pearson Education Incorporated; 2006.

50. Gow D, Rothwell J, Hobson A, Thompson D, Hamdy S. Induction of long-term plasticity in human swallowing motor cortex following repetitive cortical stimulation. Clin Neurophysiol. 2004;115(5):1044–51.

51. Wallace DA, Beard DJ, Gill RHS, Carr AJ. Reflex muscle contraction in anterior shoulder instability. J Shoulder Elbow Surg. 1997;6(2):150–5.

52. Borsa PA, Sauers EL, Lephart SM. Functional training for the restoration of dynamic stability in the PCL-injured knee. J Sport Rehabil. 1999;8(4):362–78.
53. Lephart SM, Giraldo JL, Borsa PA, Fu FH. Knee joint proprioception: a comparison between female intercollegiate gymnasts and controls. Knee Surg Sports Traumatol Arthrosc. 1996;4(2):121–4.
54. Lephart SM, Pincivero DM, Giraldo JL, Fu FH. The role of proprioception in the management and rehabilitation of athletic injuries. Am J Sports Med. 1997;25(1):130–7.
55. Edgerton VR, Tillakaratne NJK, Bigbee AJ, de Leon RD, Roy RR. Plasticity of the spinal neural circuitry after injury. Annu Rev Neurosci. 2004;27:145–67.
56. Holmich P. Adductor-related groin pain in athletes. Sports Med Arthro Rev. 1997; 5(4):285–91.
57. Zhang J, Yang R, Pendlebery W, Luo P. Monosynaptic circuitry of trigeminal proprioceptive afferents coordinating jaw movement with visceral and laryngeal activities in rats. Neuroscience. 2005;135(2):497–505.
58. Zhang JD, Luo PF, Pendlebury WW. Light and electron microscopic observations of a direct projection from mesencephalic trigeminal nucleus neurons to hypoglossal motoneurons in the rat. Brain Res. 2001;917(1):67–80.
59. Zhang JD, Pendlebury WW, Luo PF. Synaptic organization of monosynaptic connections from mesencephalic trigeminal nucleus neurons to hypoglossal motoneurons in the rat. Synapse. 2003;49(3):157–69.
60. Hamdy S, Aziz Q, Rothwell JC, Hobson A, Barlow J, Thompson DG. Cranial nerve modulation of human cortical swallowing motor pathways. Am J Physiol Gastro Liver Phys. 1997;35(4):G802–8.
61. Hamdy S, Aziz Q, Rothwell JC, Hobson A, Thompson DG. Sensorimotor modulation of human cortical swallowing pathways. J Physiol Lond. 1998;506(3):857–66.

16. Compensatory Strategies and Techniques

Susan G. Butler, Cathy A. Pelletier,
and Catriona M. Steele

Abstract The management of dysphagia usually begins with compensatory strategies and techniques, which are intended to improve swallowing function in an immediate but temporary manner. These techniques allow the patient to obtain their safest but least restrictive level of oral intake. In this chapter, we explore three main types of compensatory intervention for dysphagia: postural modifications; texture modification and thickened liquids; and sensory enhancements.

Introduction

Compensatory strategies and techniques such as postural modifications, texture modifications/thickened liquids, and sensory enhancements are used to *compensate* for dysphagia, especially aspiration, so that patients can obtain their safest but least restrictive level of oral intake. It is important that speech language pathologists evaluate each patient's dysphagia during an instrumental examination, either videofluoroscopic examination (VFSE) or flexible endoscopic examination of swallowing (FEES). They should then determine, based on the patient's swallowing physiology/bolus flow and cognitive status (memory, attention, and compliance), which modification is most appropriate. Correctly applied, compensatory strategies can be immediate solutions for dysphagia and aspiration.

R. Shaker et al. (eds.), *Manual of Diagnostic and Therapeutic Techniques for Disorders of Deglutition*, DOI 10.1007/978-1-4614-3779-6_16,
© Springer Science+Business Media New York 2013

Postural Modification

Postural modification can eliminate or markedly reduce patients' food or liquid aspiration as demonstrated during a VFSE or FEES. Alternatively, postural modifications may be implemented during an instrumental assessment to effect immediate change in swallowing physiology and bolus flow dynamics. The most common postural modifications include chin tuck, head turn, head lean, side lying, supraglottic swallow, and super supraglottic swallow (Table 16.1). The chin tuck is the most researched and probably the most frequently utilized postural modification; however, the others have all received attention in the literature and also can be appropriate modifications for dysphagia.

With patients who aspirate, clinicians should attempt postural modifications first to eliminate or decrease aspiration, thus maintaining as normal a diet as possible. If postural modifications are not successful or a patient is not a good candidate for them, then food texture and/or liquid viscosity modifications should be instituted to control the aspiration. Postural modifications should be attempted first because, although food/liquid modifications can be successful in eliminating aspiration, they are often associated with dehydration, malnutrition, and decreased quality of life. However, the patient's abilities to follow commands, insight, memory, and lack of impulsivity are all important determinants in whether postural modifications can be consistently and reliably used to eliminate aspiration. Frequently, both postural and food/liquid modifications are needed to eliminate aspiration.

Chin Tuck: Chin tuck is often used to compensate for a delayed pharyngeal response that contributes to aspiration risk before the swallow. A classic example of when the chin tuck may be successful is when a bolus (often thin liquid) is observed, via VFSE or FEES, to spill into the laryngeal vestibule and trachea before initiation of the swallow. A chin tuck widens the vallecular space, allowing a longer bolus spill time into the vallecula while the swallow is initiated. A chin tuck also minimizes the laryngeal vestibule opening, moving the larynx slightly up and forward while bringing the epiglottis closer to the laryngeal vestibule entrance. In addition, a chin tuck maneuver allows the base of the tongue to approximate the posterior pharyngeal wall. All of these changes yield enhanced airway protection before and during the swallow. Given a chin tuck changes the pharyngeal and laryngeal dimensions [1], the possible positive or negative effects of the changes (e.g., widening of the vallecular space or narrowing of pyriform sinuses) should be evaluated relative to its effects on food or liquid residue.

Table 16.1. Postural modifications to treat oropharyngeal dysphagia.

Postural modification	Problem targeted by modification	Physiologic rationale[a]	Studies investigating modification
Chin tuck	Delay in swallowing initiation/pharyngeal response	Widens vallecular space allowing for a larger reservoir for bolus to spill prior to swallow initiation	[1, 2, 46–57]
Head turn	Unilateral oropharyngeal weakness	Directs bolus flow down stronger side of pharynx	[46, 52, 54, 58]
Head tilt	Unilateral oropharyngeal weakness	Directs bolus flow down stronger side of pharynx	[46, 52, 54]
Side lying	Unilateral oropharyngeal weakness	Directs bolus flow down stronger side of pharynx-utilizing gravity	[46, 54, 59]
Supraglottic swallow	Delayed and/or decreased airway protection	Voluntary breath hold results in true vocal fold closure	[47, 55–57]
Super supraglottic swallow	Delayed and/or decreased airway protection	Effortful breath hold results in true and false vocal fold closure as well as arytenoid to base of epiglottis approximation [60–62]	[60–62]

[a]Note: the primary rationale of all postural modifications is to decrease or eliminate aspiration and improve the efficiency of bolus flow.

Reports in the literature vary as to how best to implement the chin tuck. Some instruct patients to perform the chin tuck by dropping their head forward to their chest, while others instruct patients to keep their neck straight and tuck their chin in and down just slightly. Steele and colleagues found that the cue, "tuck your chin so that it touches your chest and so that you can see your knees," was effective in eliciting an optimal chin tuck angle [2] to eliminate aspiration [1]. When assessing the effectiveness of the chin tuck modification, it may be worthwhile to try the second method if the first does not eliminate aspiration. How well the chin tuck eliminates aspiration must be instrumentally assessed. In some patients, the chin tuck results in more severe aspiration. Given that silent aspiration is more prevalent than aspiration with a throat clear or cough, an instrumental exam will allow the clinician to assess the usefulness of the chin tuck while trying to achieve the patient's safest but least restrictive diet level.

Head Turn/Head Lean: Head turn and head lean are used to compensate for unilateral oropharyngeal weakness that results in marked residue in the vallecula and/or pyriform sinuses of the affected side and also frequently contributes to the risk of aspiration during and/or after the swallow. When conducting a VFSE, the unilateral oropharyngeal weakness and corresponding residue are best appreciated in the anterior-posterior view, while the aspiration is often most easily observed in the lateral view. When conducting a FEES, the superior view provides assessment of both-sided residue and aspiration. In cases of unilateral oropharyngeal weakness or residue, the head turn modification involves turning the head as far to the weak side as possible. The patient is then cued to swallow the food or liquid on the strong (unaffected) side of their mouth and throat. By turning the head in this manner, the weak side of the pharynx is largely closed off and diverts the food/liquid to the strong side of the pharynx, with the goal of decreasing vallecular and pyriform sinus residue and aspiration.

Recently, it has been reported that the head turn may result in improved upper esophageal sphincter opening duration [3] during the swallow, allowing improved bolus flow from the pharynx into the esophagus. Accordingly, if pyriform sinus residue is noted during an instrumental swallowing evaluation, the head turn may be an effective postural modification to improve the efficiency of the swallow.

The head *lean* can also be used for unilateral pharyngeal weakness and associated residue and/or aspiration. In this maneuver, the patient leans his or her head to the strong (unaffected) side and then swallows the food/liquid on the strong side of the mouth and throat, to keep the bolus away from the weak side. Sometimes, a clinician can increase the effectiveness of the head lean by having the patient lean his or her head and body to the strong side, while propped on an elbow. When unilateral oropharyngeal weakness is identified, the clinician may need to test both the head turn and the head lean to determine which modification is best. Some clinicians will incorporate both strategies by having a patient turn to the weak side and then lean his or her head forward, toward the strong side, to obtain the most effective bolus flow.

Side Lying: Side lying is used to compensate for unilateral oropharyngeal weakness that results in marked residue on one side of the pharynx and/or aspiration. Conventional wisdom dictates that the patient lies with the stronger side down, so that gravity combined with the intact pharyngeal contraction will propel the bolus down the stronger side of the pharynx and into the esophagus, thus keeping the bolus away from the airway. There are many versions of side lying: lying with the head flat and in line with the body; lying with the head resting on a pillow; and staying propped up on an elbow with the head supported by a hand. In general, the side lying position is attempted when the swallowing problem is so severe that a simple head turn or head lean will not eliminate aspiration. The effectiveness of the side lying position can be assessed during VFSE, as the patient lies on the table used to conduct esophagrams, and/or FEES; however, many find the FEES is easier to conduct with the patient in the side lying position. This allows ample time to determine which positions are most effective, without excessive radiation exposure.

Supraglottic and Super Supraglottic Swallow: The supraglottic swallow is primarily used to compensate for delayed and/or decreased vocal fold closure that causes aspiration. However, the super supraglottic swallow also increases the duration of base of tongue to posterior pharyngeal wall pressure and approximation. To perform the supraglottic swallow, the patient is cued to: (1) take a deep breath, (2) hold the breath, (3) swallow, and then (4) release the swallow into a cough. The breath hold prior to the swallow aims to achieve true vocal fold closure before the swallow, to eliminate aspiration before or during the swallow. The cough performed at the completion of the swallow clears any residue (i.e., penetration) from the true or false vocal folds that may have entered the laryngeal vestibule during the swallow and could be aspirated once the patient opens the vocal folds and inhales.

The super supraglottic swallow is similar to the supraglottic swallow, but employs extra effort. The patient is cued to: (1) take a deep breath, (2) hold the breath *with effort*, (3) swallow *hard*, and then (4) release the swallow into a cough. The extra effort with breath holding provides greater airway protection via true and false vocal fold closure and arytenoid to base of epiglottis approximation (i.e., narrowing of the entrance into the laryngeal vestibule).

The supraglottic and super supraglottic swallow are among the more difficult postural modifications to teach patients. For some patients with cognitive dysfunction, the four steps may be difficult to implement; however, providing written instructions is often helpful. Further, patients often reflexively release the breath hold as they initiate the swallow, resulting in an open airway and eliminating the effectiveness of the modification. Endoscopic biofeedback can be helpful in teaching the supraglottic and super supraglottic swallows. During a session, the clinician instructs the patient to maintain vocal fold/laryngeal closure before the initiation of "white-out" (i.e., pharyngeal phase of swallow). Another common problem in the correct use of the supraglottic swallows is that patients, especially in the beginning, have difficulty mastering the release of the swallow into a cough. Patients often erroneously complete the swallow, inhale/exhale, and then cough. Inhaling/exhaling before will likely result in aspiration if food/liquid was present on the vocal folds.

Another important point to consider is patient fatigue. Thus, a patient may demonstrate the successful use of a super supraglottic swallow, as shown by elimination of aspiration, based on a few single swallows during a VFSE; however, can the patient maintain this throughout a meal? FEES, given its ability to test a person through an entire meal, may be the best way to assess the success of the supraglottic or super supraglottic swallow for functional eating. If a patient cannot successfully implement the supraglottic swallow through an entire meal due to fatigue, the clinician may recommend more frequent, smaller meals. Finally, potential cardiovascular effects (i.e., supraventricular tachycardia, premature atrial contractions, and premature ventricular contractions) of implementing the supraglottic or super supraglottic swallow need to be considered/monitored especially in patients with stroke and/or coronary artery disease [4].

In Summary: Postural modifications can be an excellent way to address dysphagia; however, their success requires the patient's strict adherence to the postural modification recommended. Clinicians should look for opportunities to instruct patients, their medical staff, and caregivers in the use—and importance—of the targeted postural modification to help assure compliance. Compliance may also be improved by reviewing the instrumental swallowing evaluation with patients and their caregivers. Additionally, clinicians may offer visual cues (signs to remind patients) and check back frequently to assure the postural modification is still appropriate and being implemented correctly.

A postural modification is generally considered a temporary solution to compensate for a swallowing problem. Patients may use these modifications while their swallowing is spontaneously recovering and/or while they are engaged in a program of strength/resistance training to improve the oropharyngeal musculature. However, the ultimate goal is to transition patients from the needed postural modifications to a safe eating/drinking scenario that is as normal as possible. Instrumental exams such as the VFSE or FEES are objective ways to determine if a patient's swallowing ability has improved such that a postural modification is no longer warranted.

Key Messages

- Postural modifications are used to eliminate penetration/aspiration and improve efficiency of oropharyngeal bolus flow.
- Postural modifications are often attempted before initiation of texture/viscosity modifications, because thickening liquids or modifying food textures can result in dehydration and malnutrition sequelae.
- Patients must demonstrate, at a minimum, relatively good cognitive ability, memory, and compliance to recommendations for postural techniques to be employed successfully.
- Postural modifications should only be used as long as needed. Instrumental re-evaluations are helpful in identifying when a postural modification is no longer warranted.

Texture Modification and Thickened Liquids

Texture modification is commonly used to address both safety and efficiency concerns in swallowing [5]. This technique is grounded in the idea that specific components of dysphagia are related to difficulties managing the flow of liquids through the oropharynx. With thin liquids, a patient may have difficulty controlling the flow of thin liquids in the mouth (leading to premature spillage into the pharynx), or they may have difficulty engaging airway protection in a timely manner. In these situations, it is logical to try slowing the flow of the liquid by thickening it to a nectar- or honey-thick consistency. By contrast, if a patient has difficulty clearing thick substances (e.g., solid foods, puddings, and purees) from the pharynx, then it makes sense to alter the texture of these items to promote easier flow and clearance. Solid foods can be pre-processed by chopping, grinding, mincing, or combining with sauces; puddings and purees can be thinned to aid pharyngeal clearance.

These general principles have been applied to the formulation of diet texture recommendations for patients with dysphagia. Unfortunately, it is difficult to standardize the texture and flow properties (viscosity) of foods and liquids for people with dysphagia. One approach to thickening is to use a powdered thickener at the bedside or in the dining room. This approach is vulnerable to variation across mixers [6], and the viscosity of the product is also likely to change over time. Cornstarch-based thickeners are particularly prone to thickening over time [7]. Gelatin-based thickeners are prone to thinning in warm temperatures. Different liquids will interact with the thickening powder in different ways, so that the end products differ [7–11]. For example, adding the same amount of thickening powder leads to a thinner end product when the liquid is high-fat milk than when the liquid is skim milk. The fat content of the milk interferes with the bonding ability of the thickening powder [8, 9, 11]. Consequently, one cannot assume that a single thickening recipe can be applied to all liquids.

An alternative to bedside or tableside thickening is to prepare thickened liquids ahead of time in a facility kitchen according to strict recipes. This method may be subject to similar concerns regarding end-product viscosity, due to the common practice of chilling and re-warming foods that are pre-prepared on patient trays. Alternatively, several food companies sell pre-prepared thickened liquids, which commonly come in either nectar-thick or honey-thick viscosities. However, strict guidelines regarding these target viscosities do not exist, and the viscosity of two "nectar-thick" liquids from different companies may differ substantially. Similarly, even within the product line of a single company, viscosity may differ quite widely across different liquids (e.g., milk, apple juice, orange juice) [7, 12]. Pre-thickened products are vulnerable to the influences of temperature on viscosity. Furthermore, shaking or stirring a pre-thickened liquid may change its viscosity. In North America, preliminary viscosity boundaries for four levels of liquid were proposed in the National Dysphagia Diet [13]. Similar classification systems also have been proposed in the United Kingdom and Australia [14]. Regardless of the classification system in place, clinicians need to be aware that the industry tolerance for variations in viscosity within a labeled class is quite large. For this reason, clinicians may need to specifically evaluate clinical signs of tolerance with different thickened products, paying attention to issues such as temperature and standing time as sources of possible variation. Care should also be taken to develop standard recipes within an institution to guide on-site preparation of thickened liquids using different thickening products and liquids.

One practical approach to understanding dietary viscosity and texture differences in a particular facility is to conduct a mapping exercise. Most clinicians will not have access to industrial rheometers or to engineers or food scientists who can conduct proper tests of viscosity or other food texture properties. However, two simpler options can help to confirm the similarity in flow characteristics across different liquids on a kitchen's menu.

In the "line-spread" test, calibrated volumes of a liquid are placed in a cylinder at the center of a plastic plate marked with concentric circles at 0.5 cm intervals, radiating out from the center [15, 16]. When the cylinder is lifted, the liquid will flow, and measures of average flow distance can be taken at fixed time intervals in four quadrants of the display. A Bostwick consistometer [17] is a commercially available device that functions in a similar manner; liquid samples are initially contained in a holding chamber, and then flow along the bottom of a rectangular chamber marked with a ruler showing 0.5 cm distances when a gate is released. For accurate results, the devices must be level, and proper cleaning is required to eliminate soapy films or other residues on the devices that may alter liquid flow. For both methods, the initial volume and height of the sample must be carefully controlled to ensure valid measures. A practical suggestion for clinicians seeking to understand the flow characteristics of liquids available in their facilities is to undergo a mapping exercise, in which the entire menu cycle is characterized using these devices. Similarly, either commercial products used for instrumental swallowing examination, or products made following recipes can be mapped to items on the facility menu using these tools. Given the need for proper cleaning and methodological rigor, these devices do not lend themselves to use for monitoring of liquid flow on a daily basis.

When determining the best viscosity for a patient, clinicians need to be aware that barium products used in the VFSE are likely to differ in viscosity from regular liquids [18]. This dilemma is unavoidable and means that texture recommendations arising from the VFSE are generalizations. Barium not only alters viscosity, but density and flavor as well. One way to limit this concern is to use barium of a standard density across all stimuli in the examination. For example, the Varibar product line uses a 40 % w/v density across different viscosity levels (nectar, thin honey, thick honey, and pudding). Clinicians should follow the manufacturer's instructions regarding the amount of water to be added and mixing, to achieve the desired density. One study has shown that aspiration is more common when more diluted solutions are used [19]. When clinicians are preparing stimuli for a VFSE, they should use a balance to measure the proportion of barium to achieve a constant weight-to-volume ratio. Mixing barium suspension or barium powder with variable amounts of water, or with other foods and liquids, is an off-label use of these products. If an adverse event were to occur with the use of a custom-mixed barium preparation, the clinician needs to be aware that they have used the product in a manner other than that specified by manufacturer guidelines.

Clinicians need to be aware that patients often dislike thickened liquids and foods with modified textures. The literature suggests that this can result in two major consequences. First, a patient may be non-compliant with diet texture recommendations [20]. A person may choose to drink thin liquids against recommendations, or eat foods not recommended by the clinician. The potential consequences include aspiration, leading to respiratory consequences, or choking, resulting in an emergency situation. Clinicians should do their best to inform the patient about these risks, so that the patient can make an informed choice. It is also acceptable for a clinician and a facility to refuse to facilitate or equip a patient to take these risks, meaning that the facility will not provide easy access to the products in question.

A second risk associated with disliking texture-modified foods and liquids is the possibility that the patient will not drink or eat them, leading to inadequate nutritional intake. The literature suggests that the available fluid content of thickened liquids is equivalent to that of non-thickened liquids [21], but that patients on texture-modified diets are at risk of malnutrition and dehydration [22, 23].

Clinicians are often curious about whether it is safe for patients with dysphagia to ingest water orally, even when they are prescribed a thickened-liquid diet. The rationale for allowing water intake is that water, by itself, is relatively harmless to the respiratory system [24]. The Frazier Rehabilitation Hospital in Louisville, Kentucky, allows all patients some oral intake of water, regardless of their dysphagia status. Anecdotal reports from this hospital show no increase in the rate of pneumonia compared to similar facilities [25]. However, there are few studies of water protocols in the literature [26] and their findings remain inconclusive. Studies concur that fluid intake will probably increase with the use of water protocols. Most protocols specify a need for heightened vigilance in oral care, to limit the possibility of aspirating pathogenic bacteria during water swallowing. This is probably a critical component of free water protocols; however, oral care is important for all patients with dysphagia.

Key Messages

- Thickened liquids may be helpful when a patient has difficulty controlling the flow of thin liquids, leading to premature spillage and pre-swallow aspiration.
- Thinner items may be helpful for patients who show residue after the swallow.
- Thickeners interact in different ways with different liquids and are susceptible to the influence of time and temperature, making it hard to achieve similar end products.
- Barium stimuli should be prepared according to standardized recipes to ensure similarity from test to test.

Sensory Enhancement

Placing food or liquid in the mouth results in the experience of multiple sensations simultaneously. Even just the sight and smell of food will stimulate a host of metabolic reactions along the gastrointestinal tract [27–31]. Although it is known that sensory input is important to elicit a swallow, quantifying the sensory input and the specific motor response(s) involved has been more challenging. In particular, what type and intensity of sensory input is required to evoke more normative swallow behaviors in oropharyngeal dysphagia? Will one type of sensory input be enough to trigger a swallow? Or must it occur in combination with other sensations? Answers to these questions are difficult because the sensory input of food and liquid is inherently multi-factorial.

One of the most elusive problems in dysphagia treatment is how to reliably trigger a swallow reflex. A delayed pharyngeal swallow is common in pharyngeal dysphagia, and it increases the risk of penetration and aspiration. Decreased oral sensory input may increase oral transit time and lead to a loss of bolus control. This may result in oral leakage, food left in the mouth after swallowing, increased oral preparatory time, or spillage into the hypopharynx prior to the swallow.

During oral preparation and the act of swallowing, individuals perceive several types of sensations. Somatosensory perception includes temperature, pressure, touch, location in space (proprioception), and pain (nocioception). Somatosensory perception also involves the chemosenses, i.e., olfaction and gustation. Taste and smell are called chemosenses because a chemical reaction must occur for perception to occur. Our experience of *flavor* (as sensory scientists would call it) depends not only on taste and smell but a sensation called chemesthesis, or irritation of the mucosa [32]. Examples of chemesthesis include the sensation of hotness from a chili pepper or the coolness of menthol. Chemesthesis is mediated by the trigeminal nerve that innervates the fungiform papillae on the anterior two thirds of the tongue. Carbonation is another property of liquids that is not perceived by mechanoreceptors but via chemesthesis. The bubbles in a carbonated beverage are converted into carbonic acid [33]. The composite perception of taste, smell, and chemesthesis creates the *flavor* experience when eating and drinking [34].

There are five known basic taste qualities, e.g., sweet, salty, sour, bitter, and umami [35, 36]. Umami is a Japanese term that connotes a savory, meaty type of taste, which is derived from the glutamate family. All five of these taste qualities can be perceived throughout the tongue, although specific taste receptors may have preferential responses to particular taste stimuli. The idea that only certain areas of the tongue can perceived sweet, salty, bitter, or sour [37] is incorrect and was refuted in 1974 [38].

The sense of smell is categorized in two ways. Orthonasal aroma is perceived by sniffing or smelling the air outside of the nose. Retronasal aroma is the perception of volatiles (chemicals that tend to vaporize or evaporate quickly at low temperatures) that arise from food or liquid in the mouth. These chemicals provide an aroma that is sensed by their transport via the nasopharynx to the olfactory epithelium. Plugging the nose when food, liquid, or medicine is placed in the mouth greatly reduces retronasal aroma. Retronasal aroma is important to food identification. Interestingly, studies have documented that the sense of smell can begin to deteriorate as early as the fourth decade, while taste remains quite robust [39–41].

How might any of these somatosensory sensations influence swallowing? Could one or more be useful to increase the swallowing reflex or elicit more normative swallowing behaviors? Three possible ways to enhance sensory input and thus improve pharyngeal dysphagia are tactile stimulation (see Fig. 16.1), sour bolus, and carbonation (see Table 16.2).

Unfortunately, all of these techniques have only been shown to have a short-lived effect on swallowing [42–45]. More normative swallowing behaviors have been observed with these techniques during VFSEs when

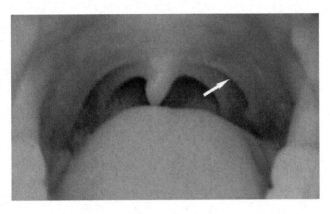

Fig. 16.1. *Arrow* indicates location of anterior faucial pillar where thermal-tactile stimulation is to occur.

compared to a swallow without the stimuli. However, no evidence has been reported that continuous use of the techniques results in positive benefits throughout a meal or rehabilitates swallowing physiology long term. To date, there are no studies supporting the benefit of carbonated beverages over time and thermal-tactile stimulation appears to be beneficial only for the first few swallows post-stimulation [42, 45]. The use of sour taste is beneficial only when the sourness (citric acid concentration) is very high. A more palatable sweet–sour taste did not decrease penetration or aspiration in one small study with nursing home residents [44]. The only taste consistently associated with improved swallowing physiology is an unpalatable, highly sour stimulus such as found in lemon juice. This product is clearly not an appropriate treatment stimulus. Consequently, at this time, none of these sensory enhancement strategies is recommended to treat oropharyngeal dysphagia.

Key Messages

- The act of eating and drinking evokes many chemically evoked sensations simultaneously such as taste, retronasal aroma, and chemesthesis.
- There is no evidence to date that thermal-tactile stimulation will provide a long- term benefit to improve a delayed swallowing response.
- Carbonation is perceived by chemesthesis, not mechanoreceptors.

Table 16.2. Sensory enhancements to treat oropharyngeal dysphagia.

Strategy	Targeted physiology	Procedure	Expected results
Thermal-tactile stimulation	Delayed swallow reflex	Using a cold laryngeal mirror stroke each anterior faucial pillar in an upward fashion 5–6×. Instruct to dry swallow or provide small amount of water	Faster swallow reflex [45]
Sour taste	Delayed swallow reflex, decreased oral transit	Provide small bolus of lemon juice, then present small volumes of water until swallow initiation looks slow; repeat sequence of stimuli	Faster swallow initiation and oral transit time [63]
Carbonation	Delayed swallow reflex	Provide carbonated beverage	Faster swallow reflex [42]

- Palatable lemon products do not improve swallowing. Only a very high citric acid taste, similar to lemon juice, has improved oropharyngeal dysphagia.

In conclusion, compensatory strategies offer a *temporary* solution to dysphagia. Patients with dysphagia and aspiration should periodically undergo instrumental reevaluation to determine if their diet can be upgraded to a less restrictive form of oral intake and without use of compensatory strategies. While compensatory strategies are often helpful, their effectiveness should be instrumentally evaluated in each patient, as sometimes a compensatory strategy can worsen bolus flow and aspiration. Finally, patients should be evaluated to see whether they can participate in, and benefit from, an intervention that will potentially rehabilitate their underlying dysphagia.

Acknowledgments We thank Karen Potvin Klein, MA, ELS (Research Support Core, Wake Forest University Health Sciences) for her editorial contributions to this chapter.

References

1. Welch MV, Logemann JA, Rademaker AW, Kahrilas PJ. Changes in pharyngeal dimensions effected by chin tuck. Arch Phys Med Rehabil. 1993;74(2):178–81.
2. Steele CM, Hung D, Sejdic E, Chau T, Fraser S. Variability in execution of the chin-down maneuver by healthy adults. Folia Phoniatr Logop. 2011;63(1):36–42.
3. McCulloch TM, Hoffman MR, Ciucci MR. High-resolution manometry of pharyngeal swallow pressure events associated with head turn and chin tuck. Ann Otol Rhinol Laryngol. 2010;119(6):369–76.
4. Chaudhuri G, Hildner CD, Brady S, Hutchins B, Aliga N, Abadilla E. Cardiovascular effects of the supraglottic and super-supraglottic swallowing maneuvers in stroke patients with dysphagia. Dysphagia. 2002;17(1):19–23.
5. Garcia JM, Chambers IV E, Molander M. Thickened liquids: practice patterns of speech-language pathologists. Am J Speech Lang Pathol. 2005;14(1):4–13.
6. Glassburn DL, Deem JF. Thickener viscosity in dysphagia management: variability among speech-language pathologists. Dysphagia. 1998;13(4):218–22.
7. Garcia JM, Chambers IV E, Matta Z, Clark M. Viscosity measurements of nectar- and honey-thick liquids: product, liquid, and time comparisons. Dysphagia. 2005;20(4):325–35.
8. Sopade PA, Halley PJ, Cichero JAY, Ward LC. Rheological characterisation of food thickeners marketed in Australia in various media for the management of dysphagia. I: water and cordial. J Food Eng. 2007;79:69–82.
9. Sopade PA, Halley PJ, Cichero JAY, Ward LC, Hui LS, Teo KH. Rheological characterization of food thickeners marketed in Australia in various media for the management of dysphagia. II: milk as a dispersing medium. J Food Eng. 2008;84:604–15.

10. Garcia JM, Chambers IV E, Matta Z, Clark M. Serving temperature viscosity measurements of nectar- and honey-thick liquids. Dysphagia. 2008;23(1):65–75.
11. Sopade PA, Halley PJ, Cichero JAY, Ward JD, Liu J, Varliveli S. Rheological characterization of food thickeners marketed in Australia in various media for the management of dysphagia. III: fruit juice as a dispersing medium. J Food Eng. 2008;86:604–15.
12. Steele CM, Van Lieshout PH, Goff HD. The rheology of liquids: a comparison of clinicians' subjective impressions and objective measurement. Dysphagia. 2003;18(3): 182–95.
13. Association AD. National dysphagia diet: standardization for optimal care. Chicago: American Dietetic Association; 2002.
14. Cichero JAY, Atherton M, Bellis-Smith N, Suter M. Texture-modified foods and thickened fluids as used for individuals with dysphagia: Australian standardised labels and definitions. Nutr Diet. 2007;64:S53–76.
15. Mann LL, Wong K. Development of an objective method for assessing viscosity of formulated foods and beverages for the dysphagic diet. J Am Diet Assoc. 1996;96(6): 585–8.
16. Nicosia MA, Robbins J. The usefulness of the line spread test as a measure of liquid consistency. Dysphagia. 2007;22(4):306–11.
17. Germain I, Dufresne T, Ramaswamy HS. Rheological characterization of thickened beverages used in the treatment of dysphagia. J Food Eng. 2006;73:64–74.
18. Steele CM, Cichero JA. A question of rheological control. Dysphagia. 2008;23(2): 199–201.
19. Fink TA, Ross JB. Are we testing a true thin liquid? Dysphagia. 2009;24(3):285–9.
20. Colodny N. Dysphagic independent feeders' justifications for noncompliance with recommendations by a speech-language pathologist. Am J Speech Lang Pathol. 2005;14(1):61–70.
21. Sharpe K, Ward L, Cichero J, Sopade P, Halley P. Thickened fluids and water absorption in rats and humans. Dysphagia. 2007;22(3):193–203.
22. Finestone HM, Foley NC, Woodbury MG, Greene-Finestone L. Quantifying fluid intake in dysphagic stroke patients: a preliminary comparison of oral and nonoral strategies. Arch Phys Med Rehabil. 2001;82(12):1744–6.
23. Finestone HM, Greene-Finestone LS, Wilson ES, Teasell RW. Malnutrition in stroke patients on the rehabilitation service and at follow-up: prevalence and predictors. Arch Phys Med Rehabil. 1995;76(4):310–6.
24. Effros RM, Jacobs ER, Schapira RM, Biller J. Response of the lungs to aspiration. Am J Med. 2000;108(Suppl 4a):15S–9.
25. Panther K. The Frazier free water protocol. Perspectives (American Speech-Language Hearing Association Special Interest Division 13: Swallowing and Swallowing Disorders). Dysphagia. 2005;14:4–9.
26. Garon B, Engle M, Ormiston C. A randomized control study to determine the effects of unlimited oral intake of water in patients with identified aspiration. J Neurol Rehabil. 1997;11:139–48.
27. Katschinski K. Nutritional implications of cephalic phase gastrointestinal responses. Appetite. 2000;34:189–96.

28. Konturek SJ, Konturek JW. Cephalic phase of pancreatic secretion. Appetite. 2000;34:197–205.

29. LeBlanc J. Nutritional implications of cephalic phase thermogenic responses. Appetite. 2000;34:214–6.

30. Powley TL. Vagal circuitry mediating cephalic-phase responses to food. Appetite. 2000;34:184–8.

31. Teff K. Nutritional implications of the cephalic-phase reflexes: endocrine responses. Appetite. 2000;34:206–13.

32. Green BG. Chemesthesis: pungency as a component of flavor. Trends Food Sci Technol. 1996;7:415–20.

33. Dessirier JM, Simons CT, Carstens MI, O'Mahoney M, Carstens E. Psychophysical and neurobiological evidence that the oral sensation elicited by carbonated water is of chemogenic origin. Chem Senses. 2000;25:277–84.

34. Pelletier CA. Chemosenses, aging and oropharyngeal dysphagia. Top Geriatr Rehabil. 2007;23(3):249–68.

35. Chaudhari NL, Landin AM, Roper SD. A metabotropic glutamate receptor variant functions as a taste receptor. Nat Neurosci. 2000;3:113–9.

36. de Araujo IE, Kringelbach ML, Rolls ET, Hobden P. Representation of umami taste in the human brain. J Neurophysiol. 2003;90:313–9.

37. Smith DV, Margolskee RF. Making sense of taste. Sci Am. 2001;284:32–9.

38. Collings VB. Human taste response as a function of locus of stimulation on the tongue and soft palate. Percept Psychophys. 1974;16(1):169–74.

39. Cowart BJ. Relationships between taste and smell across the life span. Ann N Y Acad Sci. 1989;561:39–55.

40. Schiffman SS. Taste and smell losses in normal aging and disease. J Am Med Assoc. 1997;278(16):1357–62.

41. Weiffenbach JM, Kurihara K, Suzuki N, Ogawa H. Human sensory function for taste is robust across the life-span. Olfaction and Taste XI. Tokyo: Springer; 1994. p. 551–3.

42. Bulow M, Olsson R, Ekberg O. Videoradiographic analysis of how carbonated thin liquids and thickened liquids affect the physiology of swallowing in subjects with aspiration on thin liquids. Acta Radiol. 2003;44:366–72.

43. Logemann JA, Pauloski BR, Colangelo L, Lazarus C, Fujiu M, Kahrilas PJ. Effects of a sour bolus on oropharyngeal swallowing measures in patients with neurogenic dysphagia. J Speech Hear Res. 1995;38:556–63.

44. Pelletier CA, Lawless HT. Effect of citric acid and citric acid-sucrose mixtures on swallowing in neurogenic oropharyngeal dysphagia. Dysphagia. 2003;18(4):231–41.

45. Rosenbek JC, Robbins J, Willford WO, et al. Comparing treatment intensities of tactile-thermal application. Dysphagia. 1998;13(1):1–9.

46. Rasley A, Logemann JA, Kahrilas PJ, Rademaker AW, Pauloski BR, Dodds WJ. Prevention of barium aspiration during videofluoroscopic swallowing studies: value of change in posture. AJR Am J Roentgenol. 1993;160(5):1005–9.

47. Nagaya M, Kachi T, Yamada T, Sumi Y. Videofluorographic observations on swallowing in patients with dysphagia due to neurodegenerative diseases. Nagoya J Med Sci. 2004;67(1–2):17–23.

48. Lewin JS, Hebert TM, Putnam Jr JB, DuBrow RA. Experience with the chin tuck maneuver in postesophagectomy aspirators. Dysphagia. 2001;16(3):216–9.

49. Logemann JA, Gensler G, Robbins J, et al. A randomized study of three interventions for aspiration of thin liquids in patients with dementia or Parkinson's disease. J Speech Lang Hear Res. 2008;51(1):173–83.

50. Shanahan TK, Logemann JA, Rademaker AW, Pauloski BR, Kahrilas PJ. Chin-down posture effect on aspiration in dysphagic patients. Arch Phys Med Rehabil. 1993;74(7):736–9.

51. Robbins J, Gensler G, Hind J, et al. Comparison of 2 interventions for liquid aspiration on pneumonia incidence: a randomized trial. Ann Intern Med. 2008;148(7):509–18.

52. Ertekin C, Keskin A, Kiylioglu N, et al. The effect of head and neck positions on oropharyngeal swallowing: a clinical and electrophysiologic study. Arch Phys Med Rehabil. 2001;82(9):1255–60.

53. Castell JA, Castell DO, Schultz AR, Georgeson S. Effect of head position on the dynamics of the upper esophageal sphincter and pharynx. Dysphagia. 1993;8(1):1–6.

54. Logemann JA, Rademaker AW, Pauloski BR, Kahrilas PJ. Effects of postural change on aspiration in head and neck surgical patients. Otolaryngol Head Neck Surg. 1994;110(2):222–7.

55. Bulow M, Olsson R, Ekberg O. Videomanometric analysis of supraglottic swallow, effortful swallow, and chin tuck in healthy volunteers. Dysphagia. 1999;14(2):67–72.

56. Bulow M, Olsson R, Ekberg O. Videomanometric analysis of supraglottic swallow, effortful swallow, and chin tuck in patients with pharyngeal dysfunction. Dysphagia. 2001;16(3):190–5.

57. Bulow M, Olsson R, Ekberg O. Supraglottic swallow, effortful swallow, and chin tuck did not alter hypopharyngeal intrabolus pressure in patients with pharyngeal dysfunction. Dysphagia. 2002;17(3):197–201.

58. Logemann JA, Kahrilas PJ, Kobara M, Vakil NB. The benefit of head rotation on pharyngoesophageal dysphagia. Arch Phys Med Rehabil. 1989;70(10):767–71.

59. Drake W, O'Donoghue S, Bartram C, Lindsay J, Greenwood R. Eating in side-lying facilitates rehabilitation in neurogenic dysphagia. Brain Inj. 1997;11(2):137–42.

60. Logemann JA, Pauloski BR, Rademaker AW, Colangelo LA. Super-supraglottic swallow in irradiated head and neck cancer patients. Head Neck. 1997;19(6):535–40.

61. Lazarus C, Logemann JA, Gibbons P. Effects of maneuvers on swallowing function in a dysphagic oral cancer patient. Head Neck. 1993;15(5):419–24.

62. Lazarus C, Logemann JA, Song CW, Rademaker AW, Kahrilas PJ. Effects of voluntary maneuvers on tongue base function for swallowing. Folia Phoniatr Logop. 2002;54(4):171–6.

63. Logemann JA, Pauloski BR, Colangelo L, Lazarus C, Fujiu M, Kahrilas PJ. Effects of a sour bolus on oropharyngeal swallowing measures in patients with neurogenic dysphagia. J Speech Hear Res. 1995;38(3):556–63.

17. Rehabilitative Maneuvers and Exercise

Justine Joan Sheppard

Abstract Habilitation and rehabilitation in pediatric dysphagia considers deficiencies in underlying competencies for swallowing, the developmental skills that comprise mature eating and swallowing function, the motivation to eat and interactive eating pragmatics. This chapter reviews intervention strategies for these deficiencies. Maneuvers and exercise are considered for which there is empirical support that demonstrates treatment efficacy for dysphagia in sucking, drinking, eating solid food and saliva control.

Introduction

Rehabilitation and habilitation for oropharyngeal dysphagia in infants and children include swallowing function for saliva, drinking, eating, and taking oral medications. For each function there is a developmental sequence that begins in infancy and, in typical development, ends in early childhood when mature, independent, functionally effective patterns emerge. At maturity the skills are sufficiently robust for children to engage successfully in the variety of environments to which they are exposed.

Typical development of swallowing function may be disrupted by a variety of conditions including developmental disability, gastroesophageal and gastrointestinal disorder, cardiopulmonary disorder, renal disease, neurological conditions, and anatomical anomalies [1]. In addition, there is a high prevalence of dysphagia in infants and children who were born prematurely [2]. Oropharyngeal dysphagia may be associated with multiple etiologies [3] and present with multiple contributing causes [4]. The disorder could be chronic and lifelong or transient, resolving with treatment within a developmental period. Furthermore, the topography

R. Shaker et al. (eds.), *Manual of Diagnostic and Therapeutic Techniques for Disorders of Deglutition*, DOI 10.1007/978-1-4614-3779-6_17,

of the disorder and response to treatment may vary with the severity of the dysphagia involvement [5]. Treatment may occur in a variety of settings, from neonatal intensive care units to schools, each with its own therapeutic constraints and primary therapeutic objectives [6, 7]. Given this range of concerns, treatment efficacy research has been selective. Therefore, the clinician is well advised to be thoughtful when generalizing research results among subpopulations and settings.

Oropharyngeal dysphagia affects swallowing and eating function in a variety of ways. Underlying *sensory motor physiology* may be impaired, thereby affecting eating effectiveness and efficiency directly. Coordination, strength, and precision of movement in oral and/or pharyngeal swallowing and respiratory, upper extremity, and postural controls that support swallowing and eating may be affected. When these sensory motor impairments occur prior to acquisition of developmental skills for eating and swallowing, they interfere with emergence of skill. Physiological and functional deficiencies typically co-occur in infants and young children and may be sufficiently severe to interfere with airway protection, growth, and nutrition.

Acquisition of the complex, developmental sequence of *skills and subskills* involved in swallowing and eating may be delayed or disrupted in the absence of underlying physiological issues. Medical and psychological disorders and environmental conditions that interfere with the child's access to the timely and sufficient experiences for learning eating skills will tend to result in functional deficiencies. See Table 17.1 for the developmental progression of eating skills and subskills that culminate in mature swallowing and feeding function [8]. In the typical child, interrelationships among the developmental skills facilitate their sequential emergence. Once the sequence has been disrupted, however, it is often necessary to train each of the skills. The developmental cascade triggered in typical development by exposure to new foods, utensils and eating environments is seen infrequently in these children.

The development of *motivation for eating*, the willingness to engage in eating, and *eating pragmatics*, the social and context-dependent behaviors that sustain the eating experience, are grounded in the child's anticipation of positive experience—ease of eating, comfort, and hunger satiation. When negative experiences and dysphagia occur, motivation and pragmatics may be insufficient to support adequate nutrition, hydration, and the timely and sufficient experience for acquisition of skills and underlying competency [9].

Satisfactory treatment outcomes for pediatric dysphagia are associated closely with gaining the motivation to participate in eating

Table 17.1. The developmental progression of eating skills and subskills culminating in mature swallowing and feeding function (Reprinted from Sheppard [8]).

Milestone eating skill	Swallowing and feeding subskills	Related postural and manipulative subskills
Sucking	Suck–swallow–breathe coordination for nipple feeding	Alerting, orienting head and mouth toward food and opening mouth
		Semi-reclining postural alignment and stabilization
	Expression-suction balance needed for a specific nipple system	Holding hands on breast/bottle during sucking
	Oral grasp and containment of nipple and fluid	Strength and stamina for task
	Ability to expel nipple from mouth	
	Generalization of sucking skills/performance to different nipples, feeding partners and independence	
Transition Feeding from nipple to spoon	Adjustment of oral initiation of the reflexive swallow and pharyngeal phase swallowing dynamics to accommodate changing oral and pharyngeal anatomy	
	Swallow–breathe coordinations for larger and more viscous boluses	
	Removing food from spoon, containing and transferring into place for swallowing	
	Ability to expel food	

(continued)

Table 17.1. (continued)

Milestone eating skill	Swallowing and feeding subskills	Related postural and manipulative subskills
Spoon feeding variety of foods that do not require mastication	Transition of swallow dynamics from suck–swallow to propulsion swallow Sensory tolerances for variety of food tastes and textural coarseness Ability to contain and process coarser and more viscous food and transfer into place for swallowing Tongue propulsion forces for more viscous and larger boluses	Transition from semi-reclining to upright postural alignment and stabilization Increasing participation in feeding with upper body movement toward approaching bolus Independence strategies—holding food in hand while controlling oral participation (beginning finger-feeding)
Biting	Alignment of mandible and maxilla for severing Crushing force onset and offset for biting Ability to contain and expel pieces	Independence strategies—self-feeding with fingers
Chewing	Mouth opening timing, size, and shape adjustments for bolus characteristics and techniques of the feeder Ability to contain, collect, and transport for mastication and expelling Ability to coordinate mandible, tongue, and cheek movements for mastication Ability to control cyclical crushing force onset and offset Judgment of swallow-ready consistency Tongue propulsion dynamics for progression of increasing levels of chewing difficulty Tongue propulsion forces for more viscous and larger boluses	

Drinking from cup and straw	Lip and cheek coordination for maintaining mouth on cup or straw Ability to sip Sequential sip–swallow Ability to contain and control a low viscosity/low cohesiveness bolus Ability to time initiation of swallow for the faster moving liquid bolus	Head–neck postural alignment and control for cup/straw drinking Independence strategies—holding cup or straw in hand while controlling oral participation
Independence	Coordinating/controlling skilled, simultaneous hand–mouth functions Pacing size of bolus Pacing rate of food intake Alternating foods and food and liquid Maintaining acceptable, age-appropriate neatness	Upper body and upper extremity control Maintaining utensils and food on tray/table

exercise and the appropriate pragmatics for socially successful eating experiences. In clinical practice, engagement of the child in exercise and rehabilitative maneuvers is dependent on successful management of these behavioral issues. The close developmental and functional relationships among underlying competency, skills, motivation, and pragmatics are seen in typical development and in pathology. They account for the description of pediatric dysphagia as, "pediatric swallowing and feeding disorder," and the broad range of interdisciplinary concerns in its rehabilitation [10].

Experience-dependent brain plasticity results in critical and sensitive periods in development that support acquisition and performance of movement behaviors. During these periods there is vulnerability for neuronal change and mapping of brain structures in response to extrinsic and intrinsic sensory experience and related motor responses. The child's sensory and motor experiences influence the onset and duration of the critical period [11, 12]. While the age ranges for critical and sensitive periods related to swallowing and feeding have not been determined, it is apparent clinically that specialized strategies are needed to support older children for whom the natural developmental course in acquisition and mastery of these skills and behaviors has been disrupted and/or whose experiences have been atypical.

In pediatric as in adult dysphagia disorders, rehabilitation maneuvers and strategies are selected to address the particular disorder profile. Axioms in pediatric dysphagia rehabilitation are (a) medical issues that may be contributing or co-occurring should be resolved or managed so as to minimize discomfort that the child may associate with eating. This is especially important as aversive experience associated with eating has been found in children to result in phagophobia, eating refusal [13], deficient motivation for eating, atypical eating pragmatics, and delayed development of eating skill [6, 8, 14]; (b) Airway protection issues that may impact on respiratory health and pulmonary integrity should, when suspected, be ruled out prior to initiating rehabilitation. If deficiencies exist they must be considered in the rehabilitation plan [15, 16]; and (c) Maintaining growth, nutrition, and hydration are primary considerations that are supported by the rehabilitative program.

It is the purpose of this chapter to review rehabilitative maneuvers and exercises that have been proposed for improving pediatric swallowing and feeding disorders as it affects eating and saliva control. This is a selective review. The strategies that are included are those for which research studies have found statistically significant treatment effects or are well supported by clinical reasoning and published case results.

Rehabilitation

The functional aims of rehabilitative maneuvers and exercise are (a) to improve the physiology of swallowing as reflected in swallowing effectiveness and feeding efficiency; (b) to advance acquisition of developmental skills needed for mature swallowing function for food, medications and saliva, and the motivation and pragmatic skills that support these activities; and (c) to promote positive health outcomes for the ongoing nutrition and pulmonary function [10, 17–19].

Stages of Skill Acquisition

Acquiring new skill follows a course from emergence to mastery to retention. Those stages also occur when improving performance for an already acquired skill [20, 21].

Early learning. Acquisition of a new skill begins with experiencing and responding to new environmental demands, for example, a nutritive nipple, a cup, spooned food, or chewable foods. This is the "early learning" stage of the task during which there is trial and error and error correction that results in inconsistency among task repetitions and "practice" sessions. During this stage, the child develops sensory tolerances for the task, an essential support for motivation to participate [6, 8, 22].

Intermediate learning. In the "intermediate learning" stage the child has advanced his/her ability. Motor coordinations are more consistent and errors are reduced. However, those improvements are confined largely to familiar practice conditions: environment, eating partners/feeders, foods, bolus size, eating rate, etc. As in early stage learning, retention is fragile and dependent on ongoing practice.

Advanced learning. In the "advanced learning" stage, skills are habituated enough so the child can practice in a variety of unfamiliar performance conditions. In this stage of learning, the child learns to sustain the skills with a variety of eating partners, in a variety of eating environments, and with a variety of unfamiliar foods. It is characteristic of the growing child that his/her food and liquid intake increases to support growing nutritional needs, while the duration of the mealtime continues to be approximately the same. In this stage capabilities are developed for increasing eating efficiency and swallowing larger and more viscous boluses. Skills are retained by ongoing engagement in the activities. In some instances additional "booster" training may be needed.

Rehabilitative Maneuvers and Exercises

Research in interventions for pediatric swallowing and feeding disorder addresses sucking habilitation and habilitation and rehabilitation for eating solid food and liquid from cup or straw and controlling saliva.

Sucking Habilitation

Sucking refers to nipple feeding from breast or bottle. Preterm infants are the primary population for which the effectiveness of rehabilitation maneuvers and exercise strategies for sucking function have been tested. Functional outcomes for sucking habilitation include both breast and bottle feeding; however, most experimental studies address only bottle feeding. Studies consider the effectiveness of non-feeding strategies for improving function, referred to in this population as oral motor interventions (OMI), and maneuvers that are applied during nipple feeding.

Oral motor interventions. OMI that have been studied are non-nutritive sucking (NNS) elicited by conventional pacifier, NNS entrained by a pacifier that provided patterned, orocutaneous stimulation to mimic the temporal organization of normal NNS, and combined modalities of peri- and intra-oral stimulation routines (OSR) and conventional NNS. There have been two evidence based systematic reviews of use of OMI in preterm infants. Arvedson et al. [17, 18] reviewed studies of OSR and conventional NNS. They concluded that the strategies showed promise for improving swallowing physiology and acquisition of oral feeding, but, because of mixed results, they advise the clinician to consider their use carefully. A systematic review of NNS by Pinelli and Symington (2005) had reached the same conclusions. The clinician can consider these strategies for improving sucking in older infants with the caveat that results may differ.

Conventional-non-nutritive sucking (C-NNS). Normal NNS is seen as a precursor to oral feeding in preterm infants [11, 23]. C-NNS is an exercise that provides the infant with a non-feeding nipple (pacifier) on which to suck. The exercise has been tested on preterm infants as young as 26 weeks gestational age (GA) [24, 25]. Various applications of the modality include providing the pacifier during tube feedings for a limited time or for the duration of the tube feeding and providing the pacifier prior to oral feeding alone or combined with an OSR. Treatment durations were variable, ranging from 10 to 40 days [18]. When C-NNS was used prior to initiating oral feeding, positive outcomes were achieved in the physiological characteristics of nutritive sucking once oral feeding was initiated. When C-NNS was used for 5 min immediately prior to oral feeding, there were positive effects on volume consumed and time to complete feeding that persisted when tested 1 week following the end of treatment [26].

C-NNS at the breast has been used to facilitate the onset of breast feeding. In this maneuver, the breast is pumped until empty before the infant is offered the nipple. This exercise resulted in improved transition to breast feeding and longer breastfeeding duration per feeding session [27, 28].

Entrained non-nutritive sucking. Typical C-NNS consists of bursts of 6–12 suck cycles followed by a pause for swallowing and breathing. The sucks occur at a rate of approximately 2 per second. Barlow and colleagues [11, 23] found preterm infants who experienced sucking with a non-nutritive nipple programmed to pulsate in a pattern that mimicked typical NNS improved their C-NNS and oral feeding as compared to untreated control infants. They refer to this exercise as entrained-non-nutritive sucking (E-NNS). The E-NNS treatment was made available to infants who, at approximately 32 weeks gestational age, did not demonstrate rhythmic C-NNS or nutritive sucking. The infants received E-NNS for 3 min during tube feedings for 7–10 days. This treatment improved patterning of C-NNS and increased the percent of feeding taken orally.

Oral stimulation routines. Peri- and intra-oral stimulation routines were tested on preterm infants as an isolated intervention and in combination with C-NNS. OSR as an isolated strategy resulted in significant, positive effect on nutritive suck [29]. Fucile and colleagues [25] provided a detailed description of a routine consisting of 15 min of stimulation applied to external and internal cheeks and lips, gums, and tongue followed by 3 min of C-NNS [25]. This treatment resulted in earlier initiation of oral feeding and earlier discharge from hospital [25, 30]; however, the effect was greater in the early learning stage for acquisition of nutritive suck (1–2 oral feedings per day) than the later learning stage (6–8 oral feedings per day) [24].

Feeding maneuvers and exercise. Feeding exercises and swallowing maneuvers that have been considered for preterm infants are, frequency of oral feeding opportunities, oral (cheek and chin) support, external pacing and infant regulation of initiation of feeding and amount consumed.

Increased feeding experience. Feeding experience was defined as the number of oral feeding opportunities an infant received from the age that oral feeding began. A feeding was counted, regardless of amount of intake, if the infant was removed from the incubator, swaddled, and offered a nipple feeding. Three groups of infants, stratified by severity of medical complications, tested this functional practice effect. Regardless of level of medical complication, infants with higher daily average feeding experience achieved oral feeding in fewer days than those with comparable medical complexity who had less experience, and they were discharged from hospital sooner [31].

Semi-demand feeding. The timing and amount of feeding vary among NICUs and patients from least flexible, "scheduled interval feeding," for which there is a preset schedule and prescribed amount to be ingested by the infant, to most flexible schedule, "ad libitum feeding," which begins in response to the infants hunger cues and ends when the infant indicates satiation [7]. Semi-demand feeding is feeding that is initiated when hunger cues occur in response to periodic testing and ends when the infant has completed a prescribed volume. Semi-demand feeding is a middle ground that has been found to shorten the time to achieving full oral feeding by 5 days [32].

External pacing. Transitional sucking, an abnormal pattern seen in preterm infants with respiratory difficulties, is characterized by insufficient coordination of breathing, sucking, and swallowing. In addition, arrhythmic breathing occurs in the pauses between bursts of sucking [33]. Infants exhibiting this pattern suffer from apnea and bradycardia during feeding. In external pacing (EP) the feeder regulates an infant's sucking and breathing coordination by removing the nipple from the mouth after 3–5 sucks and imposing a 3–5 s pause before returning the nipple to the mouth.

Law-Morstatt et al. [33], in their study of EP, conducted rigorous training for the adults who were to feed the infants. Treatment duration for infants was 2–3 weeks during which all feedings for study infants were paced. These infants exhibited significant decrease in bradycardia episodes and more efficient sucking at discharge from the hospital as compared to infants with similar problems who were not paced.

See Table 17.2 for a review of intervention strategies for sucking.

Eating Solid and Liquid Foods

Rehabilitative maneuvers and exercises for failures in age-appropriate acquisition of swallowing and feeding skills are divided

Table 17.2. Intervention maneuvers and exercises for initiating and improving sucking function in preterm infants in the Neonatal Intensive Care Unit.

Strategy type	Citations	Maneuvers and exercises/ swallowing problem	Procedure for implementing strategy
Oral motor (prefeeding) intervention	Pinelli and Symington (2005); Arvedson et al. [17, 18]; Nyqvist et al. [28]; Nurayanan et al. [27]	Conventional nonnutritive sucking. Used for infants with emerging abilities for nonnutritive sucking and oral feeding	A pacifier is provided for sucking during tube feedings or prior to oral feeding as part of an oral stimulation routine Breast nipple is offered after breast milk has been pumped
	Barlow et al. [11]; Poore et al. [23]	Entrained nonnutritive sucking Used for infants who have failed to develop adequate nonnutritive sucking and suck–swallow patterns	A pacifier that has been modified to pulsate at a rate that simulates the pattern of nonnutritive sucking bursts and pauses is provided for 3-min epochs.
	Fucile et al. [25]; Rocha et al. [30]	Oral stimulation routine with conventional nonnutritive sucking Used for infants with emerging abilities for oral feeding	Massage using fingers is applied to external and internal cheeks, upper and lower lip, upper and lower gum and lateral borders and mid-blade of tongue for a total of 12 min. The oral stimulation is followed by 3 min of conventional non-nutritive sucking

(continued)

Table 17.2. (continued)

Strategy type	Citations	Maneuvers and exercises/swallowing problem	Procedure for implementing strategy
Sucking maneuvers and exercise	Pickler et al. [31]	Frequency of oral feeding Used for infants with emerging abilities for oral feeding	Infants for whom oral feeding has started are removed from the incubator, swaddled, and offered a nipple feeding with number of experiences from "2 or less" to "more than 6.5" daily. More frequent oral feeding resulted in fewer days to full oral feeding and discharge
	McCain et al. [32]	Semi-demand feeding Used for infants with emerging abilities for oral feeding	The infant is fed the prescribed amount of feeding when hunger cues, which are tested at scheduled intervals, are apparent and fed a prescribed amount of formula
	Law-Morstatt et al. [33]	External pacing Used for infants with respiratory disease and 'transitional sucking pattern' who are experiencing bradycardia or respiratory symptoms (coughing, choking apnea) or fatigue during oral feeding	During nipple feeding the feeder removes the nipple from the infant's mouth every three to five sucks and imposes a 3–5 s breathing pause. This continues throughout the feeding

generally into those that address motivation and pragmatics of eating, such as feeding refusal and disruptive eating behaviors, those that address advancing the developmental skills, such as failure to advance from nipple feeding to drinking from a cup or from eating puree or mashed food to chewing, and those that address physiological impairments, such as aspiration, excess residual in pharynx after swallowing, and dribbling of food and saliva.

The advantages of addressing behavior, development, and physiologic problems simultaneously as a means for achieving optimum therapy outcomes have been discussed [6, 8, 34]. Better treatment results have been achieved in both behavior and skills in school-aged, developmentally disabled children when these issues were addressed simultaneously as opposed to sequentially [34]. However, in this review, rehabilitative strategies for movement behaviors are discussed separately from those for affective behaviors according to the intended outcomes in the studies.

Movement Behaviors

Studies of rehabilitative interventions for improving movement and skill have considered effectiveness of non-feeding strategies, referred to as oral motor exercise (OME), and interventions that occur during feeding, referred to as oral sensory-motor therapy and consistent functional practice (CFP).

Oral motor exercise. The term, oral motor exercise, refers to various rehabilitative maneuvers and exercises that are implemented in other than swallowing activities. Arvedson and colleagues provided an evidence-based systematic review of the effects of OME on pediatric swallowing [17]. They describe three categories of OME: (a) active OME in which the patient performs a task and experiences the mentation and sensations that are associated with initiation, movement, and outcomes of the activity. Active OME are noneating exercises that are practiced with the expectation of a rehabilitative effect on swallowing or feeding function [17, 35]. Training exercises for increasing tongue or respiratory muscle strength are examples of active OME that has been found useful for rehabilitation in adult-onset dysphagia disorders that 'have' been found, but have not yet been tested on children [36–38]. (b) Passive OME includes massage and passive range of motion in which the patient experiences sensations and body movements imposed by the clinician [35]. In general the desired patient response is passive acceptance of the input without specific movement. (c) Sensory applications is a subset of passive exercise, in which sensory agents such as cold or electrical stimulation are applied to structures for specific physiological effects, such as reducing delay in initiation of swallow [39, 40]. When considering use of OME, it is important to differentiate those modalities for which effects have been durable, i.e., rehabilitative, from those that had transient, i.e., compensatory.

Oral appliance therapy. Oral appliance therapy (APT) is an OME that involves use of a custom-made, palatal appliance designed to facilitate jaw stabilization or tongue mobility. APT is an active OME, which means the child responds to the stimulus device with changes in muscle activity in the mouth. When the appliance design is configured to stimulate jaw stabilization, it facilitates mouth closure, i.e., lip closure, high jaw position, and tongue maintenance within the dental arch. When grooves and beads are added to the palatal surface of the appliance, it continues to facilitate the closed mouth posture in addition to facilitating exploratory tongue movement.

APT was tested for effectiveness in children with cerebral palsy and moderate severity dysphagia [5]. The appliance was worn for 1 year throughout the night or, when not acceptable for nighttime use, for periods of 20 min or more when awake. The outcome measures were improved eating skills as measured by the Functional Feeding Assessment subtest of the Multidisciplinary Feeding Profile [41], and growth [42]. Significant functional improvements were seen in spoon feeding, biting, and cup-drinking after the first 6 months of the treatment during which the appliance design was intended to facilitate jaw stabilization. Improvement in chewing was seen after the second 6-month period, during which the appliance design was modified to facilitate tongue exploration. A second year follow-up found improvements were retained whether or not the appliance continued to be used, although additional improvement did not occur. Significant change in weight or height did not occur [43].

Oral stimulation routines. Oral and perioral stimulation routines are experienced as passive exercise. The effectiveness of OSR in this older population has been tested in studies using multiple stimulus modalities including stroking, rubbing, stretching, and applications of ice and vibration. When dosage was specified, treatment duration, was 10–15 min, five times a week, for 14 weeks [17]. Stimuli were applied to specific anatomical areas depending on the intended effects. Subjects were developmentally disabled and multiply handicapped children. The objectives were to improve oral muscle tone, facilitate more normal oral responses to OSR, improve biting and chewing, reduce dribbling of food, and reduce tongue thrusting and tonic bite patterns. In a single subject study, there was a significant reduction in tongue thrusting when eating solid foods. However, the gain was not maintained 2 weeks post treatment. In other studies, improvements in eating function and weight gain were inconsistent among subjects and not significant where controls were available.

Oral sensory-motor therapy. Oral sensory-motor therapy, also oral sensorimotor therapy (OST) is an approach in which the sensory array associated with functional oral motor task is managed therapeutically to facilitate acquisition of new skill or, in an already acquired skill, to improve task efficiency and quality of performance and reduce movement errors [44]. Passive OME can be included as a prefeeding routine; however, the essential element in OST exercise is structured sensory experience during function. The sensory elements consist of a combination of modalities. For example, an eating task could include static elements, such as proprioceptive sensation from ideal postural alignments and exteroceptive sensation from postural supports and dynamic sensory elements such as the speed and trajectory of the spoon as it moves toward, enters, and is withdrawn from the mouth and the points of contact and pressures exerted within the mouth. Compensatory sensory maneuvers, such as modifying food viscosity and bolus size for ease of swallowing, can be incorporated into the exercise, or those elements can be used as rehabilitation maneuvers to increase the difficulty of the task gradually.

The basic treatment principles for OST are (a) the sensory maneuvers are selected for their expected physiologic effects on the patient's specific motor impairments [35]; (b) optimum, postural alignment and postural support are considered throughout the exercise; (c) all exercises are conducted in the context of the target task, thereby adhering to the principle of "specificity of training" [17, 35]; (d) when possible, developmental skills and subskills are taught in the sequence in which they are acquired in typical development; and (e) the difficulty of the exercise can be increased or decreased by altering the sensory maneuvers [44].

OST was tested in two studies of children with cerebral palsy who had moderately impaired eating. In those studies a 7-min exercise was conducted immediately prior to the midday meal. In three exercise routines, maneuvers were implemented to improve agility and strength in lips, tongue, or mandible during an ingestion task. The difficulty of that task was advanced as the child improved [45–49]. Progress was measured by the Functional Feeding Assessment subtest of the Multidisciplinary Feeding Profile [41]. Significant changes in eating competence were seen for spoon feeding, biting, and chewing [46] and there was a decrease in the time taken to eat puree in a group of subjects which had demonstrated aspiration on videofluoroscopic swallowing study (VFSS) at the beginning of the study [49].

A study of OST combined with thermal stimulation used VFSS to test effects of an OST exercise program on pharyngeal phase of swallowing. The six subjects, two of whom were adults, had intellectual and developmental disability and dysphagia. All had one or more signs of pharyngeal phase swallowing impairment. Each received a baseline and three follow-up VFSSs at 4-month intervals. The baseline VFSS "cookie swallow" revealed aspiration in two subjects, multiple swallows to clear the pharynx, prolonged pharyngeal transit time, and residue in valleculae and pyriform sinuses. Rehabilitation maneuvers used during feeding targeted lip closure, chewing, and lateral tongue movement. Thermal stimulation for initiation of the swallowing reflex was included in the therapy routine [39]. Follow-up VFSS after 4, 8, and 12 months found progressive improvements in pharyngeal phase of swallowing in all subjects. Reductions were seen in aspiration, pharyngeal transit time, residue, and number of swallows needed to clear the pharynx. Gains continued for all subjects throughout the study, although thermal stimulation was discontinued for three of the subjects following the 8-month VFSS.

Consistent functional practice. CFP is a descriptive term for functional practice of the target skill with consistent technique and routine as a means of improving underlying physiological capabilities for performance, acquiring new skills and subskills, and improving eating efficiency in previously learned skills. Specificity of training is the guiding principle for this strategy, whereby practice of the target task is the primary mechanism for advancing motor capability [20, 21]. The difference between OST and CFP is the focus on the sensory structure of the task for optimizing learning in OST and the emphasis on the movement structure of the task for optimizing learning in CFP. In CFP the exercises address the deficient task components and accommodate the individual physiologic limitation. In CFP practice strategies can differ depending on whether the child is at an early, intermediate, or advanced level of learning for the particular skill or subskill targeted in the exercise [22].

The concept of task specificity as applied to eating refers not only to the movement dynamics of the task and its variability from moment to moment, but also to environmental structures, postural alignments, postural stability and mobility, the sensory experiences preceding during and following the task, self-feeding, and active acceptance of the bolus as well. Head neck alignment, seating alignment and support, eating surfaces, utensils, the movement gesture for active acceptance of the approaching bolus, and the self-regulation of ingestion in self-feeding are examples of the detail that is planned and controlled in CFP in order to provide an optimum learning experience [6, 22, 44, 50].

A static CFP model, one in which the exercise difficulty was not advanced as capabilities improved, was tested in a study of the effects of consistent food presentation on oral motor capabilities. The subjects were children with cerebral palsy and quadriplegic distribution of impairments [50]. A robotic device was used to assure consistent food presentation. The device was activated by the child to bring food to mouth and allow the child to take the food from the spoon. This condition was compared to hand delivered dependent feeding. Within condition comparisons were made between those children with and without speech with the assumption that those without speech had more severe oral motor involvement. Oral motor competencies and postural control during eating were tested using the Schedule for Oral-Motor Assessment [51]. Significant improvements occurred overall in postural and oral-motor control during eating and in specific control for lip and jaw movement, and, in the nonspeaking subjects, in mastication and swallowing for puree. Skills continued to improve based on interim assessments during the 3-month intervention period. The children transferred skills gained by robotic feeding to hand feeding. Some deterioration in improved functions was seen in the post-intervention period during which all feedings were delivered by hand. However, this occurred only in tests using hand feeding and not in tests using the robotic device. Although postural control is considered to be an integral part of swallowing and eating competency, it is viewed generally as a variable to be controlled rather than one to be studied. Notable, significant improvements were seen to result from CFP in postural control as well as mastication and use of lips and jaw in the absence of exercises that targeted these areas specifically [50].

Included in a multifaceted program as the strategy for acquiring and advancing skills, CFP was found to be effective for advancing from tube feeding to oral feeding in two single case studies. In that study, the difficulty of functional practice was advanced systematically to support maturation of skills, as well as improvement of underlying competency [6] (Table 17.3).

Table 17.3. Intervention maneuvers and exercises for improving swallowing function for solid and liquid food.

Citations	Maneuvers and exercises/functional swallowing objective(s)	Procedure
Gisel and Alphonce [5]; Haberfellner et al. [42]; Gisel et al. [43]	Oral appliance therapy	A customized palatal appliance is constructed to be worn during sleep or intermittently during the day when not engaged in eating
	To improve performance of existing eating and drinking skills	
Arvedson et al. [17, 18]	Oral stimulation routines	Various sensory modalities are applied to peri- and intra-oral sites. These include stroking, rubbing, stretching, ice and vibration applied when not engaged in eating
	To improve performance of existing eating and drinking skills	
Gisel [45]; Sheppard [22]	Oral sensory-motor therapy	The sensory structure of the functional eating task is selected and controlled to facilitate learning new skills and improving competencies for existing skills
	To improve existing eating and drinking skills and advance development of skills that have not yet emerged	
Pinnington and Hegarty [50]; McKirdy et al. [6]; Sheppard [22]	Consistent functional practice	The movement components of exercises, selected to develop specific eating task components and developmental skills, are practiced as fixed eating routines
	To improve existing eating and drinking skills and advance development of skills that have not yet emerged	

Affective Behaviors, Motivation, and Pragmatics

It was found that 85 % of children referred to an interdisciplinary team for swallowing and feeding disorder had behavioral eating disorder associated with dysphagia alone or in combination with neurological conditions, structural abnormalities, cardiorespiratory problems and metabolic dysfunction [4]. Inappropriate behaviors associated with eating can be attributed to disorders of state regulation and caregiver–infant reciprocity, infantile anorexia, sensory food aversions, post-traumatic feeding disorder, feeding disorder associated with a concurrent medical condition, and complex behavioral feeding disorders caused by a combination of these problems [19]. Successful intervention depends on accurate diagnosis and management of ongoing causes [19], in addition to recognition of interactive dynamics during feeding that may be maintaining the abnormal behavior patterns [52]. Approaches that address the existing medical, neuromotor, and behavioral issues in an integrated manner have been advocated as optimum for children presenting with complex swallowing and feeding disorder [1, 6, 8, 34].

There is substantial research and clinical practice literature that considers behavioral modification strategies as a means for improving motivation and inducing eating in children with food refusal and dysphagia [10]. Rehabilitation maneuvers and exercises are described that have been found to be useful across disorder categories for shaping motivation for eating and the interactive dynamics that will support participation in rehabilitative exercise and increase oral intake [6, 10].

Escape Extinction

Maintenance of eating refusal and related behaviors in children are thought to result from the reinforcing effect of ending the eating experience. Escape extinction (EE) describes maneuvers by which children's habitual behaviors are not permitted to end eating. Not removing the cup or spoon until the child permits food to be placed in his/her mouth, used alone and in combination with reinforcement strategies, has been found to increase food intake [10, 53]. A "feedback" system in which a child can see the number of bites that must be accepted has been successful for improving both motivation and pragmatics during transition from tube to oral feeding in 'two school-age children.' [6]. Gains have been retained after EE strategies were faded.

Escape Extinction Paired with Other Strategies

Piazza [10] reviewed studies of the effectiveness of pairing EE with other behavioral treatment maneuvers for achieving increased food acceptance and reduction of behaviors that are inappropriate for supporting eating. Maneuvers that have been found to be effective are (a) pairing preferred and non-preferred foods in a single bite or blended [54]; (b) "reducing response effort"—beginning with empty spoon and gradually increasing bite sizes [55]; (c) "texture fading"—beginning with accepted food consistency and gradually increasing food texture and (d) providing positive reinforcement for successful efforts [6, 53]. In some children EE combined with other maneuvers is more effective than EE alone. However, use of maneuvers without EE have been found to be ineffective for improving behaviors or food acceptance [10] (Table 17.4).

Saliva Swallowing

Difficulties with saliva swallowing occur when there are deficiencies in controlling saliva in the mouth, initiation of swallowing as saliva accumulates or pharyngeal clearance of saliva [56]. This issue has been addressed in the literature for children with cerebral palsy. Although pharyngeal phase involvement for saliva swallowing has been noted [57], drooling has been associated primarily with deficiencies in oral preparatory and oral initiation phases of swallowing, specifically use of negative pressure (suction) in bolus formation and the latency between suction and bolus propulsion for initiation of swallow. Furthermore, in some children ability to collect and hold the saliva on the tongue and ability to close lips were found to be associated with drooling [58].

The frequency of typical saliva swallowing has been associated with rate of saliva flow [59]. A study of frequency of saliva swallowing in typically developing and developmentally disabled children pre- and post-eating found significant differences between the two test times and between the two groups, with higher swallowing frequency seen post-eating than pre-eating. Developmentally disabled children in this test group had lower mean swallowing frequency pre-eating and higher mean frequency post-eating [60]. Clinical experience suggests that developmentally disabled children who tend to cough after finishing eating do not increase post-eating saliva swallowing frequency over the baseline pre-feeding rate. Saliva swallowing frequency in children with

Table 17.4. Rehabilitation maneuvers and exercise for improving motivation for eating and eating pragmatics.

Citation	Maneuvers and exercises/functional Swallowing objective(s)	Procedure
Piazza [10]; McKirdy et al. [6]	Escape extinction (EE) To reduce food refusal and facilitate participation in eating exercise	Escape extinction procedures vary depending on the child's capabilities and the severity of the problem. Food is presented in a dependent or independent task. The presentation method may be non-removal of the spoon at the lips or food provided for self-feeding. Reinforcement is withheld and instructions/models are repeated until acceptance meets the required standard. The eating session ends when a preset amount of a given food is actively accepted
McKirdy et al. [6]	Visual information feedback (plus EE) To reduce food refusal, facilitate participation in eating exercise, and increase swallowing for food	Manipulable objects, such as pegs/peg board, ring stack, blocks are presented with the eating task to inform child of the number of bites or sips and swallows required to complete the task. Removal of one object indicates that the child's effort was satisfactory and one less repetition is needed for completion. A task can consist of one or more repetitions
Patel et al. [53]; McKirdy et al. [6]; Schmidt and Wrisberg [21]	Reinforcement (plus EE) To reduce food refusal, facilitate participation in eating exercise, and increase swallowing for food	Reinforcement as motivator for increasing the occurrence of desired response is provided to the child immediately following its occurrence, e.g., taking the food into the mouth, swallowing the food, or increasing amount of intake. The selected reinforcement must be motivating to the child. The reinforcement schedule is changed as the child advances from early learning to advanced learning stages

(continued)

Table 17.4. (continued)

Citation	Maneuvers and exercises/functional Swallowing objective(s)	Procedure
Piazza [10]	Mixing preferred and non-preferred foods (plus EE) To reduce food refusal, facilitate participation in eating exercise, and increase swallowing for food	Preferred taste foods are combined (blended) with gradually increasing amounts of the non-preferred or unfamiliar food. "Texture fading" applies this strategy for introducing progressively coarser food textures
Piazza [10]	Reducing response effort (plus EE) To reduce food refusal, facilitate participation in eating exercise, and increase swallowing for food	The difficulty or effort associated with eating is reduced by compensations, i.e., reducing the size of the bolus, bolus viscosity, or pace of bolus presentation

cerebral palsy who drool is lower than that of children with cerebral palsy who do not drool [61]. Sochaniwskyj and colleagues concluded that drooling resulted from a combination of inefficient and infrequent swallowing. Treatment programs for saliva control typically include both oral motor and swallowing exercise and behavioral modification strategies.

Oral Motor Exercises

An evidence-based systematic review of the effectiveness of OME for improving pediatric swallowing disorders included articles that studied effects on drooling [17]. In this context OME refers to exercise in which saliva swallowing is not the target task. The authors noted mixed results for positive change. A review follows of two studies that used OME in combination with other maneuvers to improve drooling. Those studies were selected because they included more subjects and control groups.

An OME program combined the use of an orthopedic chin cup for stabilizing the mandible in an elevated position and approximating the lips with exercises for improving voluntary lip and tongue movements, blowing, and sucking. Active exercises included blowing candles, musical toys, bubbles and balloons, and sucking straws and ice. Treatment duration for three experimental groups ranged from 9 to 14 months. In addition, this study design included behavioral strategies and CFP of saliva swallowing (see below). The children were 6–18 years of age. The two groups that used the chin cup did better than the group that participated in the active OME only. All the experimental groups did better than the control group [62].

An OME program was combined with the use of EMG auditory feedback, that signaled contraction of the orbicularis oris and infra-hyoid muscles; and with visual feedback from a mirror. The children, who were 6–18 years old, were taught to turn the auditory signal on and off with muscle contraction and subsequently with lip puckering, lip approximation, sucking, blowing, and swallowing. Multiple baselines compared the effectiveness of the OME with the use of external cueing for swallowing and auditory EMG feedback to indicate a successful swallow. In this study the most significant reduction in drooling occurred after OME. A nonsignificant increase in drooling rate and drop in frequency of swallowing had occurred at follow-up, 1 month after treatment [63].

Behavioral Treatments

Van der burg and colleagues reviewed the literature on behavioral treatments for drooling. Those maneuvers aimed to reduce drooling by manipulation of events preceding or following the drooling. Treatment targets that have been studied were swallowing, wiping chin, head control, mouth closure, length of time without drooling, and performing a self-control routine. In these studies strategies were combined to achieve reduced drooling. Outcomes have been positive, but evaluation of the effectiveness of these interventions is hampered by the inconsistency in the definition of drooling, the limited number of subjects in the studies and, in some studies, failure to test retention of skill after treatment was terminated [64, 65]. It is noteworthy for treatment that behavioral strategies were reduced systematically as the children improved in order to allow them to substitute natural contingents for the behavioral maneuvers.

Antecedent techniques. Instruction and cuing for swallowing are maneuvers that aim to prevent the occurrence of drool. Typically instruction will target the behaviors that are assumed to reduce drooling, for example, swallowing when wetness is noted, keeping mouth closed, and holding head upright. Cueing, used to remind the child to swallow periodically, has included periodic verbal cueing to "suck and swallow" [62] and use of an electronic device to cue the child to swallow on a preset schedule. Electronic cueing devices may have outputs that are visual, auditory, or vibratory. Time intervals for cueing ranged from 15 s to 5 min [63, 64].

Consequent techniques. Consequent techniques consist of maneuvers that provide feedback of adequacy of saliva control or of a related targeted behavior, such as swallow or lip closure [22]. Feedback may be neutral, that is neither positive nor negative, as occurs in the use of a mirror for self-management of drooling. Feedback has been combined with positive or negative reinforcement or punishment [62, 64]. For example, praise, edibles, and token rewards have been used as positive reinforcement while "time-out" as a form of withdrawal of attention was used as a negative reinforcement strategy. Punishment has included reprimand for drooling, repeat of instruction for swallowing, and requirement for repeated mouth wiping. Typically, the use of negative reinforcements and punishment for failure were used in conjunction with positive reinforcement for success.

Consistent functional practice. CFP for saliva control involves habituation and generalization of control, as it occurs naturally, when the child is focused on another function. Typically, controls were taught in a therapeutic environment and transferred to school [62, 63] and home [65]. CFP for saliva control is illustrated here by a study that incorporated CFP exercise with antecedent and consequent maneuvers

Self-management treatment (SMT). In SMT the child was trained to swallow and wipe his/her chin in response to sensations of saliva accumulation or drooling. During training, instruction and reinforcement were paired with CFP of saliva control during the child's daily educational and recreational activities.

SMT was studied in ten children with developmental disability in a short-term residential setting [65]. Training occurred in 3 daily 90 min sessions concurrent with the child's daily activity, 5 days weekly for 3 weeks. Practice validity was achieved with both self-monitoring and the use of recreational and educational equipment and materials that were supplied for each child by their teacher and parents [65]. The outcome measure was progressively longer time intervals before drooling occurred, beginning at one time interval below the child's baseline latency or at a minimum of 30 s. The child was instructed in the exercise routine—to check their chin for wetness, swallow and wipe their chin dry, and the target interval for staying dry. A mirror was provided. Positive verbal comment or a sticker was given for self-initiation of the exercise routine and for achieving the target time interval. Negative verbal comment and restatement of the instructions followed failure to initiate the exercise when saliva was drooled onto the chin. The activity was generalized to home for short practice intervals on weekends. At the end of the treatment, all of the children remained dry for 30–60 min. Three children retained their gains at 6 and 24 week follow up. Seven children regressed but retained improvements over baseline (Table 17.5).

Summary

Therapeutic intervention for infants and children with dysphagia is threefold. It includes strategies for improving the motivation and pragmatic behaviors that support the child's eating and participation in swallowing therapy, exercise for advancing the developmental skills for mature swallowing function, and exercise for improving underlying neuro-motor competencies for swallowing. Etiologies, levels of involvement, comorbidities, developmental levels, and treatment settings are among the variables that are considered in selecting appropriate

Table 17.5. Rehabilitation maneuvers and exercise for improving saliva swallowing.

Citations	Maneuvers and exercises/functional swallowing objectives	Procedures
Harris and Dignam [62]	Oral motor exercise To improve non-swallowing coordination in oral structures	Voluntary lip, jaw, or tongue movements and respiratory control are practiced in non-swallowing functional activities, such as blowing candles, bubbles, balloons and musical toys and sucking straws and ice, and in voluntary range-of-motion for lip pucker and approximation
Koheil et al. [63]	External cuing To improve timing for initiating saliva swallowing and feedback that swallow has occurred	Cuing systems used to initiate saliva swallowing have included verbal cuing—"suck, swallow" and electronic timing devices with visual, auditory, or vibratory outputs. Surface EMG on suprahyoid muscles signals the occurrence of a swallow with an auditory signal
Harris and Dignam [62]; van der Burg et al. [64]	Instruction To improve awareness of saliva accumulation and postures that have been associated with better control	Instructions used to heighten awareness include swallowing when wetness is detected, keeping mouth closed, and holding head upright
Harris and Dignam [62]	Feedback To improve awareness of the adequacy of saliva management during a specific interval	Feedback strategies include use of a mirror and verbalization to inform the child of their achieving (or failing) saliva control for a designated time target
Harris and Dignam [62]	Reinforcement and punishment To motivate use of strategies for improving saliva control	Reinforcement and punishment for achievement on well-defined saliva control tasks is provided on a systematic schedule immediately following the task performance
Harris and Dignam [62]; Koheil et al. [63]; van der Burg et al. [65]	Consistent functional practice To improve the biomechanics of saliva swallowing	A consistent practice routine for saliva swallowing is conducted while child is engaged in daily activities, thus developing the awareness and ability to control saliva while attention is directed otherwise. Consistency in structure of the practice routine and achievable targets, feedback, and reinforcement facilitate learning

treatment strategies. Advancing capabilities in order to keep up with age-related increases in nutritional need and maintain swallowing-related respiratory health are the primary considerations that guide the clinical choices for treatment objectives and rehabilitative strategies. Although this chapter is limited in its focus to rehabilitative maneuvers and exercise, in pediatric intervention compensatory strategies are typically integrated with rehabilitation/habilitation to support the desired health-related outcomes while advancing skills, underlying competencies, and eating pragmatics.

References

1. Field D, Garland M, Williams KE. Correlates of specific childhood feeding problems. J Paediatr Child Health. 2003;39:299–304.
2. Lefton-Greif MA, Arvedson JC. Pediatric feeding and swallowing disorders: state of health, population trends, and application of the International Classification of Functioning, Disability, and Health. Semin Speech Lang. 2007;28(3):161–5.
3. Cooper-Brown L, Copeland S, Dailey S, et al. Feeding and swallowing dysfunction in genetic syndromes. Dev Disabil Res Rev. 2008;14:147–57.
4. Burklow KA, Phelps AN, Schultz JR, McConnell K, Rudolph C. Classifying complex pediatric feeding disorders. J Pediatr Gastroenterol Nutr. 1998;27(2):143–7.
5. Gisel E, Alphonce E. Classification of eating impairments based on eating efficieny in children with cerebral palsy. Dysphagia. 1995;10:268–74.
6. McKirdy LS, Sheppard JJ, Osborne ML, Payne P. Transition from tube to oral feeding in the school setting. Lang Speech Hear Serv Sch. 2008;39:249–60.
7. Sheppard JJ, Fletcher KR. Evidence-based interventions for breast and bottle feeding in the Neonatal Intensive Care Unit. Semin Speech Lang. 2007;28(3):204–12.
8. Sheppard JJ. Motor learning approaches for improving negative, eating-related behaviors and swallowing and feeding skills in children. In: Preedy VR, editor. International handbook of behavior, diet and nutrition. London: Springer; 2011.
9. Hadders-Algra M. The neuronal group selection theory: promsing prinnciples for undrstanding and treating developmental motor disorders. Dev Med Child Neurol. 2000;42:707–15.
10. Piazza CC. Feeding disorders and behavior: what have we learned? Dev Disabil Res Rev. 2008;14:174–81.
11. Barlow SM, Finan DS, Lee J, Chu S. Synthetic orocutaneous stimulation entrains preterm infants with feeding difficulties to suck. J Perinatol. 2008;28:541–8.
12. Hensch TK. Critical period regulation. Annu Rev Neurosci. 2004;27:549–79.
13. Okada A, Tsukamoto C, Hosogi M, et al. The study of psycho-pathology and treatment of children with phagophobia. Acta Med Okayama. 2007;61(5):261–9.
14. DiScipio WJ, Kaslon K. Conditioned dysphagia in cleft palate children after pharyngeal flap surgery. Psychosom Med. 1982;44(3):247–57.

15. Lefton-Greif MA, McGrath-Morrow SA. Deglutition and respiration: development, coordination and practical implications. Semin Speech Lang. 2007;28(3):166–79.

16. Cass H, Wallis C, Ryan M, Reilly S, McHugh K. Assessing pulmonary consequences of dysphagia in children with neurological disabilities: when to intervene? Dev Med Child Neurol. 2005;47:347–52.

17. Arvedson JC, Clark H, Lazarus C, Schooling T, Frymark T. The effects of oral-motor exercises on swallowing in children: an evidence-based systematic review. Dev Med Child Neurol. 2010;52(11):1000–13.

18. Arvedson JC, Clark H, Lazarus C, Schooling T, Frymark T. Evidence-based systematic review: effects of oral motor interventions on feeding and swallowing in preterm infants. Am J Speech Lang Pathol. 2010;19:321–40.

19. Chatoor I. Diagnosis and treatment of feeding disorders in infants, toddlers, and young children. Washington, DC: Zero to Three; 2009.

20. Schmidt RA, Lee TD. Motor control and learning, a behavioral emphasis. 3rd ed. Champaign: Human Kinetics; 1999.

21. Schmidt RA, Wrisberg CA. Motor learning and performance, a problem-based approach. 3rd ed. Champaign: Human Kinetics; 2004.

22. Sheppard JJ. Using motor learning approaches for treating swallowing and feeding disorders: a review. Lang Speech Hear Serv Sch. 2008;39:227–36.

23. Poore M, Zimmerman E, Barlow SM, Wang J, Gu F. Patterned orocutaneous therapy improves sucking and oral feeding in preterm infants. Acta Paediatr. 2008;97(7):920–7.

24. Fucile S, Gisel E, Lau C. Effect of oral stimulation program on sucking skill maturation of preterm infants. Dev Med Child Neurol. 2005;47:158–62.

25. Fucile S, Gisel E, Lau C. Oral stimulation accelerates the transition from tube to oral feeding in preterm infants. J Pediatr. 2002;141:230–6.

26. Hill AS. The effects of nonnutritive sucking and oral support on the feeding efficiency of preterm infants. Newborn Infant Nurs Rev. 2005;5(3):133–41.

27. Nurayanan I, Mehta R, Choudhury DK, Juin BK. Sucking on the "emptied" breast: non-nutritive sucking with a difference. Arch Dis Child. 1991;66:241–4.

28. Nyqvist KH, Sjolden P-O, Ewald U. The developmetn of preterm infants' breastfeeding behavior. Early Hum Dev. 1999;55(3):247–64.

29. Gaebler CP, Hanzlik JR. The effects of a pre-feeding stimulation program on preterm infants. Am J Occup Ther. 1996;50:184–93.

30. Rocha AD, Moreira ME, Pimenta HP, Ramos JR, Lucena SL. A randomized study of the efficacy of sensory-motor-oral stimulation and non-nutritive sucking in very low birthweight infant. Early Hum Dev. 2007;83:385–8.

31. Pickler RH, Best A, Crosson D. The effect of feeding experience on clinical outcomes in preterm infants. J Perinatol. 2009;29:124–9.

32. McCain GC, Gartside P, Greenberg J, Lott JWA. A feeding protocol for healthy preterm infants that shortens the time to oral feeding. J Pediatr. 2001;139:374–9.

33. Law-Morstatt L, Judd DM, Snyder P, Baier RJ, Dhanireddy R. Pacing as a treatment technique for transitional sucking patterns. J Perinatol. 2003;23:483–8.

34. Bailey RL, Angell ME. Effects of an oral-sensory/oral-motor stimulation/positive reinforcement program on the acceptance of nonpreferred foods by youth with physical

and multiple disabilities. Physical Disabilities: Education and Related Services. 2006;24(1):41–61.

35. Clark H. Neuromuscular treatments for speech and swallowing: a tutorial. Am J Speech Lang Pathol. 2003;12:400–15.

36. Robbins J, Kays SA, Gangnon RE, et al. The effects of lingual exercise in stroke patients with dysphagia. Arch Phys Med Rehabil. 2007;88:150–8.

37. Burkhead LM, Sapienza CM, Rosenbek J. Strength-training exercise in dysphagia rehabilitation: principles, procedures and directions for future researh. Dysphagia. 2007;22(3):251–65.

38. Pitts T, Bolser D, Rosenbek J, Troche M, Okun MS, Sapienza CM. Impact of expiratory muscle strength training on voluntary cough and swallow function in Parkinson disease. Chest. 2009;135:1301–8.

39. Helfrich-Miller KR, Rector KL, Straka JA. Dysphagia: its treatment in the profoundly retarded patient with cerebral palsy. Arch Phys Med Rehabil. 1986;67:520–5.

40. Clark H, Lazarus C, Arvedson JC, Schooling T, Frymark T. Evidence-based systematic review: effects of neuromuscular electrical stimulation on swallowing and neural activation. Am J Speech Lang Pathol. 2009;18:361–75.

41. Kenny DJ, Koheil RM, Greenberg J, et al. Development of a multidisciplinary feeding profile for children who are dependent feeders. Dysphagia. 1989;4:16–28.

42. Haberfellner H, Schwartz S, Gisel E. Feeding skills and growth after one year of intraoral appliance therapy in moderately dysphagic childen with cerebral palsy. Dysphagia. 2001;16(2):83–96.

43. Gisel E, Haberfellner H, Schwartz S. Impact of oral appliance therapy: are oral skills and growth maintained one year after termination of therapy? Dysphagia. 2001;16(4): 296–307.

44. Sheppard JJ. The role of oral sensorimotor therapy in the treatment of pediatric dysphagia. Perspectives on Swallowing and Swallowing Disorders (Dysphagia). 2005;14(2):6–10.

45. Gisel E. Interventions and outcomes for children with dysphagia. Dev Disabil Res Rev. 2008;14:165–73.

46. Gisel E. Oral-motor skills following sensorimotor intervention in the moderately eating-impaired child with cerebral palsy. Dysphagia. 1994;9(3):180–92.

47. Gisel E. Effect of oral ssensorimotor treatmenton measures of growth and efficiency of eating in the moderately eating-impaired child with cerebral palsy. Dysphagia. 1996;11(1):48–58.

48. Gisel E, Applegate-Ferrante T, Benson J, Bosma JF. Oral-motor skills following sensorimotor therapy in two groups of moderately dysphagic children with cerebral palsy: aspiration vs nonaspiration. Dysphagia. 1996;11(1):59–71.

49. Gisel E, Applegate-Ferrante T, Benson J, Bosma JF. Effect of oral sensorimotor treatment on measures of growth, eating efficiency and aspiration in the dysphagic child with cerebral palsy. Dev Med Child Neurol. 1995;37(6):528–43.

50. Pinnington L, Hegarty J. Effects of consistent food presentation on oral-motor skill acquisition in children with severe neurologiccal impairment. Dysphagia. 2000;15(4): 213–23.

51. Reilly S, Skuse D, Mathisen B, Wolke D. Schedule for oral-motor assessment (SOMA): methods of validation. Dysphagia. 1995;10:192–202.

52. Piazza CC, Fisher WW, Brown KA, et al. Functional analysis of inappropriate mealtime behaviors. J Appl Behav Anal. 2003;36:187–204.

53. Patel MR, Piazza CC, Martinez CJ, Volkert VM, Christine MS. An evaluation of two differential reinforcement procedures with escape extinction to treat food refusal. J Appl Behav Anal. 2002;35(4):363–74.

54. Mueller MM, Piazza CC, Patel MR. Increasing variety of foods consumed by blending non preferred into preferred foods. J Appl Behav Anal. 2004;37:159–70.

55. Kerwin ME, Ahearn WH, Eicher PS, Burd DM. The costs of eating: a behavioral economic ananlysis of food refusal. J Appl Behav Anal. 1995;228(3):245–60.

56. Sheppard JJ. Salivation and saliva control in children, more than just drooling. Pediatric Feeding and Dysphagia Newsletter. 2003;4(1):1–2.

57. Jongerius PH, van Hulst K, van den Hoogen FJ, Rotteveel JJ. The treatment of posterior drooling by botulinum toxin in a child with cerebral palsy. J Pediatr Gastroenterol Nutr. 2005;41:351–3.

58. Lespargot A, Langevin M-F, Muller S, Guillemont S. Swallowing distrubances associated with drooling in cerebral-palsied children. Dev Med Child Neurol. 1993;35:298–304.

59. Kapila YV, Dodds WJ, Helm JF, Hogan WJ. Relationship between swallow rate and salivary flow. Dig Dis Sci. 1984;26(6):528–33.

60. Sheppard JJ, Guglielmo A, Burke L, Leone AM, Gross K. Frequency of swallowing in typically developing and developmentally delayed children before and after eating. AAMR 128th Annual Meeting, Philadelphia, 2004.

61. Sochaniwskyj AE, Koheil RM, Bablich K, Milner M, Kenny DJ. Oral motor functioning, frequency of swallowing and drooling in normal children and in children with cerebral palsy. Arch Phys Med Rehabil. 1986;67(12):866–74.

62. Harris MM, Dignam PF. A non-surgical method of reducing drooling in cerebral-palsied children. Dev Med Child Neurol. 1980;22:293–9.

63. Koheil RM, Sochaniwskyj AE, Bablich K, Kenny DJ. Biofeedback techniques and behaviour modification in the conservative remediation of drooling by children with cerebral palsy. Dev Med Child Neurol. 1987;29:19–26.

64. van der Burg JJW, Didden R, Jongerius PH, Rotteveel JJ. Behavioral treatment of drooling: a methodological critique of the literature with clinical guidelines and suggestions for future research. Behav Modif. 2007;31:573–93.

65. van der Burg JJW, Didden R, Engbers N, Jongerius PH, Rotteveel JJ. Self-management treatment of drooling: a case series. J Behav Ther Exp Psychiatry. 2009;40:106–19.

18. Compensatory Strategies and Techniques

Claire Kane Miller and J. Paul Willging

Abstract Management and treatment of feeding and swallowing disorders in infants and children is complex due to the multitude of etiologies and interacting variables that may be present in any given situation. The underlying causes of dysphagia in the pediatric population are both congenital and acquired and include an array of structural, neurologic, cardiorespiratory, genetic, systemic, and metabolic conditions. Feeding and swallowing difficulties may evolve or intensify secondary to medical complications, physiologic abnormalities, or ongoing environmental factors that, singly or in combination, impair progression of normal feeding and swallowing behavior. Inadequate recognition and management of pediatric feeding and swallowing dysfunction has serious implications including potential malnutrition, chronic respiratory disease, disruption of oral motor/feeding skill development, and extended use of nasogastric or gastrostomy tube feedings. Lack of dysphagia treatment, delayed initiation of treatment, or the use of inappropriate treatment approaches may all contribute to prolonged dysphagia and potentially untoward consequences. Thus, thorough dysphagia diagnostic evaluation, accurate identification of oral and pharyngeal swallowing physiology and dysfunction, and appropriate selection of compensatory and rehabilitative interventions is essential to maximize each child's potential for a satisfactory outcome. A multidisciplinary approach in the differential diagnosis and management of pediatric feeding and swallowing problems is essential in the identification and management of problems that may occur across multiple systems.

The goals of dysphagia therapy in infants and children are thus dependent upon the constellation of issues present and are comprised of

R. Shaker et al. (eds.), *Manual of Diagnostic and Therapeutic Techniques for Disorders of Deglutition*, DOI 10.1007/978-1-4614-3779-6_18, © Springer Science+Business Media New York 2013

techniques to modulate responses to sensory stimulation and to facilitate increased oral motor control for successful and safe oral intake. The underlying paradigm of pediatric dysphagia treatment is comprised of direct rehabilitative maneuvers/exercises as discussed in Chap. 17 and/or the use of compensatory techniques and strategies. Compensatory strategies include changes in positioning for feeding, sensory stimulation techniques, the use of specialized feeding equipment, and the implementation of specific behavioral approaches focusing on the development of positive and productive feeder/child interactions. Compensatory techniques may be used singly or in combination by the dysphagia clinician at various points in the treatment plan; the use is specific and based on the responses of each patient. The end result of pediatric dysphagia therapy may not always be full oral feeding, and this concept should be discussed and understood early on in the treatment plan by the dysphagia clinician. The following chapter will focus on the application of compensatory strategies and techniques to assist with treatment of oral sensory, oral motor, and pharyngeal phase dysfunction. Available evidence to support the use of the compensatory strategies and techniques in the treatment of specific conditions is summarized. Continued research to establish a robust evidence base for the use of treatment approaches in pediatric feeding and swallowing practice is needed to establish best practice guidelines.

Overview of Compensatory Dysphagia Treatment Techniques in Pediatrics

Overall, empiric data regarding the use of compensatory strategies and subsequent treatment outcomes in the pediatric dysphagia population is limited. Virtually all of the results reported in the literature have been based upon retrospective review of patient treatment and outcome as opposed to prospective, randomized clinical trials. Clearly, the feasibility of employing clinical trials (treatment/no treatment) is difficult with the pediatric population due to the undesirable option of withholding treatment for infants and children with feeding and swallowing difficulties.

The approaches to dysphagia treatment in the pediatric population are dependent on the child's oral sensory, oral motor, and airway protection/swallowing function status. Clearly, the clinician must have thorough knowledge of the child's overall medical and developmental status, as well as airway protection ability during non-nutritive and nutritive swallowing conditions to determine the appropriate treatment approaches and goals of intervention. Treatment interventions may be direct as well as compensatory in nature, though the use of compensatory strategies may predominate in some cases secondary to the child's developmental level, medical status, and the nature of the dysphagia. Definition and specific application of the compensatory techniques in the treatment of pediatric dysphagia will be described in the remainder of the chapter.

Alterations in Positioning

Establishing optimal positioning during non-nutritive peri oral and intraoral stimulation for oral alerting prior to feeding, as well as during oral feeding trials, is basic to facilitating coordinated oral motor movements and swallowing safety [1, 2]. Postural modifications differ depending on the type of muscle tone abnormality present. In addition, variations in infant positioning may be needed to help facilitate coordination of respiration and swallowing during feeding. For example, prone or side-lying positioning in infants with retrognathia (posteriorly placed mandible) and resultant posterior displacement of the tongue may help to facilitate more anterior tongue positioning and decrease the likelihood of increased, problematic respiratory effort with feeding attempts [2, 3]. Infants with increased muscle tone may have excessive head and neck extension which interferes with efficient feeding. Such infants may position from positional adjustments that facilitate neutral positioning of the head and neck. As infants mature, the degree of maturation in head, neck and trunk control as well as underlying muscle tone will determine what positioning option for feeding is most appropriate. If there are significant issues with muscle tone and motor control that become evident with maturity, specialized adaptive seating to maintain optimum positioning for feeding will be necessary. The characteristics of muscle tone and resulting posture are interrelated with the infant's state, physiologic control, and oral motor control during feeding and therefore the choice of positioning must be individualized [2]. Considerations for positioning are summarized in Table 18.1.

Table 18.1. Positions for infant feeding and rationale.

Type of position	Rationale
Cradle	Traditional "standard" position, infant is "cradled" in feeder's arms, with midline orientation of the trunk with neutral alignment of the head and neck
	Alterations can easily be make to bring infant in more upright positioning as needed
En face	Infant is positioned in feeder's lap and facing feeder, feeder's hand supports head
	Maximal control of head is possible, assists with decreasing excessive head extension during feeding
	Difficult to provide adequate trunk control
Side-lying	Infant is positioned on feeder's lap in side-lying with trunk straight and well-supported
	Feeder must take care not to allow head to move into excess extension in this position
	May be helpful in bringing retracted tongue forward
Supine on lap	Feeder positions infant on lap—facilitates keeping the trunk straight and well-supported, and keeps the head in a neutral position

Adapted from Wolf and Glass [2].

Use of Specialized Feeding Equipment

There is a wide variety of specialized feeding equipment accessible for use in pediatric dysphagia treatment that includes numerous bottle, nipple, cup, and utensil options. Clinical efficacy data to support the use of specific feeding equipment is limited, and therefore clinician expertise and judgment generally guides the selection of the type of equipment used. Clinical decisions are based on the sensory and motor dysfunction present combined with the infant or child's responses during implementation of specialized feeding equipment options.

Sensory Stimulation Techniques

As in adults, sensory stimulation techniques including modification of bolus consistency, bolus placement, volume, temperature, and taste may be implemented in pediatric dysphagia treatment. A description and rationale for commonly used sensory stimulation techniques is summarized below.

Altering Fluid Viscosity

Increasing the viscosity of liquid to assist with the maintenance of airway protection during swallowing is a common interventional strategy used in pediatric dysphagia treatment for a wide variety of conditions; however, the efficacy across different disorders has not been systematically studied [4]. There is a need to standardize methods of thickening in dysphagia practice as lack of standardization has resulted in different degrees of thickening between practitioners and caretakers [5–7].

The rationale supporting the use of increased liquid viscosity and thus the slower bolus flow is to allow a greater amount of time for the infant or child to control the bolus intraorally so as to achieve airway closure prior to bolus arrival in the hypopharynx and swallowing initiation [1, 4]. Therefore, infants or children demonstrating difficulty with oral control and/or a delayed pharyngeal swallowing response with subsequent threat of inadequate airway protection may benefit from the use of thickened fluids. Further study is required to confirm this rationale for use and to determine the efficacy of using thickened fluid in the treatment of varied dysphagia conditions specific to infants and children. In the pediatric population, medical and nutritional consultation is mandatory prior to altering the viscosity of fluid regardless of condition to confirm that the infant or child's caloric and/or fluid requirements will not be compromised. The possible effects of various thickening agents on the digestive system in infants have not been systematically studied [4].

Bolus Modification: Volume, Texture, Taste, Temperature

Volume, texture, taste, and temperature modifications to solid and liquid boluses are commonly used in pediatric dysphagia practice. Research focusing on bolus volume and consistency in children and adults suggests that swallow behavior may differ depending upon the degree of volume as well as consistency type of the bolus [8, 9]. Specific alterations of bolus consistency, taste, temperature, viscosity have been shown to have an effect on swallow function in adults by numerous investigators [10–15]. Similar empirical evidence is needed to define changes in swallowing dynamics in infants and young children in both normal and disordered populations. The use of strong flavor input (carbonation, citrus, spicy, salty, sour) to facilitate a timely and efficient oral and pharyngeal swallowing response in pediatric patients is primarily anecdotal in nature. Changes in bolus volume, flow, temperature, and texture will be described in compensatory treatment approaches.

Alternating Liquid and Solid Bolus Presentations

Alternating liquid boluses with solid boluses may also assist with clearance of pharyngeal residue in some cases. In addition, pediatric patients with conditions involving altered speed of esophageal motility, such as repaired tracheoesophageal fistula/esophageal atresia, may benefit from alternating fluid boluses with solid boluses to assist with bolus transfer, though the clinical efficacy of this strategy has not been systematically studied.

Non-nutritive Oral Sensory Stimulation

Sensorimotor stimulation techniques for infants and children include tactile input to the body, orofacial, and intraoral area, encouragement of non-nutritive sucking on pacifiers, oral exploration using commercially available oral sensory toys, and oral care/tooth brushing. The rationale for implementation of non-nutritive oral sensory stimulation is to heighten sensory awareness and facilitate motor action, and to prevent oral aversion, facilitate sucking, and promote development of oral motor skills necessary to transition to oral feedings [1, 16–18]. Specifically, the efficacy of non-nutritive sucking has been found to significantly decrease length of hospital stay for preterm infants. Evidence to support the use of other oral and nonoral sensorimotor interventions has also been reported [18].

Application of Compensatory Strategies and Sensory Stimulation Techniques

There has been a growing trend in research with a focus on the efficacy of dysphagia interventions in specific populations with common medical diagnoses. Such an approach allows definition of specific variables and the effect of interventions, thus facilitating the identification of clinical pathways for best practice. For example, the recent investigations of the efficacy of non-nutritive stimulation and the associated positive effects provide evidence that supports treatment goals and interventions [17–19].

Structural Etiologies of Pediatric Dysphagia: Compensatory Strategies and Techniques for Treatment

Anatomic abnormalities in any of the structures of the aerodigestive tract have the potential to disrupt the feeding and swallowing process, and include choanal atresia or stenosis, cleft lip/palate, craniofacial anomalies, and congenital defects of the larynx, trachea, or esophagus such as laryngomalacia, bilateral vocal cord paralysis, laryngeal cleft, tracheoesophageal fistula, and esophageal atresia. Many genetic syndromes include structural abnormalities that result in pediatric dysphagia. Table 18.2 summarizes the structural etiologies that contribute to pediatric dysphagia, the potential effect on feeding and swallowing, and suggested compensatory techniques and strategies.

Cleft Lip/Palate and Craniofacial Anomalies

Cleft lip and palate are the most common congenital defects of the face and the fourth most common birth defect. Infants with syndromic and non-syndromic cleft lip and palate and craniofacial anomalies frequently have feeding issues which are of immediate concern and warrant consultation. The feeding problems will reflect the type and severity of the cleft, and will vary depending upon whether the cleft is of the lip or palate, and if it is unilateral, bilateral, complete, or incomplete. The feeding problems that ensue include inadequate oral suction during feeding, lengthy feeding times, nasal regurgitation, excessive air intake, and inadequate volume of oral intake [20–22]. Infants born with cleft lip/palate in conjunction with syndromes, sequences, or associations have a higher likelihood of oral phase difficulty in combination with pharyngeal swallowing dysfunction because of cranial nerve abnormalities or neuromotor components that may be present [23]; compensatory strategies for addressing pharyngeal phase dysfunction will be discussed later in this section.

Compensatory treatment interventions for infants with cleft lip/palate include modification of nipple and bottle types, positioning alterations, oral facilitation techniques, and modifications in the feeding method,

Table 18.2. Structural etiologies of pediatric dysphagia and use of compensatory strategies/techniques.

Structural issue	Effect on feeding/swallowing	Compensatory strategy/technique
Cleft lip ±palate Craniofacial anomalies	Oral phase dysfunction Nasopharyngeal reflux Poor coordination of suck/swallow	Modification of nipple/bottle Assistance with flow—feeder assisted Regulation of flow by feeder Modification of positioning
Choanal stenosis—unilateral	Difficulty with coordination of respiration, sucking, swallowing	Surgical intervention as necessary may alleviate feeding issues Pacing of intake to regulate speed of intake, facilitate coordination of respiration/swallowing
Laryngomalacia	Poor coordination of suck, swallow, respiration	Upright positioning Pacing by feeder to regulate rate of intake Nutritional interventions—increase caloric density of fluid Increased viscosity of fluid may assist with airway protection Surgical intervention as necessary in severe cases may alleviate feeding issues
Vocal fold paralysis	Difficulty with airway protection during swallowing	Increased viscosity of fluid may assist maintenance of airway protection Use of effortful swallow may help to assist with supraglottic closure for airway protection Upright positioning

Laryngotracheal anomalies	Difficulty with airway protection during swallowing	Alter viscosity of fluid
	Sensory and/or motor abnormalities impacting pharyngeal phase	Alter texture of solids
		Alternate solids/liquids to assist with pharyngeal clearance
		Use modified supraglottic swallowing sequence to assist with airway closure and clearance of residue
		Use of effortful swallow may assist with recruiting supraglottic structures for closure
Esophageal issues	Impaired esophageal motility resulting in globus sensation	Improve oral phase efficiency for adequate bolus preparation prior to swallowing
		Alternate solids and liquids to assist with clearance
		Maintain upright positioning during and after feeding
		Sham feedings

such as the use of feeder-assisted squeezing in synchrony with the infant's sucking efforts to assist with fluid delivery. Feeding obturators are also used in some centers to provide a separation of the nasal cavity from the oral cavity to help eliminate regurgitation of liquids into the nose. Most reports regarding the efficacy of the varied treatment interventions for infants and toddlers with cleft lip, cleft palate, and craniofacial anomalies are from case studies, though there is increasing availability of empiric evidence to guide practice [24–26].

Modification of Nipple and Bottle Types

There are a variety of specialized nipples and bottles available to facilitate the feeding process in infants with cleft lip/palate. When considering what nipple or bottle system to use to help the infant compensate during the feeding process, there are multiple parameters to consider. The characteristics of commonly used nipples and bottle systems are listed in Table 18.3. The type of nipple chosen is based on the type of cleft present and the infant's oral motor/feeding skills. Several classifications of clefts exist though the system proposed by Kernahan and Stark in 1958 has gained the most universal acceptance. This system recommends that clefts be classified based on embryologic development into two basic categories: clefts of the primary (hard) palate and clefts of the secondary (soft) palate with the incisive foramen as the dividing point. A modification of this system allows identification of cleft severity. Based on the segments involved, the extent of the cleft is classified as complete, incomplete, bilateral, or unilateral [20]. Infants with a minimal or incomplete cleft of the soft palate may occlude the cleft with the base of the tongue during sucking, and will not require any modification of the nipple. In contrast, infants with a complete cleft of the hard and soft palate will have more difficulty feeding as the open cavity does not provide a palatal surface for compression of the nipple and negative pressure generation needed for efficient sucking. The nipple must be pliable enough to release breast milk or formula with limited compression and without creation of suction while providing an appropriate degree of proprioceptive input to stimulate sucking. The clinician should understand that the degree of nipple pliability is related to flow rate. That is as the flow rate is increased, the ability to coordinate sucking, swallowing, and respiration may be disrupted.

As with all infants, the nipple shape should provide adequate contact between the nipple and tongue for adequate compression. Broad, flat nipples may be advantageous for infants with isolated cleft lip as they

Table 18.3. Specialized feeding equipment for infants with cleft lip/palate.

Type of equipment	Rationale
Special Needs ® Feeder (formerly Haberman and Mini-Haberman Feeder)	The nipple is designed to release milk from infant compression efforts, so suction is not required
	The nipple is soft and pliable with one-way valving component that prevents rapid fluid flow and opens only when infant sucks
	The nipple designed for assistive squeezing
	Flow control can be regulated by feeder
	Mini special needs feeder is designed for smaller or premature infants with cleft lip/palate
Soft Cup ™ Advanced Cup Feeder—Medela	The cup is made of soft pliable silicone and is contoured
	A control valve, with self-filling cup-like reservoir with flow rate, is controlled by the feeder
	Active sucking is not required
Pigeon nipple/bottle	Nipple has one side with thick wall for placement against roof of mouth and one side with a thin wall for the infant to suck
	The bottle is soft and compressible, allowing assisted feeding
	The nipple can be used with other bottles
Mead Johnson Cleft Palate Nurser	Soft, compressible bottle is easily squeezed
	It is fitted with a cross-cut nipple
	A standard nipple can be used with a modified hole as necessary

may conform to the cleft and help to prevent excessive intake of air during sucking. The nipple size chosen should be based upon the length needed to provide adequate contact between the nipple and tongue to facilitate effective tongue movements. Nipple length can vary substantially, and therefore the selection of an appropriate nipple is individualized to each particular infant's needs. The size of the nipple hole and type of nipple hole (single hole, cross-cut, "Y" shape) will determine flow rate. The size of nipple holes and thus flow rate may vary widely across different styles of nipples, and therefore, matching the infant's sucking is important. A flexible plastic squeeze bottle or plastic bottle liner may be used with a variety of nipples to assist with fluid delivery during feeding; this will be discussed later in the Chapter.

Positioning

Positioning the infant with a cleft palate in an upright position (60°) allow gravity to assist with posterior fluid flow and help to prevent nasal regurgitation that may occur secondary to the cleft palate [1, 2, 20]. The infant's head should be supported in a neutral position, with arms forward, trunk in midline, and the hips flexed. Placing the infant in a semi-reclined or supine position increases the potential for formula entry into the nasopharynx resulting in nasal regurgitation, sneezing, and coughing. However, side-lying or supine positioning may be feasible for infants with craniofacial anomalies that involve retrognathia and resultant glossoptosis [3]. In such cases, the alteration in positioning facilitates anterior positioning of the tongue, alleviating upper airway obstruction during feeding.

Oral Facilitation Techniques

Oral motor techniques to facilitate the oral phase may include lip, cheek, and jaw support provided by the feeder [24, 27]. The infant's jaw can be stabilized by placement of the feeder's middle finger under the infant's chin, and the index finger between the chin and lower lip, thus providing a stable platform for active movements of the tongue, lips, and cheeks [2]. Cheek support, provided by gentle placement of the feeder's index or middle finger and thumb on each side of the cheeks, facilitates lip closure. Placement of the thumb and index or middle finger on the sucking pads applying gentle pressure may help to provide cheek stability and improve lip seal. For some infants, combined use of cheek and jaw support may assist with approximation of the lip on the nipple and increased sucking efficiency [2, 28, 29].

Modification of Feeding Method

Assisted feeding in conjunction with specialized cleft palate nipples/bottles has been shown to be an effective facilitative feeding strategy [30, 31]. Assisted feeding requires the feeder to provide careful assistive squeezing of the bottle and/or nipple in synchrony with the infant's sucking efforts. Modulating or pacing the assistive squeeze in rhythm with the infant's movements and reactions is postulated to assist with maintaining a coordinated swallow and respiratory pattern [32]. If assistive squeezing during feeding is recommended as a compensatory feeding strategy by the clinician, care should be taken to ensure that the parent/caretaker understands the rationale and is able to demonstrate this method effectively and independently during feeding.

Feeding Obturators

A feeding obturator consists of an acrylic plate, inserted into the infant's mouth, fitting over the palatal defect, thus closing the defect and maintaining a seal between the nasal and oral cavities. There are differing views regarding the use of feeding appliances in facilitation of oral feeding in the cleft palate infant. There are some centers that routinely recommend the use of the feeding obturator vs. other appliances in cases of infants with severe feeding problems. The benefits of the obturator are to provide a stable base for the infant to compress the nipple during sucking efforts, thereby improving feeding efficiency. Disadvantages of the obturator include the expense, potential difficulty in insertion of the appliance, problems with maintaining proper placement, irritation to the oral tissues, and the frequent need to replace the obturator to accommodate growth of the infant [20].

Congenital and Acquired Laryngeal and Tracheal Conditions

Complex airway conditions associated with dysphagia in pediatric patients include congenital or acquired subglottic stenosis, glottis stenosis, laryngotracheal stenosis, laryngeal webs or atresia, and tracheal lesions. Congenital subglottic stenosis is relatively rare, and usually occurs in combination with genetic conditions or laryngeal abnormalities including vocal fold paralysis, laryngeal web, laryngeal atresia, subglottic hemangioma, tracheomalacia, and tracheal stenosis [33]. Acquired conditions are more frequent and include subglottic and/or tracheal stenosis as a result of prolonged endotracheal intubation or trauma, hypopharyngeal stenosis secondary to trauma or ingestion, or vocal fold paralysis as a result of recurrent laryngeal nerve injury.

Laryngotracheal Reconstruction

Necessary surgical interventions to repair and expand the airway may have an effect on the laryngeal functions necessary for effective airway protection during swallowing [33, 34]. Therefore, strategies and techniques to assist with development of compensatory swallowing function are often necessary, and may include use of a modified supraglottic swallowing sequence, alternation of solid and liquid bolus intake during feeding, modification of bolus taste, temperature or volume, and possibly altering liquid viscosity [35].

Modified Supraglottic Swallowing Sequence

The supraglottic swallowing sequence may be efficacious in assisting with swallowing function in patients undergoing procedures that involve alteration of the laryngeal anatomy [35]. Use of a series of simple picture card sequences to assist with teaching the steps for a supraglottic closure sequence may be beneficial with patients who demonstrate an appropriate developmental comprehension level. The modified sequence is composed of five steps: gentle cough/throat clear prior to taking bolus; oral "holding" of the bolus prior to swallow initiation; effort to hold breath prior to swallow initiation and during bolus transfer; swallow, followed by gentle cough/throat clear. Use of an appropriately thickened fluid bolus to assist patients with maintenance of bolus control when learning the supraglottic swallowing sequence may be helpful in that the thickened liquid will have slower transit into the hypopharynx and allow patients more time to achieve compensatory airway closure prior to swallowing [35].

Modification of Bolus Consistency, Taste, and Temperature

Patients undergoing laryngeal reconstruction may experience post-operative swallowing discomfort. Modification of bolus viscosity offering very easy to manage, or non-chew, smooth consistencies is often of assistance in facilitating ease of swallowing during initial oral intake. As in any situation where there may be throat pain or discomfort during swallowing, thick boluses or difficult to manage foods such as stringy meats or chips with sharp edges that require more oral manipulation and effortful swallowing to manage should be avoided [35]. Use of strong but pleasant flavors (citrus, sour, spicy) and variation in bolus temperature may heighten sensory input, and help with facilitating swallowing onset and overall swallowing efficiency in the post-operative period [35].

Congenital Laryngeal Anomalies

Other laryngeal anomalies such as choanal atresia, vallecular cyst, laryngomalacia, vocal fold paralysis, and laryngeal web may create upper airway obstruction that significantly interferes with oral feeding attempts. Feeding difficulties commonly accompany vallecular cysts; a well-recognized cause of upper airway obstruction in infants and children. Once identification and excision of the vallecular cyst occurs, feeding difficulties typically resolve. Additionally, surgical correction of choanal atresia alleviates the respiratory issues impacting successful oral feeding.

Laryngomalacia is the most common laryngeal anomaly, and may cause significant inspiratory stridor which increases with the respiratory effort of infant feeding. Severe cases require surgical intervention (supraglottoplasty) to relieve the upper airway obstruction. There is a wide variation in the degree of associated airway obstruction, and laryngomalacia typically resolves by 18 months of age.

In cases of mild-to-moderate laryngomalacia whereby surgical intervention is not required, strategies such as slowing liquid flow rate to decrease overall swallowing frequency and respiratory effort may be helpful. Change in flow rate can be accomplished by using a slower flow nipple, or by changing the viscosity of the fluid. Provision of imposed breaks or pause intervals during feeding may provide the infant with additional time for ventilation during feeding [32].

Vocal fold paralysis is the second most frequent cause of upper airway obstruction in the pediatric population [36]. Congenital bilateral vocal fold paralysis usually results in with the vocal folds in midline position. This position poses an obstruction that may be life-threatening and require a tracheostomy. Although bilateral vocal fold paralysis may occur in isolation, it often occurs in conjunction with other developmental anomalies of the central nervous system, including Chiari malformation type II, hydrocephaly, and cerebral agenesis; conditions whereby pediatric dysphagia is likely. Acquired vocal fold paralysis may occur secondary to an infectious process, endotracheal intubation, or injury to the recurrent laryngeal nerve following surgery for repair of thoracic or cardiovascular anomalies [37]. In such cases, deglutitive airway protection may be compromised and defined through an instrumental assessment of swallowing performed after the cardiac surgical procedure. Assessment of swallowing function and deglutitive airway protection includes the effect of compensatory strategies as described above. As compensatory techniques facilitate safe swallowing, a feeding treatment plan can be devised, incorporating appropriate use of strategies for each patient.

Pediatric laryngectomy is rare, but is indicated in patients secondary to conditions such as tumor, severe recurrent respiratory papillomatosis, or caustic ingestion. Pre-operative counseling with the family and patient is required to describe the resultant anatomic and physiologic changes that will affect communication and swallowing. Compensatory strategies such as the use of soft, easy to manage foods post-operatively may assist with ease of swallowing in the immediate post-operative period should any discomfort be present.

Esophageal Conditions

Infants born with esophageal atresia and/or tracheoesophageal fistula/ TEF, esophageal stricture or web, or vascular rings who undergo surgical repair may have persisting esophageal dysphagia with accompanying clinical signs and symptoms of swallowing difficulty or refuse to eat or drink. Narrowing in the esophagus at the site of the tracheoesophageal fistula repair may slow esophageal transit and result in symptoms of dysphagia. In addition, significant esophageal dysmotility may be present with continued dysphagia [38]. Treatment strategies may include alternation of solids and liquid consistency to assist with esophageal motility, upright positioning during and after oral feeding to assist with promoting motility, and emphasis on adequate oral preparation (sufficient chewing prior to transferring for swallowing) of solid boluses to help facilitate esophageal transit [1].

In some cases, oral feeding may be delayed for weeks or months until surgery can be performed on the esophagus, or until recovery is complete. Lack of exposure to oral feeding over a prolonged time period has been linked to the development of oral aversion; infants with esophageal conditions requiring npo for extended time periods may be at risk [39]. Compensatory strategies to help avoid the development of oral aversion include early provision of oral input and stimulation, as well as the implementation of sham feedings (oral feeds which are drained or suctioned from the blind end of the esophagus [2]). The use of the early oral sham feeds has been reported to be useful in provision of nutritive oral input needed to establish and maintain nutritive suck-swallow skills and therefore facilitates continued progress of oral motor skills for feeding [39].

Aortic arch anomalies compress the esophagus or trachea in varying degrees, and the clinical presentation in infants and children may include gagging and vomiting, solid food refusal, and preference for intake of soft solids and liquids [40]. Resistance or refusal to swallow solids may occur secondary to the impingement on the esophagus, and surgery to alleviate the obstruction will likely improve the symptoms of dysphagia. In cases where surgery is not recommended, compensatory strategies may include assisting the child in developing efficient chewing skills to ensure adequate bolus preparation prior to swallowing to expedite passage of the bolus through the esophagus. In addition, alternating of sips of liquid with intake of solids may help facilitate esophageal motility and overall clearance. Discouraging oral intake while in supine positioning and encouraging upright positioning during and following oral feeding are recommended.

Colonic interposition is a surgical option in pediatric patients who require esophageal replacement secondary to long gap esophageal atresia, severe caustic ingestion injury, epidermolysis, or tumor [41]. Supplemental gastrostomy tube feeds are likely necessary post-operatively for several months while oral feedings are being established. However, restoration of oral intake is possible, and implementation of compensatory dysphagia treatment strategies may assist with this transition. Patients are typically started on a clear liquid diet and subsequently advanced as tolerated. Age-appropriate oral motor skills, and in particular, efficient chewing skills, is of particular importance for adequate bolus preparation to ease bolus passage through the esophagus. Focus on developing strength and efficiency of chewing skills by use of first crunchy but easily dissolvable foods may be one treatment strategy. Allowing adequate intervals between bites to assist with clearance, alternation of liquids/solids, and avoiding foods that are stringy or that require extensive oral manipulation prior to swallowing are advised. Task-specific oral motor exercises to develop strength and efficiency of chewing skills as described in Chap. 17 may be indicated.

Cricopharyngeal achalasia is a relatively rare disorder in infants and children, characterized by inability to relax the upper esophageal sphincter to accommodate bolus passage during swallowing. The diagnosis is often delayed as the incidence is rare and the condition is not often recognized initially [42]. The etiology of cricopharyngeal achalasia in the pediatric population remains unknown. It has been diagnosed in patients with neurologic defects including Chiari malformation and myelomeningocele, but also has been reported to occur in isolation [42]. Signs and symptoms of cricopharyngeal achalasia include choking and nasopharyngeal reflux during feeding, coupled with recurrent respiratory infections and pneumonia presumably secondary to swallowing dysfunction and subsequent aspiration. Fluoroscopic observation of swallow function will reveal a characteristic narrowing on the posterior pharyngeal wall with enlargement of the hypopharynx [43]. Management options include balloon dilatation of the upper esophagus, botulinum toxin, and cricopharyngeal myotomy [42–44]. Dysphagia therapy may be necessary in cases where the children have developed oral aversion and/or feeding resistance [45]. Treatment strategies may include both oral sensory and oral motor strategies in combination with behavioral intervention techniques, discussed later in this chapter.

Neurologic Etiologies: Compensatory Strategies and Techniques

Neurologic impairment secondary to cortical dysfunction, abnormalities in the brainstem, or injury to the cervical spinal cord may compromise the strength and efficiency of the oropharyngeal and esophageal phases of swallowing. Strength and efficiency of oral motor movements, oral sensory awareness and discrimination, coordination of airway protection, and postural control and overall alertness for feeding may be affected. Neurologic issues are the most common etiology of pediatric feeding and swallowing disorders and include anoxic encephalopathy, cerebral palsy, vascular accidents, tumors, Chiari malformations, cranial nerve abnormalities, myopathies, muscular dystrophy, and genetic syndromes involving the cranial nerves responsible for the sensory and motor functions fundamental to safe and efficient feeding and swallowing.

Infants and children with neurologic conditions are known to have a high incidence of oral motor, oral sensory, and pharyngeal swallowing dysfunction [1]. Oral phase issues include problems with sensory awareness and organization, as well as difficulty with movements of the jaw, tongue, lips, cheeks, and palate that are necessary for efficient oral feeding. Oral hypersensitivity or hyposensitivity may be present, as well as limitations in oral motor actions characterized by jaw extension or thrust, tongue retraction or protrusion, limited tongue mobility, lip retraction, or pursing or tonic bite reaction [1, 2, 29]. Tongue base retraction for effective bolus transfer and initiation of swallowing may be delayed or absent, and there may be failure to initiate a swallow in severe cases. Delayed swallowing response, reduced strength of pharyngeal contraction, laryngeal penetration, aspiration, and silent aspiration are all factors that require assessment and management. Strategies to manage oral and pharyngeal dysfunction associated with neurologic conditions include: positional adaptations and feeding equipment modifications, combinations of oral sensorimotor stimulation and exercises, altering liquid viscosity and texture modifications, and implementation of supplemental nutrition via enteral feedings as necessary.

Positioning Adaptations and Considerations

Consideration of overall muscle tone (hypertonicity, hypotonicity, and fluctuating tone), body posture, and positioning is key to maximizing oral motor function for feeding. Ensuring that the infant or child with abnormal muscle tone is positioned in a stable, well-supported position is necessary prior to initiation of oral sensory or motor facilitation techniques. Positioning recommendations are individualized for each child depending upon the orthopedic, medical, respiratory, and neurologic components present. Input from an occupational or physical therapist to assist in determining the most appropriate positioning for oral feeding is beneficial. Characteristics of an optimal feeding position should include orientation of the head and extremities in the body midline, neutral symmetric shoulder position, and neutral anterior-posterior alignment of the head and neck. A variety of positions as well as equipment may be used to facilitate appropriate body positioning during feeding, including infant seats, wedges, and bolster chairs. Strapping or vesting options are available to assist with trunk control. Specific head control options include head rests, side supports, and circumference head rests [29]. Equipment options are widely varied and must be prescribed specifically for the individual patient.

Slight flexion or extension of the neck providing an alteration in swallow physiology may have therapeutic benefit in some cases. For example, slight extension of the head and neck may assist with posterior oral transit as opposed to anterior loss of oral presentations in patients with severe oral dysfunction. In other cases, positioning that encourages slight neck flexion may assist with generation of pressure for a more efficient swallow in some cases. The specific swallowing maneuvers associated with positioning are discussed in Chap. 17.

Oral Sensorimotor Stimulation Techniques

Oral sensorimotor strategies encompass the use of proprioceptive input, tactile, gustatory, visual, sensory, and auditory information to manage the sensory and motor limitations that may be interfering with feeding. Table 18.4 summarizes possible compensatory strategies and treatment options to help with management of limiting oral motor patterns including lip retraction or pursing, tongue protrusion, jaw thrust or retraction, tonic bite reflex, tongue retraction, and limited tongue and lip movements. Specific exercises and swallowing maneuvers are discussed in Chap. 17.

Table 18.4. Oral sensorimotor stimulation techniques.

Problem	Possible factors	Type of oral dysfunction	Compensatory strategy/technique
Oral facial hypertonia	Neurologic injury	Increased muscle tone results in abnormal movement patterns of the orofacial structures	Optimum positioning during feeding
			Firm input, pressure in orofacial area, monitor responses, adjust
Oral facial hypotonia	Neurologic injury	Low muscle tone results in abnormal movement patterns	Optimum positioning during feeding
	Myopathy	Open mouth posture	Compensatory tactile, vibratory input to the orofacial area
			Feeder places thumb and index finger on cheeks to assist with lip seal
Orofacial weakness, unilateral, bilateral	Neurologic injury, CVA Hemifacial microsomia	Orofacial asymmetry Pocketing of oral food residue	Food placement to stronger side Use of alerting flavors to increase oral sensory input
		Effortful chewing	Use of easy to manage solids, requiring less masticatory effort
Lack of spontaneous, anticipatory mouth opening	State of alertness Neurologic injury Feeding refusal/resistance	Problems with initiating feeding, unable to place spoon or nipple intraorally	Use arousal techniques as appropriate Attempt to elicit rooting reflex in infants Touch/pressure to gums Tactile input to perioral area, if appropriate, tactile input with spoon to lips

Tongue protrusion	Hypotonia	Difficult to maintain placement of nipple or spoon on body of tongue	Postural support—head neutral or slightly flexed
	Hypertonia	Results in anterior loss of food, liquid	Feeder places one hand on child's jaw, and finger under chin, tactile input with nipple or spoon onto tongue Use of tactile input downward pressure with nipple to improve central grooving and facilitate sucking Narrow, shallow bowl spoon with placement onto the body of the tongue, providing downward pressure (slight) may help to facilitate posterior tongue movements for bolus transfer
Tongue retraction	Abnormalities in muscle tone	Tongue is pulled into or falls into posterior portion of oral cavity Poor contact between tongue and nipple leading to inefficient sucking	Positioning to ensure head/neck alignment Tactile input to the tongue to encourage forward positioning
	Retrognathia	Poor contact of spoon onto tongue, resulting in deposit of food in anterior sulcus	Use of longer nipple to provide greater contact with the tongue and facilitate more effective tongue movements Use of gentle downward pressure of spoon onto tongue body to provide tactile input and facilitate more efficient movements of the tongue for bolus transfer

(continued)

Table 18.4.   (continued)

Problem	Possible factors	Type of oral dysfunction	Compensatory strategy/technique
Tongue tip elevation	Decreased tone and stability in head, neck, trunk Oral aversion/resistance	Position of tongue tip prevents proper positioning of nipple intraorally, prevents placement of spoon onto tongue body	Positioning to ensure forward head flexion and promote downward positioning of tongue tip Use of tactile input with gentle downward pressure to encourage downward positioning of tongue to facilitate presentation of nipple or spoon
Lack of central grooving of tongue in response to nipple	Abnormal muscle tone in tongue, retraction	Lack of channel for smooth fluid transfer for swallowing Ineffective sucking pattern, poor suction	Facilitate central grooving via proprioceptive input Choose firm, straight nipple for provision of tactile input to encourage central grooving
Limited tongue movements	Abnormal tone Cranial nerve damage Inexperience with oral feeding	Lack of range and strength of tongue movements necessary for efficient sucking and/or anterior-posterior transfer of pureed, mastication of solids	Sensory input to facilitate motor movements Oral sensory stimulation may include use of vibration for tactile input, use of texture such as crunchy, but immediately dissolvable solids to stimulate biting and lateral tongue movements, varied tastes, varied temperatures to increase sensory input and facilitate motor action
Excessive jaw movements	Low orofacial tone Facial weakness Compensation for abnormal tongue movements	Lack of stable base for tongue movements results in inefficient oral phase	Feeder provides external support by placing finger under jaw during bottle or spoon presentations Gentle pressure under the mandible, use as little external support as possible to allow development of internal stability

| Tonic bite reflex | Neurologic | Bite reflex occurs with tactile input, child may bite on nipple, spoon, and not release | Do not attempt to pull spoon or nipple from oral cavity as tonic reflex will intensify
Apply gentle input at temporomandibular joint to encourage relaxation of jaw
Use coated spoon to assist with removal and protect dentition |
| Nasopharyngeal reflux | Neurologic, lack of velopharyngeal closure during swallowing
Structural—cleft palate | Velopharyngeal port remains open during swallowing (normally tightly closed during swallowing) resulting in nasopharyngeal reflux of food, liquid | Upright positioning to promote posterior transfer and minimize nasopharyngeal reflux
Thickened liquid may result in lesser degree of nasopharyngeal reflux |

Altering Liquid Viscosity/Bolus Modification

Alterations in liquid viscosity and in bolus consistency, taste, and temperature may be effective compensatory strategies, depending on the situation. Thickening liquids may assist with modulation of liquid intake in terms of volume and facilitate oral control, oral transfer, and airway protection with swallowing as discussed previously. Bolus modification by selection of food textures based upon oral motor skill ability is recommended to maximize oral control as well as swallowing safety. For example, patients with primarily anterior-posterior tongue movements for transfer of smooth pureed foods may tend to continue with this predominant transfer pattern even if a small food lump requiring oral manipulation is mixed into the familiar smooth pureed mixture. Transferring the lump for swallowing without adequate oral preparation will likely result in a protective, gagging response, and possibly lead to future resistance and aversion. Bolus modifications selected by the clinician should be based upon the oral motor and oral sensory discrimination skills that are present. The bolus modification should be appropriate in facilitation of movements needed for bolus manipulation and transport. For example, lateral placement of a crunchy, but immediately dissolvable solid may assist with stimulating lateral tongue movements necessary for development of chewing skills for manipulation. Though not empirically proven, the use of alerting flavors, varied temperature, and the tactile input of the solid may provide additional sensory stimulation to facilitate the oral motor action appropriate for developmental level.

Premature Infants, Medically Complex Infants, Cardiorespiratory Issues

Cardiorespiratory compromise with oral feeding trials is reflected in an infant's inability to initiate or sustain a coordinated respiration pattern with appropriate oxygen saturation levels during sucking and swallowing efforts [46]. The respiratory effort expended during feeding efforts may result in accompanying apnea or episodes of bradycardia. In particular, premature infants, and infants with co-morbidities such as cystic fibrosis, congenital heart disease, and infants with bronchopulmonary dysplasia are likely to have associated cardiorespiratory issues associated with oral feeding efforts. Premature infants with bronchopulmonary dysplasia have been shown to have low sucking pressure and sucking frequency, as well as short sucking burst durations, and low feeding efficiency coupled with prolonged deglutition apnea [47]. The primary concern for the clinician is preservation of cardiorespiratory stability. This can be accomplished by working with members of the NICU team to establish an appropriate treatment plan focused on the transition to oral feeding appropriate.

Compensatory strategies used by the dysphagia clinician in the neonatal intensive care unit may include: position alteration, non-nutritive oral sensorimotor stimulation, initiation of nutritive feeding trials, input with nipple/bottle selection, recommendations in regard to changes in the flow rate of liquid during nutritive feeding trials, and provision of imposed pause intervals during feeding to regulate the rate of an infant's intake during feeding. The infant's gestational age, medical status, and physiologic stability should be considered prior to implementation of a feeding plan. Generally, infants who are 34 weeks gestation and greater, without significant medical co-morbidities, with ability to maintain state regulation (ability to reach and maintain a quiet, alert state) and demonstrate appropriate oral reflexes (rooting, non-nutritive sucking), may be appropriate for initial assessment of non-nutritive oral motor skills and eventually, transition to nutritive feeding [1, 2]. The time interval for transition to full oral feeding will vary and the volume of oral feeding is gradually increased based upon the infant's performance during oral feeding trials. Prior to initiation of oral feeding, the infant's digestive system tolerance of the feeding, maintenance of an appropriate respiratory rate (~20–50 breaths per minute), and ability to tolerate physical handling and transitions without signs of stress should be considered.

Positioning considerations include maintaining overall flexion, with orientation of the head and extremities to the body midline, keeping the shoulders symmetric and forward, hips flexed, and maintaining neutral anterior-posterior alignment of the head and neck. Swaddling the infant during the feeding trials assists with maintaining stability and midline positioning.

The presence of oral reflexes (root, suck, swallow), management of oral secretions, non-nutritive initiation of sucking, as well as the strength and rhythmicity of sucking are assessed. The pediatric SLP may provide an oral sensorimotor program initially, with focus upon provision of pleasant orofacial, perioral, and intraoral tactile input and presentation of the pacifier during tube feedings [19]. If the infant demonstrates rooting and suck/swallow reflexes non-nutritively and ability to maintain physiologic stability, initiation of oral feeding trials may be appropriate. With the agreement of the medical team, the therapist may begin with initiation of nutritive stimulation. Introduction of very small tastes of breast milk or formula either on the pacifier, or alongside the pacifier by use of a 1 mL syringe or via flexible dropper in a slow careful fashion, may be appropriate. The taste stimulation is controlled and limited to very small amounts, thereby providing taste exposure, and miniscule amounts of fluid to transfer for swallowing. The infant's responses should be monitored closely to assess any stress reaction such as increased heart or respiratory rate. As suck/swallow competence with small amounts of nutritive intake is established, gradual increases in volume can be made. Communication should occur with the medical team prior to proceeding with any changes in oral volume. A small 1–3 mL syringe may be placed inside the nipple to allow the clinician to control the amount of formula contained in the nipple, so as not to overwhelm the infant during the initial nutritive trials. Subsequent determination of flow rate and volume of intake is made based upon the infant's responses and physiologic reaction; all feeding recommendations are made in conjunction with the medical team in the NICU.

Nipple and bottle selection should match the particular infant's oral structure and function. There is no single nipple or bottle that is considered or has been proven to be the most advantageous. The pliability of the nipple, shape, size, length, and hole type and size are all factors that must be considered on an individual basis. The infant's ability to maintain lip approximation on the nipple, to demonstrate tongue cupping around the nipple, and to initiate sucking and active compression of the nipple are considerations in nipple selection.

The use of external pacing during oral feeding trials may assist the infant in maintaining a coordinated suck-swallow-respiration pattern and help to minimize feeding-related apneic episodes. The therapist imposes breaks or pauses for respiration in the nutritive suck-swallow cycle by breaking suction or tilting the bottle downward to stop the flow of liquid, while maintaining contact of the nipple to the infant's lip. Continued research in identification of respiratory phase patterns and apneic pause during swallowing will provide objective evidence to support the use of pacing as a feeding strategy.

Metabolic/Inflammatory Processes

Metabolic abnormalities such as glycogen storage disease or disorders of nitrogen, amino acid, carbohydrate, or fatty acid metabolism may require implementation of special feeding regimens. Severe allergies and inflammatory processes such as esophagitis present a similar scenario in terms of the food restrictions imposed, with allowance of only a very restricted range of solid foods, or intake of elemental formula in the absence of any solid food intake. If oral intake restrictions occur during critical periods for oral motor skill acquisition, subsequent delays in oral motor skill development, oral aversion, and significant feeding refusal behavior may develop [48–50]. In addition, prior to diagnosis, there may be a period of time whereby the child may experience discomfort associated with eating, which may result in feeding refusal or the tendency to develop maladaptive feeding behaviors, such as selective food intake or behavioral resistance to feeding.

The most common eosinophilic gut disease is eosinophilic esophagitis; a chronic, inflammatory, immunoallergic disease [51]. The incidence and prevalence of eosinophilic esophagitis in infants, toddlers, and children is increasing [52–54]. Specific feeding dysfunction characterized by maladaptive feeding behaviors (i.e., feeding refusal, selective intake), as well as oral motor skill dysfunction, has been described in several investigations [53, 55–58]. In addition, there are increasing numbers of infants and children who present with numerous and severe food allergies and are restricted to oral intake of a very narrow range of items which may limit exposure to varied tastes and textures during critical times for oral motor skill development.

At times, even after diagnosis and treatment of the underlying medical condition, the pediatric patient may persist with feeding refusal, texture avoidance, or failure to progress forward in treatment. The dysphagia clinician as well as other professionals involved in patient care can assist in several ways to help prevent the development of oral aversion during periods of restricted oral intake and can also implement appropriate treatment strategies during the re-introduction of solids into the oral diet. Provision of oral sensorimotor programs including recommendations for oral care/tooth brushing on a daily basis with input to all regions of the mouth, including the tongue, hard palate, gums, and all tooth surfaces, provides consistent tactile input into the oral cavity and may help to prevent development of oral aversion. Treatment strategies may include individualized sessions focusing on development of oral motor mechanics necessary for manipulation of food textures and oral sensory activities, or group treatment sessions to introduce peer models to encourage imitation of oral intake. Maintaining regular, structured meal and snack routines within the allowable food range should be emphasized. Implementation of behavioral reinforcement techniques is effective in combination with compensatory feeding strategies.

Feeding Issues and Management in Children with Genetic Syndromes

Feeding and swallowing problems accompany genetic syndromes secondary to structural and neurologic factors that may be present [23]. It is beyond the scope of this chapter to discuss the possible feeding issues and interventions across all syndromes. Therefore, possible compensatory strategies for management are described for genetic syndromes likely to have accompanying dysphagia, such as Pierre Robin Syndrome, 22 q 11 Deletion Syndromes, Down Syndrome, Rett Syndrome, CHARGE syndrome, and Prader Willi Syndrome.

Pierre Robin Sequence

Pierre Robin Sequence (PRS) is one of the most recognized sequences in infants, characterized by micrognathia, glossoptosis, and often a wide "U" shaped cleft palate. PRS may occur in isolation in typically developing individuals, or as part of a multiple defect syndrome. The posterior position of the tongue creates the potential for upper airway obstruction exacerbated by the respiratory effort of feeding. Episodic or (chronic) airway obstruction may occur during sequential swallows. Possible strategies to manage feeding difficulty include prone positioning or side-lying during feeding to facilitate forward tongue positioning [3]. Feeding strategies as discussed previously for infants with cleft palate are also implemented. A patent airway is the most significant concern, and if significant upper airway obstruction is present, medical intervention will be necessary. Usually, once the airway issues are resolved, feeding difficulties in PRS are easily managed.

22q11 Deletion Syndromes

A common microdeletion of a section of chromosome 22 (22q11) is present in three clinical disorders: Velocardiofacial Syndrome, DiGeorge Syndrome, and conotruncal anomaly face syndrome. There are multiple features that accompany these disorders. Specific features that result in feeding and swallowing difficulties include cleft lip and/ or palate, other palatal anomalies (such as submucous cleft palate or velopharyngeal insufficiency), congenital heart disease, and additional anatomical laryngotracheal anomalies including vascular rings, and laryngeal web. Feeding issues may include nasopharyngeal reflux during feeding, gagging, choking, and poorly coordinated suck-swallow and respiratory phase patterns. Following instrumental examination of swallowing safety, the compensatory feeding strategies that are indicated include modifications for feeding as discussed in infants/children with cleft lip and palate, upright positioning, pacing to assist with slowing rate of oral intake, and alternation of solids/liquids to assist with pharyngeal clearance.

Down Syndrome

Infants and children with Down Syndrome may experience varied issues in feeding and swallowing. If hypotonia is present, particularly in the orofacial area, there may be decreased sucking efficiency during infancy, and later in development, decreased strength and efficiency of oral motor skills for management of solids requiring mastication. Persistence of tongue protrusion reflex may interfere with efficient sucking or with development of differentiated lingual movements necessary for development of spoon-feeding skills and emergence of chewing skills [59–61]. In addition to oral motor dysfunction, sensory feeding issues may be present, characterized by abnormal responses to tactile input that interfere with the ability to tolerate new textures of food. Compensatory treatment techniques and strategies include the use of sensorimotor interventions including bolus texture modification, altering viscosity of liquid, or the use of intense flavors to help provide oral alerting and activation of oral motor movements. The use of adaptive feeding equipment, such as easily compressible nipples and feeder assistance with jaw or cheek support to facilitate lip closure and efficiency of sucking, may be helpful. The use of relatively narrow flat spoons during spoon feeding facilitate contact of the spoon onto the body of the tongue and help to facilitate increased lip closure on the spoon for food removal. Bolus modifications may involve the use of smooth and gradually thicker consistencies as lingual control develops. The use of crunchy, easily dissolvable solids in small amounts in the context of therapy may help to stimulate lateral tongue movements and decrease the tendency toward a prominent tongue protrusion pattern.

Rett Syndrome

Rett Syndrome, a neurodevelopmental disorder affecting primarily females, is caused by a mutation on the MECP2 gene. Rett Syndrome has been associated with the occurrence of feeding problems, specifically oropharyngeal dysfunction and gastroesophageal dysmotility [62]. Rett syndrome is progressive in nature, and the dysphagia treatment approach is focused on management of the symptoms. The oropharyngeal difficulties typically involve poor tongue mobility, reduced oropharyngeal clearance, and problems with airway protection during swallowing. Compensatory management techniques may include bolus modification of textures that do not require extensive oral manipulation, and alternation of solids and liquid boluses to assist with oropharyngeal and esophageal clearance. To facilitate and maintain airway protection during swallowing, introduction of compensatory strategies such as effortful swallow, single sips of liquid as opposed to sequential swallows, or encouragement of a gentle cough to clear following swallows should be explored for effectiveness in the context of the instrumental examination.

CHARGE Syndrome

CHARGE syndrome is a genetic condition, caused by a mutation in a single gene, most often CHD7. Children with CHARGE Syndrome present with a combination of major characteristics including coloboma, choanal atresia, ear abnormalities, and cranial nerve dysfunction. There are numerous other clinical characteristics that occur with variable frequency and include heart malformations, genital abnormalities, developmental delay, and esophageal and laryngeal abnormalities. Feeding and swallowing dysfunction is known to accompany CHARGE syndrome and the issues are frequently long-term. Weak and inefficient oral phase skills for sucking and chewing, pharyngeal phase dysfunction with inadequate airway protection, and prevalence of gastroesophageal reflux secondary to cranial nerve dysfunction [63, 64]. Compensatory strategies and techniques for treatment of dysphagia include oral sensory and motor interventions, including the use of alerting oral flavors such as citrus or carbonation, bolus modifications commensurate with oral motor skill ability, and the use of verbal cues to encourage volitional lip closure and initiation of tongue movements for bolus manipulation and posterior transit. The use of an effortful swallow and alternation of liquid and solid boluses may assist with pharyngeal phase dysfunction in patients with CHARGE, as cranial nerve dysfunction may result in decreased pharyngeal contraction ability [63, 64].

Prader Willi Syndrome

Children with Prader Willi Syndrome (chromosome 15q11-q13 deletion or abnormality) present with generalized hypotonia, developmental delay, short stature, small hands and feet, and characteristic facies. The feeding issues in infancy are usually characterized by weak and inefficient oral motor skills secondary to orofacial hypotonia, which results in poor feeding endurance and inadequate oral intake volume. In contrast, in later childhood, insatiable hunger emerges coupled with food-seeking behavior and obesity [65]. Dysphagia treatment in early infancy should focus on establishing optimum positioning to facilitate sucking, choice of an appropriate nipple to assist with appropriate lip seal, and with establishing a coordinated suck-swallow sequence. Oral facilitation techniques such as provision of jaw or cheek support to assist with lip closure and sucking effort may be of benefit. Consultation with a registered dietician to determine the appropriate caloric density of formula or the need for supplemental enteral feeding is necessary in cases with severe feeding dysfunction.

Pharmacologic Treatment in Pediatric Dysphagia

Physical discomfort may further exacerbate feeding/swallowing dysfunction, and medical intervention to address such issues may facilitate a positive response to the treatment interventions employed by the dysphagia clinician. Therefore, concomitant pharmacologic treatment and dysphagia therapy may be advantageous in certain conditions. Medical interventions to assist with treatment of gastroesophageal reflux/esophagitis, delayed gastric emptying, management of oral secretions, constipation, and depressed appetite drive are described briefly in the following section.

Gastroesophageal Reflux

As discussed in previous chapters, chronic pathologic gastroesophageal reflux may lead to inflammation, esophagitis, and the potential for esophageal stricture formation in severe cases [66]. Significant and ongoing gastroesophageal reflux may contribute to feeding aversion/ resistance, swallowing dysfunction, and behavioral issues in typically developing as well as neurologically impaired children [67, 68]. The empiric use of pharmacologic agents has not been evaluated by randomized study; however, improvement in feeding behavior and swallowing function in infants and children after trials of acid suppression has been described in specific populations [69]. Infants and children who present with pediatric dysphagia and accompanying gastroesophageal reflux irritation may be more likely to respond favorably to dysphagia treatment techniques if the underlying discomfort and irritation is treated.

Delayed Gastric Emptying

Prokinetic agents (erythromycin, metoclopramide, cisapride) may improve gastric emptying and promote hunger in patients who demonstrate delayed gastric emptying and accompanying feeding refusal [70]. There are certain risks and benefits associated with each medication which require careful consideration by the practitioner even for short-term use. Children may respond favorably to the medications and may be more likely to respond to therapeutic techniques for oral aversion that involve the inclusion of foods in oral motor/feeding therapy. Subsequent improvement of oral intake volume during meals and snack intervals may also be more likely to occur.

Constipation

Persistent or severe constipation is known to impact appetite and may be a factor underlying feeding refusal/resistance and subsequent poor growth [71, 72]. Ongoing feeding refusal may result in development of feeding aversion or lack of exposure to food textures during critical times for skill acquisition. Treatment of constipation in children with associated oral motor sensory or motor issues may lead to improved responses in regard to willingness to try foods or liquids in association with motor and/or sensory strategies during dysphagia treatment. The associated increase in appetite may also facilitate a child's willingness to comply with ingestion of foods and liquids during meals in the home environment carrying over the motor and sensory strategies introduced during dysphagia treatment.

Appetite

The variables that affect appetite and satiety greatly vary among infants and children and among cultures. Regardless of etiology, persistent depression in appetite may result in inadequate volume and variety of oral intake, failure to gain weight appropriately, and impact upon normal progression of oral motor skills for feeding as a result of limited exposure to liquids and foods during critical periods for skill acquisition.

Specific to the pediatric population, infantile anorexia has been described as occurring in children between 9 and 18 months of age and is characterized by lack of hunger signals, food refusal, and acute or chronic malnutrition [73]. Other issues with appetite may arise that may be associated with prior illness or underlying medical conditions. Consideration by the practitioner of appetite stimulants such as periactin may be useful, though long-term studies of efficacy are not available. Adjustment of tube feedings as per a registered dietitian to create hunger/satiety cycles is an additional option, with presentation of oral feeding trials prior to enteral feeding. Overall, appetite may have a significant effect on an infant or child's responses to therapeutic strategies involving ingestion of oral intake and should be a consideration in the treatment plan.

Compensatory Strategies for Management of Oral Secretions

Infants and children with neurologic conditions such as cerebral palsy and significant oropharyngeal dysfunction are likely to have difficulty with management of oral secretions. This may be reflected in significant drooling, beyond the timeframe during which drooling is considered developmental in nature. In addition, children with poor oral control may have accompanying sensory and motor pharyngeal swallowing dysfunction. Patients may present with accumulated oral secretions in the hypopharynx with persistent penetration and aspiration of the secretions; significant in terms of the implications for respiratory health.

Secretion management options include oral motor strategies, medications, and surgical options. Oral motor therapy programs typically focus upon increasing sensory awareness and voluntary control of movements. The use of thermal stimulation and vibration to increase sensory input and facilitate motor action for control of secretions is frequently described, but has not been systematically studied to determine effect. The use of verbal cueing and biofeedback may be useful in establishing volitional control in selected patients within the context of oral motor therapy [74]. Medical options include anticholinergic medication and targeted injections of botulinum toxin into the salivary glands. Surgical options are available and generally considered when more conservative options have failed [75]. The surgical options include submandibular gland excision, submandibular gland duct re-routing, parotid duct ligation, or combination of the aforementioned procedures. At this time, there is no single procedure that has been determined to be the most effective.

Behavioral Issues Associated with Feeding

Regardless of the primary etiology of pediatric dysphagia, there is an increased likelihood of associated behavioral issues that present barriers to development of age-appropriate oral feeding skills in children [76]. Maladaptive feeding behaviors are varied and include behavioral resistance and refusal of oral feeding, gagging and/or vomiting in response to presentation of foods, and significant food selectivity. Pediatric feeding treatment thus encompasses sensory and motor-based approaches as discussed previously, but also behaviorally based feeding interventions, interdisciplinary feeding treatment paradigms, and family-oriented approaches [77]. Behaviorally based feeding programs are developed in conjunction with a behavioral specialist, mental health social worker, or pediatric psychologist and focus upon parent-feeding interactions, specific feeding techniques, and use of designated reinforcement strategies during oral feeding trials. A variety of behavioral interventions used to assist with weaning for tube feeding are described in the literature and involve the use of specific treatment procedures to eliminate food refusal and increase acceptance of oral intake [76, 78, 79]. The importance of appetite regulation and the involvement of the family in intervention have been described, particularly in multicomponent behavioral programs for oral aversion in children dependent upon gastrostomy feedings [80]. Continued research regarding the efficacy of specific behavioral interventions is needed.

Parent/Caretaker Training on Recommended Feeding Compensatory Strategies and Techniques

In all pediatric dysphagia treatment approaches, involvement of the parent/caretaker in setting the treatment goals and implementing the treatment strategies is a critical step in ensuring a favorable outcome. The parent/caretaker needs to learn and demonstrate success with the recommended compensatory feeding strategies and techniques so that carryover in the home environment can occur. If the family is only a passive onlooker during the treatment sessions, the likelihood of implementing direct or compensatory strategies in the home environment may be reduced. Conversely, if the parent/caretaker is actively involved in the treatment process and can demonstrate competency in the use of therapeutic strategies, carryover in the home environment and satisfactory progress toward treatment goals is likely enhanced.

Summary

There are multiple conditions that result in pediatric dysphagia and numerous professionals that are involved in aspects of the initial evaluation and the ongoing management and treatment process. [81–83] The types of medical, surgical, and therapeutic interventions utilized have a direct impact upon patient outcomes. Empirical evidence has accumulated to support the use of specific medical, surgical, and feeding interventions, though more research is needed to build a stronger evidence base for selection of specific treatment approaches. Further evidence to support interventions will lead to continued refinement of clinical pathways, and ultimately the implementation of the most effective treatment protocols.

References

1. Arvedson JC, Brodsky L. Pediatric swallowing and feeding. 2nd ed. New York: Singular Publishing; 2002.
2. Wolf L, Glass R. Feeding and swallowing disorders in infancy: assessment and management. Tucson: Therapy Skill Builders; 1992.
3. Rothchild D, Thompson B, Clonan A. Feeding update for neonates with Pierre Robin Sequence treated with mandibular distraction. Newborn Infant Nurs Rev. 2008;8:51–67.

4. Gosa M, Schooling T, Coleman J. Thickened liquids as a treatment for children with dysphagia and associated adverse effects: a systematic review. Infant Child Adolesc Nutr. 2011;3:344–50.

5. Cichero J, Jackson O, Halley PJ, et al. How thick is thick? Multicenter study of the rheological and material property characteristics of mealtime fluids and videofluoroscopy fluids. Dysphagia. 2000;15:188–200.

6. Steele CM. Searching for meaningful differences in viscosity. Dysphagia. 2005;20:336–8.

7. Stuart S, Motz J. Viscosity in infant dysphagia management: comparison of viscosity of thickened liquids used in assessment and thickened liquids used in treatment. Dysphagia. 2009;24:412–22.

8. Ruark JL, McCullough GH, Peters RL, et al. Bolus consistency and swallowing in children and adults. Dysphagia. 2002;17:24–33.

9. Ruark JL, Mills CE, Muenchen RA. Effects of bolus volume and consistency on multiple swallow behavior in children and adults. J Med Speech Lang Pathol. 2003;11:213–26.

10. Ayala KJ, Logemann JA. Effects of altered sensory bolus characteristics and repeated swallows in healthy young and elderly subjects. J Med Speech Lang Pathol. 2010;18:34–58.

11. Butler SG, Postma GN, Fischer E. Effects of viscosity, taste, and bolus volume on swallowing apnea duration of normal adults. Otolaryngol Head Neck Surg. 2004;131:860–3.

12. Ding R, Logemann JA, Larson CR, et al. The effect of taste and consistency on swallow physiology in younger and older healthy individuals: a surface electromyographic study. J Speech Lang Hear Res. 2003;46:977–89.

13. Pelletier CA, Dhanaraj GE. The effect of taste and palatability on lingual swallowing pressure. Dysphagia. 2006;21:121–8.

14. Igarahsi A, Kawasaki M, Nomura S, et al. Sensory and motor responses of normal young adults during swallowing of foods with different properties and volumes. Dysphagia. 2010;25:198–206.

15. Humbert IA, Fitzgerald ME, McLaren DG. Neurophysiology of swallowing: effects of age and bolus type. Neuroimage. 2009;44:982–91.

16. Gisel E. Interventions and outcomes for children with dysphagia. Dev Disabil Res Rev. 2008;14:165–73.

17. Boiron M, Da Nobrega L, Roux S, et al. Effects of oral stimulation and oral support on non-nutritive sucking and feeding performance in preterm infants. Dev Med Child Neurol. 2007;49:439–44.

18. Fucile S, Gisel EG, McFarland DH, et al. Oral and non-oral sensorimotor interventions enhance oral feeding performance in preterm infants. Dev Med Child Neurol. 2011;53(9):829–34.

19. Pinelli J, Symington A. Nonnutritive sucking for promoting physiologic stability and nutrition in preterm infants. Cochrane Database Syst Rev. 2005(2):CD-01071.

20. Kummer AW. Cleft palate & craniofacial anomalies: effects on speech and resonance. 2nd ed. San Diego: Singular; 2008.

21. Mizuno K, Ueda A, Kani K, et al. Feeding behavior of infants with cleft lip and palate. Acta Paediatr. 2001;91:1227–32.
22. Reid J, Reilly S, Kilpatrick K. Sucking performance of babies with cleft conditions. Cleft Palate Craniofac J. 2007;44(3):312–20.
23. Cooper-Brown L, Copeland S, Dailey S, et al. Feeding and swallowing in genetic syndromes. Dev Disabil Res Rev. 2008;14:147–57.
24. Reid J. A review of feeding interventions for infants with cleft palate. Cleft Palate Craniofac J. 2004;41(3):268–78.
25. Reid J, Kilpatrick N, Reilly S. A prospective, longitudinal study of feeding skills in a cohort of babies with cleft conditions. Cleft Palate Craniofac J. 2006;43:702–9.
26. Glenny AM, Hooper L, Shaw WC, et al. Feeding interventions for growth and development in infants with cleft lip, cleft palate or cleft lip and palate. Cochrane Database Syst Rev. 2004;(3):CD003315.
27. Einarsson-Backes L, Deitz J, Price R, Glass R. The effect of oral support on sucking efficiency in pre-term infants. Am J Occup Ther. 1994;48:490–8.
28. Hwang YS, Lin CH, Coster WJ, et al. Effectiveness of cheek and jaw support to improve feeding performance of preterm infants. Am J Occup Ther. 2010;64:886–94.
29. Morris S, Klein M. Prefeeding skills: a comprehensive resource for feeding development. Tucson: Therapy Skill Builders; 1987.
30. Shaw WC, Bannister RP, Roberts CT. Assisted feeding is more reliable for infants with cleft—a randomized trial. Cleft Palate Craniofac J. 1999;36:262–8.
31. Turner L, Jacobsen C, Humerczuk M, et al. The effects of lactation education and a prosthetic obturator appliance on feeding efficiency in infants with cleft lip and palate. Cleft Palate Craniofac J. 2001;38(5):519–24.
32. Law-Morstatt L, Judd DM, Snyder P. Pacing as a treatment technique for transitional sucking patterns. J Perinatol. 2003;23:483–8.
33. Kelchner L, Miller CK. Current research in voice and swallowing outcomes following pediatric airway reconstruction. Curr Opin Otolaryngol Head Neck Surg. 2008;16:221–5.
34. Smith LP, Otto SE, Wagner KA, et al. Management of oral feeding in children undergoing airway reconstruction. Laryngoscope. 2009;119:967–73.
35. Miller CK, Linck JL, Willging JP. Duration and extent of dysphagia following pediatric airway reconstruction. Int J Pediatr Otorhinolaryngol. 2009;73:573–9.
36. Cotton RT, Richardson MA. Congenital laryngeal anomalies. Otolaryngol Clin North Am. 1981;14:203–18.
37. Khariwala SS, Lee WT, Koltai PJ. Laryngotracheal consequences of pediatric cardiac surgery. Arch Otolaryngol Head Neck Surg. 2005;131:336–9.
38. Catalano P, DiPace MR, Caruso AM, et al. Gastroesophageal reflux in young children treated for esophageal atresia: evaluation with pH-Multichannel intraluminal impedance. J Pediatr Gastroenterol Nutr. 2011;52:686–90.
39. Golonka NR, Hayashi AH. Early "sham" feeding of neonates promotes oral feeding after delayed primary repair of major congenital esophageal anomalies. Am J Surg. 2008;195:659–62.
40. Humphrey C, Duncan K, Fletcher S. Decade of experience with vascular rings at a single institution. Pediatrics. 2006;117:e903–8.

41. Burgos L, Barrena S, Andres A, et al. Colonic interposition for esophageal replacement in children remains a good choice: 33-year median follow-up of 65 patients. J Pediatr Surg. 2010;45:341–5.

42. Brooks A, Millar A, Rode H. The surgical management of cricopharyngeal achalasia in children. Int J Pediatr Otorhinolaryngol. 2000;56:1–7.

43. Messner A, Ho AS, Malhotra PS, et al. The use of botulinum toxin for pediatric cricopharyngeal achalasia. Int J Pediatr Otorhinolaryngol. 2011;75:830–4.

44. Jain V, Bhatnagar V. Cricopharyngeal myotomy for the treatment of cricopharyngeal achalasia. J Pediatr Surg. 2009;44:1656–8.

45. Martin N, Prince J, Kane T, et al. Congenital cricopharyngeal achalasia in a 4.5 year old boy managed by cervical myotomy: a case report. Int J Pediatr Otorhinolaryngol. 2011;75:289–92.

46. Thoyre SM, Carlson JR. Preterm infants' behavioural indicators of oxygen decline during bottle feeding. J Adv Nurs. 2003;43:631–41.

47. Mizuno K, Nishida Y, Taki M, et al. Infants with bronchopulmonary dysplasia suckle with weak pressures to maintain breathing during feeding. Pediatrics. 2007;120:e1035–42.

48. Rudolph CD, Link DT. Feeding disorders in infants and children. Pediatr Clin North Am. 2002;49:97–112.

49. Kuhn D, Girolami P, Gulotta C. Feeding disorders. Int Rev Res Ment Retard. 2007;34:387–414.

50. Udall J. Infant feeding: initiation, problems, approaches. Curr Probl Pediatr Adolesc Health Care. 2007;37:374–99.

51. Putnam PE, Rothenberg ME. Eosinophilic esophagitis: concepts, controversies, and evidence. Curr Gastroenterol Rep. 2009;11:220–5.

52. Spergel JM, Brown-Whitehorn TF, Beausoleil JL, et al. 14 years of eosinophilic esophagitis: clinical features and prognosis. J Pediatr Gastroenterol Nutr. 2009;48:30–6.

53. Pentiuk SP, Miller CK, Kaul A. Eosinophilic esophagitis in infants and toddlers. Dysphagia. 2007;22:44–8.

54. Kapel RC, Miller JK, Torres C. Eosinophilic esophagitis: a prevalent disease in the United States that affects all age groups. Gastroenterology. 2008;134:1316–21.

55. Mukkada V, Haas A, Maune N, et al. Feeding dysfunction in children with eosinophilic gastrointestinal diseases. Pediatrics. 2010;126:e672–7.

56. Haas A, Maune N. Clinical presentation of feeding dysfunction in children with eosinophilic gastrointestinal disease. Immunol Allergy Clin North Am. 2009;29:65–75.

57. Robles-Medranda C, Villard F, le Gall C, Lukashok H, Rivet C, Bouvier R, Dumortier J, & Lachaux A. Journal of Pediatric Gastroenterology. 2010;50:516–520.

58. Flood EM, Beusterien KM, Amonkar MM, et al. Patient and caregiver perspective on pediatric eosinophilic esophagitis and newly developed symptoms questionnaires. Curr Med Res Opin. 2008;24:3369–81.

59. Gisel EG, Lange LJ, Niman CW. Chewing cycles in 4- and 5-year old Down's syndrome children: a comparison of eating efficacy with normals. Am J Occup Ther. 1984;38:666–70.

60. Gisel EG, Lange JL, Niman CW. Tongue movements in 4- and 5-year old Down's syndrome children during eating: a comparison with normal children. Am J Occup Ther. 1984;38:660–5.

61. Faulks D, Mazille MN, Collado V, et al. Masticatory dysfunction in persons with Down's Syndrome. Part 2: management. J Oral Rehabil. 2008;35:863–9.

62. Motil KJ, Schultz RJ, Browning K, et al. Oropharyngeal dysfunction and gastroesophageal motility are present in girls and women with Rett syndrome. J Pediatr Gastroenterol Nutr. 1999;29:31–7.

63. Dobbelsteyn C, Peacocke SD, Blake K, et al. Feeding difficulties in children with CHARGE syndrome: prevalence, risk factors, and prognosis. Dysphagia. 2008;23: 127–35.

64. Dobbelsteyn C, Marche DM, Blake K, et al. Early oral sensory experiences and feeding development in children with CHARGE syndrome: a report of five cases. Dysphagia. 2005;20:89–100.

65. McAllister CJ, Whittington JE, Holland AJ. Development of the eating behaviour in Prader-Willi Syndrome: advances in our understanding. Int J Obes. 2011;35:188–97.

66. Romano C, Chiaro A, Comito D, et al. Proton pump inhibitors in pediatrics: evaluation of efficacy in GERD therapy. Curr Clin Pharmacol. 2011;6:41–7.

67. Strudwick S. Gastroesophageal reflux and feeding: the Speech and Language Therapist's perspective. Int J Pediatr Otorhinolaryngol. 2003;67:S101–2.

68. Srivastava R, Jackson WD, Barnhart DC. Dysphagia and gastroesophageal reflux disease: dilemmas in diagnosis and management in children with neurological impairment. Pediatr Ann. 2010;39:225–31.

69. Suskind DL, Thompson DM, Gulati M, et al. Improved infant swallowing after gastroesophageal reflux treatment: a function of improved laryngeal sensation? Laryngoscope. 2006;116:1397–403.

70. Kirby M, Noel R. Nutrition and gastrointestinal tract assessment and management of children with dysphagia. Semin Speech Lang. 2007;28:180–9.

71. Erkin G, Culha C, Ozel S, Kirbiyik EG. Feeding and gastrointestinal problems in children with cerebral palsy. Int J Rehabil Res. 2010;33:218–24.

72. Chao HC, Chen SY, Chen CC, et al. The impact of constipation on growth in children. Pediatr Res. 2008;64:308–11.

73. Chatoor I, Surles J, Ganiban J, et al. Failure to thrive and cognitive development in toddlers with infantile anorexia. Pediatrics. 2004;113:e440–7.

74. Fairhurst CB, Cockerill H. Management of drooling in children. Arch Dis Child Educ Pract Ed. 2011;96:25–30.

75. Reed J, Mans CK, Brietzke SE, et al. Surgical management of drooling: a meta analysis. Arch Otolaryngol Head Neck Surg. 2009;135:924–31.

76. Linscheid TR. Behavioral treatments for pediatric feeding disorders. Behav Modif. 2006;30:6–23.

77. Davis AM, Bruce A, Cocjin J. Empirically supported treatments for feeding difficulties in young children. Curr Gastroenterol Rep. 2010;12:189–94.

78. O'Brien S, Repp A, Williams G, Christophersen E. Pediatric feeding disorders. Behav Modif. 1991;15(3):394–418.

79. Kerwin MLE. Empirically supported treatments in pediatric psychology: severe feeding problems. J Pediatr Psychol. 1999;24:193–214.

80. Byars KC, Burklow KA, Ferguson K, et al. A multicomponent behavioral program for oral aversion in children dependent on gastrostomy feedings. J Pediatr Gastroenterol Nutr. 2003;37:473–80.

81. Rudolph CD. Feeding disorders in infants and children. J Pediatr. 1994;125:S116–24.

82. Rommel N, DeMeyer A, Feenstra L, et al. The complexity of feeding problems in 700 infants and young children presenting to a tertiary care institution. J Pediatr Gastroenterol Nutr. 2003;27:75–84.

83. Burklow KA, Phelps AN, Schultz JR, et al. Classifying complex pediatric feeding disorders. J Pediatr Gastroenterol. 1998;27:143–7.

19. Special Consideration in the Evaluation of Infants and Children with Deglutitive Disorders

Neelesh Ajit Tipnis

Abstract Feeding difficulty is a common presentation of several pediatric disorders and may result from primary oral, pharyngeal, or esophageal phase dysphagia. Conditions associated with oral/pharyngeal phase dysphagia and its evaluation have been covered elsewhere. The focus of this section will be on the evaluation of conditions presenting with esophageal phase dysphagia in children.

Introduction

Feeding difficulty is a common presentation of several pediatric disorders and may result from primary oral, pharyngeal, or esophageal phase dysphagia. Conditions associated with oral/pharyngeal phase dysphagia and its evaluation have been covered elsewhere. The focus of this section will be on the evaluation of conditions presenting with esophageal phase dysphagia in children.

Conditions Associated with Esophageal Phase Dysphagia in Children

Eosinophilic Gastrointestinal Disorders

Eosinophilic gastrointestinal disorders result from the infiltration of the gastrointestinal mucosa by eosinophils, presumably as a result from allergenic stimulation of either the gastrointestinal or respiratory tracts.

R. Shaker et al. (eds.), *Manual of Diagnostic and Therapeutic Techniques for Disorders of Deglutition*, DOI 10.1007/978-1-4614-3779-6_19,
© Springer Science+Business Media New York 2013

Eosinophilic esophagitis is a condition characterized by dense eosinophilic inflammation of the esophagus (greater than 15 eosinophils per 400X high powered field) in the absence of gastroesophageal reflux disease (GERD) [1]. Typical symptoms in infants and younger children include feeding refusal, regurgitation or vomiting, and abdominal pain. Older children and adults are more typically present with esophageal dysphagia, chest pain, and food impaction.

The etiology of dysphagia in children and adults with eosinophilic esophagitis is unclear. Mucosal inflammation in eosinophilic esophagitis leads to subepithelial fibrosis and tissue remodeling [2]. Eosinophilic infiltration of the esophageal musculature may play a role in both muscle function and structure in patients with eosinophilic esophagitis and achalasia of the LES. In both, pediatric and adults with eosinophilic esophagitis, non-specific motility disturbances have been described [1, 3, 4]. Nurko et al. reported that 41% of children with eosinophilic esophagitis have abnormal esophageal manometry [5]. In a series of 42 adult patients with achalasia subjected to thoracic esophagectomy, histopathology of the distal esophagus revealed eosinophilia of the muscular layer in 52% patients [6]. Hypertrophy of the distal esophageal musculature has been reported in both adults and children with achalasia and children with eosinophilic esophagitis. Using high-frequency intraluminal ultrasonography, muscle thickness and muscle cross-sectional area (CSA) was greater in adult patients with achalasia compared to normal healthy controls [7]. Similarly, pediatric patients with achalasia of the LES had increased muscle thickness and CSA of the distal esophagus compared to healthy adult controls [8]. Children with eosinophilic esophagitis were also noted to have increase muscle and total wall thickness compared to healthy control patients [9].

The etiology of feeding difficulties in children with eosinophilic gastrointestinal disorders is multifactorial and may stem from both psychosocial and medical causes. Recently, Mukkada et al. [10] found 16.5% of children with eosinophilic gastrointestinal disorders had feeding difficulties. Seventy-six percent of these children had eosinophilia limited to the esophagus. Learned maladaptive behaviors (such as Food refusal, low volume/variety of intake, poor acceptance of new foods, spitting food out, grazing, lack of mealtime structure, requiring prompting to eat, inconsistent patterns of eating) was the most common reported symptom of disordered feeding. Oral motor skill and/or sensory deficits, and esophageal dysphagia were least common, reported in less than 20% of the cohort. Mosel et al. [11] reported significant parental stress as a key factor to be mitigated in the management of children with eosinophilic esophagitis referred to as feeding disorders program. Behavioral feeding difficulties can persist even with resolution of esophageal inflammation [10].

Gastroesophageal Reflux Disease

Gastroesophageal reflux refers to the retrograde movement of gastric contents into the esophagus. GERD refers to the condition where morbidity results from pathologic regurgitation of stomach contents into the esophagus and supra-esophageal structures. The clinical symptoms attributed to GERD are numerous and vary by age. Regardless of age, the most common cause of gastroesophageal reflux in children is a transient relaxation of the lower esophageal sphincter [12]. Exposure of esophageal mucosal surfaces to gastric contents can result in mucosal injury and/or muscle dysfunction. There is no optimal method to diagnose GERD in children, although clinical signs and symptoms, endoscopic and/or histologic findings, esophageal pH monitoring, and manometric studies have all been used. Largely, GERD remains a clinicopathologic diagnosis in children [13].

The role of gastroesophageal reflux in the development of feeding difficulties is not clear. GERD was diagnosed in 20–33% of subjects in two large retrospective studies of children with feeding disorders [14, 15]. There was no difference in the frequency of GERD in both studies among children with oral motor, oral sensory, combined oral motor/sensory, or primary behavior-related feeding disorder. However, in both studies, the criteria used to diagnose GERD were not clear. Furthermore, the effect of GERD therapy alone was not clear in either study. More recently, Weir et al. [16] prospectively evaluated 300 infants with feeding difficulties by videofluoroscopic swallow study. Aspiration occurred in 34% of these children. Silent aspiration was common in children with aspiration. Gastroesophageal reflux was present in 10% of children with asymptomatic aspiration and 26% of children with silent aspiration.

Other Causes of Esophageal Dysphagia in Children: Anatomic Abnormalities and Motor Dysfunction

Congenital abnormalities of the esophagus occur in 1:3,000 to 1:4,500 live births for esophageal atresia and esophageal duplication cysts or webs [17]. Classically, these conditions present during early infancy with feeding intolerance and vomiting. Vascular anomalies such as an aberrant subclavian artery and arterio-venous malformations can cause obstructive symptoms due to esophageal compression. Rarer are conditions that cause extrinsic compression of the esophagus by mediastinal or pulmonary structures such as tumors. Typically, surgical management mitigates the esophageal obstruction; however, dysphagia can persist post-operatively, particularly in children with esophageal atresia and duplication cysts. Causes for persistent dysphagia include stricture at surgical anastamotic sites, particularly in children with esophageal atresia, and non-specific motor abnormalities of the distal esophagus [18]. Esophageal stricture or stenosis can also complicate eosinophilic esophagitis and GERD [1, 13].

Primary motor disorders in children are uncommon. The incidence of achalasia of the lower esophageal sphincter in children was 0.18 per 100,000 person years in a European cohort [19]. The incidence of other primary esophageal motor disorders in children is not known. Both surgical myotomy and balloon dilatation of the lower esophageal sphincter have been used successfully to treat achalasia in children. Surgical myotomy is emerging as the treatment of choice for achalasia in children as laparoscopic techniques advance [20].

Suggested Evaluation of Dysphagia in Children

The course of diagnostic evaluation in a child with dysphagia should be tailored to the presenting signs and symptoms. Diagnostic choices include radiographic, endoscopic, histologic, manometric, or reflux monitoring evaluation.

Radiographic Evaluation

Fluoroscopic studies with contrast agents such as barium provide a dynamic view of the esophagus and can be used to help screen for anatomic abnormalities such as esophageal duplication cysts or webs and to identify esophageal strictures. Fluoroscopic studies also can screen for esophageal motor disorders such as achalasia of the upper and lower esophageal sphincters. Mucosal abnormalities can also be described.

Endoscopic and Histologic Evaluation

With the emergence of eosinophilic esophagitis, endoscopic and histologic evaluation of the esophagus has gained increased importance in children with dysphagia. An expert panel has established histologic criteria for the diagnosis of eosinophilic esophagitis; however, overlap of endoscopic and histologic findings of eosinophilic esophagitis with gastroesophageal reflux can occur [13]. Visible mucosal breaks are the most reliable finding for GERD in adults [21]. Histologic inflammation carries low sensitivity and specificity for GERD due to considerable overlap with other disease processes such as viral infection and eosinophilic esophagitis. Performing upper endoscopy in the setting of concomitant acid suppression therapy of 6–8 weeks duration can help differentiate eosinophilic esophagitis from GERD.

Esophageal pH and pH/Impedance Monitoring

Esophageal pH and combined pH/impedance monitoring quantifies the frequency and duration of the regurgitation of gastric contents into the esophagus. pH monitoring detects acid regurgitation into the esophagus. Impedance monitoring allows detection of gastric contents regardless of acid composition. Details of these technologies are discussed in other sections. The reflux index, the percentage of time the esophageal pH is less than 4, is the most commonly used parameter used to evaluate esophageal acidification in children [13]. Normal values for the reflux index vary by age. The utility of esophageal impedance monitoring is currently being evaluated in special pediatric populations. Normative data for the pediatric population is currently not available. The most likely use of impedance monitoring will be for the correlation of symptoms with regurgitation episodes [13].

Esophageal Motility Studies

Esophageal motility studies use multiple pressure sensors to evaluate esophageal peristalsis and the function of the upper and lower esophageal sphincter. Conversion of the pressure data into topographical isocontour color plots allows rapid evaluation of esophageal function. This technique can be combined with methods to evaluate the movement of liquid or solid bolus such as fluoroscopy or impedance to evaluate the function of the esophagus in great detail. Criteria for the diagnosis of esophageal motor disorders based on isocontour plots have been established in adults [22]. Consensus for pediatric criteria is ongoing [23]. It is likely that isocontour-based esophageal motility studies will play a greater role in the evaluation of oral and esophageal dysphagia after endoscopy and other radiographic studies have been completed.

Conclusions

Several clinical conditions can present with dysphagia symptoms in children. Careful consideration of the presenting signs and symptoms can help clinicians determine the appropriate course of diagnostic evaluation. A lack of age appropriate normative data for children requires careful interpretation of diagnostic studies.

References

1. Furuta GT, Liacouras CA, Collins MH, et al. Eosinophilic esophagitis in children and adults: a systematic review and consensus recommendations for diagnosis and treatment. Gastroenterology. 2007;133:1342–63.
2. Chehade M, Sampson HA, Morotti RA, et al. Esophageal subepithelial fibrosis in children with eosinophilic esophagitis. J Pediatr Gastroenterol Nutr. 2007;45:319–28.
3. Lucendo AJ, Castillo P, Martin-Chavarri S, et al. Manometric findings in adult eosinophilic oesophagitis: a study of 12 cases. Eur J Gastroenterol Hepatol. 2007;19:417–24.
4. Nurko S, Rosen R. Esophageal dysmotility in patients who have eosinophilic esophagitis. Gastrointest Endosc Clin N Am. 2008;18:73–89.
5. Nurko S, Rosen R, Furuta GT. Esophageal dysmotility in children with eosinophilic esophagitis: a study using prolonged esophageal manometry. Am J Gastroenterol. 2009;12:3050–7.
6. Goldblum JR, Whyte RI, Orringer MB, et al. Achalasia. A morphologic study of 42 resected specimens. Am J Surg Pathol. 1994;18:327–37.
7. Mittal RK, Kassab G, Puckett JL, et al. Hypertrophy of the muscularis propria of the lower esophageal sphincter and the body of the esophagus in patients with primary motility disorders of the esophagus. Am J Gastroenterol. 2003;98:1705–12.
8. Tipnis NA, Mittal RK. Evaluation of esophageal musculature by high frequency intraluminal ultrasonography in children with achalasia of the LES. Neurogastroenterol Motil. 2008;20 Suppl 1:26.

9. Fox VL, Nurko S, Teitelbaum JE, et al. High-resolution EUS in children with eosinophilic "allergic" esophagitis. Gastrointest Endosc. 2003;57(1):30–6.

10. Mukkada VA, Haas A, Maune NC, et al. Feeding dysfunction in children with eosinophilic gastrointestinal diseases. Pediatrics. 2010;126:e672–7. doi:10.1542/peds.2009-2227.

11. Mosel MA, Schultz LS, Silverman AH, et al. Family psychosocial dysfunction is a prominent feature in eosinophilic esophagitis presenting as pediatric feeding disorder. Gastroenterology. 2011;140:S-243–4.

12. Kawahara H, Dent J, Davidson G. Mechanisms responsible for gastroesophageal reflux in children. Gastroenterology. 1997;113:399–408.

13. Vandenplas Y, Rudolph CD, Di Lorenzo C, et al. Pediatric gastroesophageal reflux clinical practice guidelines: joint recommendations of the North American Society for Pediatric Gastroenterology, Hepatology, and Nutrition (NASPGHAN) and the European Society for Pediatric Gastroenterology, Hepatology, and Nutrition (ESPGHAN). J Pediatr Gastroenterol Nutr. 2009;49:498–547.

14. Rommel N, De Meyer AM, Feenstra L, et al. The complexity of feeding problems in 700 infants and young children presenting to a tertiary care institution. J Pediatr Gastroenterol Nutr. 2003;37:75–84.

15. Levy Y, Levy A, Zangen T, et al. Diagnostic clues for identification of nonorganic vs organic causes of food refusal and poor feeding. J Pediatr Gastroenterol Nutr. 2009;48:355–62.

16. Weir KA, McMahon S, Taylor S, et al. Oropharyngeal aspiration and silent aspiration in children. Chest. 2011;140:589–97.

17. El-Gohary Y, Gittes GK, Tovar JA. Congenital anomalies of the esophagus. Semin Pediatr Surg. 2010;19:186–93.

18. Kawahara H, Kubota A, Hasegawa T, et al. Lack of distal esophageal contractions is a key determinant of gastroesophageal reflux disease after repair of esophageal atresia. J Pediatr Surg. 2007;42:2017–21.

19. Marlais M, Fishman JR, Fell JME, et al. UK incidence of achalasia: an 11-year national epidemiological study. Arch Dis Child. 2011;96:192–4.

20. Pastor AC, Mills J, Marcon MA, et al. A single center 26-year experience with treatment of esophageal achalasia: is there an optimal method? J Pediatr Surg. 2009;44(1):349–54.

21. Vakil N, van Zanten SV, Kahrilas P, et al. The Montreal definition and classification of gastroesophageal reflux disease: a global evidence-based consensus. Am J Gastroenterol. 2006;101:1900–20.

22. Kahrilas PJ, Ghosh SK, Pandolfino JE. Esophageal motility disorders in terms of pressure topography: the Chicago Classification. J Clin Gastroenterol. 2008;42(5):627–35.

23. Goldani HA, Staiano A, Borrelli O, et al. Pediatric esophageal high-resolution manometry: utility of a standardized protocol and size-adjusted pressure topography parameters. Am J Gastroenterol. 2010;105:460–7.

Index

CPSIA information can be obtained
at www.ICGtesting.com
Printed in the USA
FSOW04n2055081116
27163FS